Praise for **Living and Dying in the USA**

"This book uses the annual, cross-sectional National Health Interview Surveys of adults aged 18+ who responded in 1986–94 and matches their responses to any death certificates filed on them in the Multiple Cause of Death file. It describes and explains how biological and socioeconomic factors in younger adults' lifestyles set the final stage for death in old age by specific medical causes. In these ways, it helps us understand why, even after three decades of Medicare, elderly Americans (the majority of all who die in the USA) live lifestyles in earlier stages that keep them alive longer if they have higher socioeconomic status in old age."

—NAN E. JOHNSON, *Florida State University, Tallahassee*

"**Living and Dying in the USA** is a unique and valuable contribution to research on social and behavioral factors associated with mortality in the United States. Its authors are three eminent demographers who bring a wealth of relevant background and experience to bear on this analysis of mortality patterns using a single national data set: the National Health Interview Survey matched to the Multiple Cause of Death file. The range of variables is large, from basic socioeconomic characteristics, to health insurance, mental health, smoking and drinking, and many others. The very large sample size permits certain analyses available nowhere else: for example, multivariate analysis of adult mortality by eight race/ethnic categories (including four Hispanic subgroups), nativity, and other sociodemographic characteristics. Along with the size and power of the data set come many intriguing findings: foreign-born African Americans have the lowest mortality of any ethnic group; net of other factors, infrequent religious attendance is consistently and significantly associated with higher adult mortality. Withal, this book is as valuable for the lines of research it suggests and the questions it leaves unanswered as for the findings it presents. It is an essential reference point for future research on adult mortality in the United States."

—CONSTANCE A. NATHANSON, *Russell Sage Foundation, New York*

"In their book **Living and Dying in the USA,** Drs. Rogers, Hummer, and Nam set out to explore the various forces that influence mortality differentials now present in the United States. Using innovative data and methods of analysis, the authors provide a snapshot picture of the relative influence of all of the major forces that have led to observed differences in the risk of death. The effects of gender, education, smoking, health insurance, employment and occupational status, ethnicity, and even religious practices are examined with respect to how each influences mortality differentials among population subgroups. This book is by far the most comprehensive and authoritative examination of adult mortality ever conducted for a single nation. Because the language is clear, the methods of analysis easily understandable, and the results easy to follow, **Living and Dying in the USA** is required reading for anyone interested in a scientifically valid snapshot of health and longevity in the United States at the dawn of the 21st century."

—S. JAY OLSHANSKY, *The University of Chicago, Illinois*

Living
AND
DYING
IN THE
USA

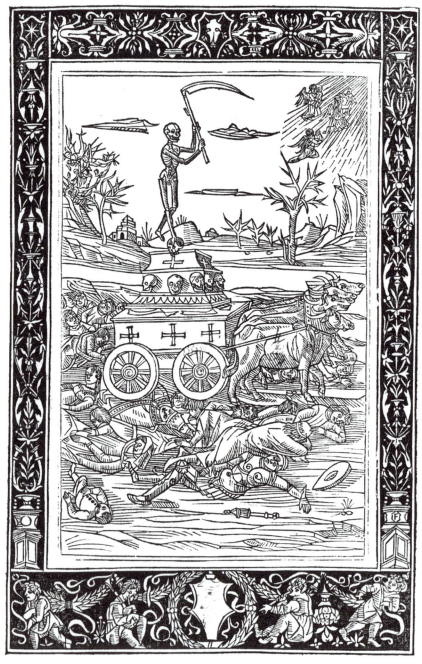

PI9107
"Triumph of Death" (illustration to *The Triumphs of Petrarch*)
Museum of Fine Arts, Boston   Harvey D. Parker Collection

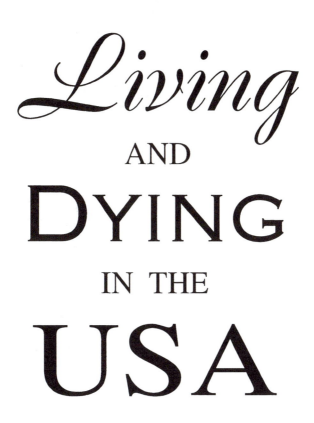

Living AND DYING IN THE USA

BEHAVIORAL, HEALTH, AND SOCIAL DIFFERENTIALS OF ADULT MORTALITY

RICHARD G. ROGERS
University of Colorado
Boulder, Colorado

ROBERT A. HUMMER
University of Texas
Austin, Texas

CHARLES B. NAM
Florida State University
Tallahassee, Florida

ACADEMIC PRESS

San Diego   London   Boston   New York   Sydney   Tokyo   Toronto

Academic Press
A Division of Harcourt, Inc.
525 B Street, Suite 1900, San Diego, California 92101-4495, USA
http://www.apnet.com

Academic Press
24-28 Oval Road, London NW1 7DX, UK
http://www.hbuk.co.uk/ap/

Library of Congress Catalog Card Number: 99-61537

international Standard Book Number: 0-12-593130-1

PRINTED IN THE UNITED STATES OF AMERICA
99 00 01 02 03 04 BB 9 8 7 6 5 4 3 2 1

To our wives and children,

Cindy, Mary, Molly, and Stacy Rogers

Dawn, Holly, and Chelsea Hummer

Marjorie and David Nam and Rebecca Giblin

CONTENTS

PART I

INTRODUCTION, OVERVIEW, AND DATA AND METHODS

1

INTRODUCTION AND OVERVIEW

2

DATA AND METHODS

PART II

DEMOGRAPHIC AND SOCIOCULTURAL CHARACTERISTICS

3

THE SEX DIFFERENTIAL IN MORTALITY

4

RACE/ETHNICITY, NATIVITY, AND ADULT MORTALITY

5

FAMILY COMPOSITION AND MORTALITY

6

RELIGIOUS ATTENDANCE, SOCIAL PARTICIPATION,
AND ADULT MORTALITY

PART III

SOCIOECONOMIC FACTORS

7

THE EFFECTS OF BASIC SOCIOECONOMIC FACTORS ON MORTALITY

8

THE EFFECT OF OCCUPATIONAL STATUS ON MORTALITY

9

HEALTH INSURANCE COVERAGE AND MORTALITY

PART IV

HEALTH CONDITIONS AND HEALTH STATUS

10

PERCEIVED HEALTH STATUS AND MORTALITY

11

FUNCTIONAL LIMITATIONS AND MORTALITY

12

MENTAL AND ADDICTIVE DISORDERS AND MORTALITY

13

CIGARETTE SMOKING AND MORTALITY

14

ALCOHOL CONSUMPTION AND MORTALITY

15

EXERCISE AND MORTALITY

16

THE INFLUENCE OF OTHER HEALTH BEHAVIORS ON MORTALITY

17

CONCLUSION

Prologue

The frontispiece shows *The Triumph of Death,* a metal-cut image with a woodcut border from the mid-15th century. It belongs to a genre that originated around the time of the plague (mid-1300s) and exhibits several common themes. Death is usually represented as a figure in black or, later, as a skeleton, armed with a bow, sword, scythe, or other weapon and riding a horse, cart, or chariot.

In this exemplar, death is seen not as frightening and horrifying, but as universal, as a law of nature. The skeleton stands atop a casket. The cart is pulled by four oxen, images of force and persistence. In its path are men and women, children and adults, as well as common people, knights, monarchs, and clergy (Olds and Williams, 1976).

The force of mortality has changed over time. Death now strikes less unexpectedly, is not as unyielding, and certainly does not attack all walks of life with equal vengeance. The force of mortality is affected by social, behavioral, psychological, and health factors.

Acknowledgments

Writing a book requires the cooperation, assistance, and input of numerous people and organizations. We have been fortunate to have an abundance of support and encouragement.

Over the years, the Population Program in the Institute of Behavioral Science and the Department of Sociology at the University of Colorado (Dr. Rogers), the Population Research Center and the Department of Sociology at the University of Texas at Austin (Dr. Hummer), and the Center for the Study of Population at Florida State University (Dr. Nam) have provided the intellectual stimulation, financial support, and needed time to complete the book.

A variety of people have offered their insights and suggestions. We thank all of the people who have read and commented on various chapters or drafts of the book, especially Parker Frisbie, Jane Menkin, Fred Pampel, Andrei Rogers, Catherine Ross, Carl Schmertmann, and Michael Wrigley. Jay Teachman provided valuable methodological and technical expertise, while Richard Cook, Starling Pullum, and James Raymer contributed computer knowledge and skills. Sarit Amir, Jacqueline Carrigan, Aurelie Cordier, Tina Fitzgerald, Patrick Kreuger, Kimberley Peters, Sameer Rajbhandary, and Rebecca Rosbenblatt created and analyzed many data sets, as well as crafted tables and figures. Thanks go to Haven Sands for initially constructing the subject and author indexes. Eileen Favorite and Nancy Mann suggested important editorial changes and refinements. And we appreciate the anonymous reviewers, who raised new issues and challenged some of our assumptions and conclusions, which caused us to rethink and rework sections and which ultimately contributed to a more cohesive and organized book.

We thank the National Center for Health Statistics (NCHS) for providing the data for these analyses. NCHS had the foresight, wherewithal, and vision to link the National Health Interview Survey (NHIS) to the Multiple Causes of Death (MCD) file through the National Death Index to create a rich resource for mortality research. This important linked data set will be analyzed for years to come. We are grateful to John Horm, who developed the methodology and who crafted the computer programs to create the NHIS-MCD. His attention to detail, concern for accuracy, and knowledge of computer-matching algorithms have contributed to a first-rate data set. Felicia LeClere's support and provocative ideas have expanded and extended the analyses in innovative ways. And Mary Grace Kovar contributed her vision and insight.

This book would not have been possible without the generous support of the National Science Foundation (NSF), the NCHS, and the National Institutes of Aging (NIA). NIA provided funding early on to develop and nurture our nascent ideas (Grant AG10113-01A2). NCHS provided the financial support to allow us to examine some of their data in-house, which provided us a better appreciation of the commitment, dedication, and organization that are involved in creating, editing, cleaning, archiving, and distributing large, nationally representative data sets. We gratefully acknowledge the hard solid work that all members of NCHS engage in to produce such high-quality data sets. NSF also provided crucial support to further develop the analyses (Grants SBR-9617905 and SBR-9617760).

Thanks go to Scott Bentley, a senior acquisitions editor at Academic Press, who has helped us along the way, has always been available to discuss emerging issues and questions, and has been a pleasure to work with.

Although many people have helped and encouraged us throughout the process, we take final responsibility for the analyses, interpretations, and conclusions reached.

PART

I

INTRODUCTION, OVERVIEW, AND DATA AND METHODS

1

INTRODUCTION
AND OVERVIEW

People of the United States enjoy one of the highest life expectancies in the world, and throughout the twentieth century their life expectancy has increased tremendously. In the context of life expectancies around the world in 1997, from 34 for Sierra Leone to 80 for Japan, the life expectancy for Americans was 76 (Population Reference Bureau 1998).

When the 20th century began, a U.S. newborn could expect to live, on average, about 49 years. By 1960, that number had risen to 70 years, and it has continued increasing to the present. Much of that increase was due to substantial reductions in infant mortality. Still, a 20-year-old in 1900 had an average of 43 years of life remaining, whereas by 1996 it had gone up to 57 years. For those reaching age 65, there was an expectation of 12 more years of life in 1900 and 18 years by 1996 (National Center for Health Statistics 1996d; Peters et al. 1998). Yet prospects of survival or death in the U.S. vary greatly for persons having different characteristics. Those at older ages have greater chances of dying and from a different pattern of medical causes than do younger people. Women do not have as high a mortality risk as men. Racial and ethnic groups vary in their mortality chances. Persons in higher educational, income, and occupational groupings have a survival advantage over those in lower socioeconomic groupings.

Through the early part of the twentieth century, mortality reductions were concentrated in infant and younger ages of the population, as infectious and parasitic diseases were more dominant. In the latter part of the century, there was a shift to dealing with chronic illnesses (especially cardiovascular diseases and cancer) that were primary causes of adult mortality.

Our book is oriented to extending our understanding of adult survival and mortality. Our study aims to examine adult mortality in the United States for a recent period of time and to account for a broad range of factors that can explain the variability that exists. As outlined more fully later, we will draw on a highly reliable national data set that incorporates a large number of relevant explanatory variables and determine the extent to which social, behavioral, and health factors shape the mortality levels of the country.

When we conceptualize the factors that might have an impact on mortality chances, we can consider factors that span social, economic, cultural, psychological, physiological, and biological aspects of existence. The biological dimension includes genetic traits, which are known to relate to certain diseases and to cellular vitality or frailty, and to sex and the aging process. The biological approach is very important for mortality research, as exemplified by such new developments as the genome project, which promises to extend the literature on genetic determinants of mortality. Although we applaud such efforts and recognize the importance of biological factors, we adopt a social science paradigm that acknowledges biological factors, but focuses on social, behavioral, and health factors. We do, however, incorporate a biological dimension through our analyses of specific causes of death.

The psychological dimension incorporates mental conditions (also linked to biological factors) and mental processes, such as attitudes and motivations that influence health care and avoidance of death (also tied to certain risk behaviors like smoking, drug use, drinking, diet, sleep, and exercise). The cultural milieu in which a person is raised and maintains in life operates to define acceptable practices of behavior that relate to health and survival.

The economic and social dimensions include levels of living, occupational pursuits, and income needed to facilitate health care (as through obtaining health insurance), as well as marriage and family characteristics and social ties to family, friends, and the community.

Clearly, no informational source exists that encompasses anything like that broad agenda. Hence, we must narrow our conceptual gaze to cover those dimensions of importance that are measurable. Even a more limited framework, with simultaneous attention to a large number of variables, can help us comprehend a great deal about patterns of adult mortality and provide a firmer base for research that will go beyond our present knowledge.

In general, several features of this book differentiate it from other discussions of factors associated with variations in mortality. First, we make use of the newest and most advanced database for studying the subject matter at hand. Second, we attempt to go significantly beyond descriptive analysis to explain the multivariate relationships existing among the various factors in our study. Third, our analysis provides a U.S. national picture of forces affecting mortality, in contrast to many of the more geographically limited studies that now exist. Fourth, we link our findings to those of other researchers and explore needed pathways of future research.

In the following paragraphs, we explicate more fully the data, analytical methods, and the strategy we use in this book to account for the relative impacts of several variables as they relate to the risks of mortality.

FACTORS RELATED TO MORTALITY

The public health and medical communities have made tremendous strides in reducing or preventing many infectious diseases: diphtheria, measles, typhoid fever, tuberculosis, and syphilis have declined substantially, and smallpox has been completely eradicated (Link and Phelan 1996). More recently, similar progress has been made in reducing chronic diseases, including heart disease and cancer (Susser and Susser 1996), as a large percentage of the general public has dealt with the hazards of smoking, excessive alcohol consumption, lack of exercise, improper diets, high cholesterol, and hypertension.

Biological research has contributed to these reductions and has also taught us more about genetically linked diseases. For example,

> The methods of recombinant DNA have led to recognition of both viral and genetic components in insulin-dependent diabetes; to the definitive tracking from person to person of HIV, tuberculosis, and other infections through the molecular specificity of the organisms; to the discovery of a herpes virus as almost certainly the agent in Karposi's sarcoma; and the drama of the familial tracking and marking of the first breast cancer gene. (Susser and Susser 1996:671)

The influence of social forces on mortality, however, has remained relatively stable or even increased over time (Hummer et al. 1998b; Link and Phelan 1995; Pappas et al. 1993; K. Smith 1996). In this book, we acknowledge that a research focus on individual risk factors captures only part of the hazard of dying. Other factors that play an important part in determining who lives and who dies each year in the United States include the family and household, social institutions, the neighborhood, and the larger community (Link and Phelan 1995; Pearce 1996). In this book, we focus mainly on factors associated with individuals, but we begin to tap into a broader set of levels by analyzing family factors.

To more fully conceptualize the many sets of factors that determine mortality, researchers must extend traditional behavioral and demographic frameworks to more complete, though more complex, models that also incorporate socioeconomic characteristics, such as education and income; family characteristics, such as marital status and family composition; and social relations, such as religious and social participation. Our book seeks to provide that extended framework by using the newest and most comprehensive mortality data source available for the United States: the National Health Interview Survey matched to the Multiple Cause of Death file through the National Death Index (NHIS-MCD).

The specific approach used in this book (see Table 1.1) focuses on the relationship between various social, behavioral, and health influences, on the one hand, and adult mortality, on the other. Where possible, we take account of the medical causes of death. We proceed with the understanding that age, sex, and race/ethnicity are fundamentally related to adult mortality (see, for example, Coale 1996; Gage 1994; Himes 1994; Rogers 1992; Rogers et al. 1996; Verbrugge 1989) and, therefore, we control for their effects throughout. We devote one chapter each to sex and race/ethnic mortality differentials; however, our data set is not detailed enough at the youngest and oldest adult ages to separately examine age effects on mortality. Throughout, then, we control for these fundamental demographic influences on mortality risk. In addition, many of our detailed models control for the effects of individuals' baseline health status, because of its interrelationships with social factors and mortality (House et al. 1988; Rogers 1995b).

Chapter by chapter, we focus on different variables at various levels of influence, highlighting the particular contributions of each. We strive for

TABLE 1.1   Factors Associated with Adult Mortality Risks

Demographic and baseline characteristics	Social and economic variables	Behavioral and health factors	Outcomes
Demographic characteristics	Socioeconomic status	Health behaviors	
Age	Education	Cigarette smoking	
Sex	Income	Alcohol drinking	
Race/ethnicity	Employment status	Exercise	
Nativity	Occupational status	Sleep	
Baseline health	Health insurance	Weight/height	Mortality outcome
		Seat belt use	Overall mortality
	Family relations		Underlying cause
	Marital status	Functional limitations	Circulatory diseases
	Family composition	Activities of Daily Living	Cancer
			Respiratory diseases
	Religious involvement and general social participation	Instrumental Activities of Daily Living	Social pathologies
		Mental and addictive disorders	
		Depression	
		Paranoia	
		Schizophrenia	

a conceptual position that highlights the mortality effects of the different variables while controlling for confounding factors. Analytically, what this means is that we are primarily concerned with the magnitude of each variable before and after the introduction of confounders, an approach that is commonly used in the mortality literature. This conceptual framework serves only as a useful guide for analyzing variables that may affect the apparent relationship between the variables in question and mortality; it is not intended to be a full causal model.

The framework (Table 1.1) differentiates factors associated with mortality risks into four main rubrics: demographic and baseline health characteristics, social and economic factors, behavioral and health factors, and mortality outcomes. Demographic characteristics include age, sex, race/ethnicity, and nativity; we also include baseline health characteristics in many of our models. Social and economic factors are thought of as quite distal to the actual biological process of dying and include indicators of socioeconomic status, family relations, and social participation. Behavioral and health factors are considered to be more proximate to mortality outcomes and include health behaviors, functional limitations, and mental and addictive disorders. Finally, the outcomes examined here include overall mortality (survive versus die) and mortality specific to underlying cause of death. These sets of variables are discussed briefly in the following three sections.

DEMOGRAPHIC AND BASELINE
HEALTH CHARACTERISTICS

Among the demographic characteristics in our study, "age" can be regarded as one of the most crucial in its relation to mortality. This is because there is a universal pattern of mortality by age that varies only moderately from group to group. In general, death rates decline from infancy to the early teen ages and increase thereafter, growing more rapidly as old age approaches (Heligman and Pollard 1980; Olshansky and Carnes 1997). At the older ages, although the mortality rates remain high, the rate of mortality increase with age slows (see Horiuchi and Wilmoth 1997, 1998). Ignoring age in an analysis of mortality would, therefore, introduce a major bias; demographers either control for age in their analyses of mortality or they conduct their analyses separately by age categories. Age is introduced as a control in all of our analyses, although the age intervals used vary from one part of the study to another.

"Sex" is a variable that we examine in its own right and as a basic control in our study. The history of mortality analysis shows that patterns of death vary between the sexes, owing to different biological functions, such as childbearing among women, intrinsic differences, and varying behaviors, such as extent of tobacco and alcohol use, in various cultures. Chapter 3 elaborates the linkage between sex and mortality and points to the essential aspects of this relationship. Likewise, "race/ethnicity" is a control variable in our analysis because mortality is seen to vary according to how peo-

ple are characterized on this dimension. We rely on the conventional categories of race and ethnicity, as determined in the NHIS and other major
data sources. We distinguish among Blacks or African Americans, Asian
Americans, Indians or Native Americans, Mexican Americans, other Hispanics (by type), and non-Hispanic Whites. These several groups have different average patterns of mortality and causes of death, although we recognize that there is a great deal of variation within as well as between those
groups. In Chapter 4, we elaborate on these distinctions, including an examination of the influence of nativity on race/ethnic mortality differential.

One additional control used in our study is "baseline health." This is
measured by seeing how respondents in the survey assess their own health.
Health status is self-reported on a five-point scale ranging from excellent to
poor. This variable does not capture all of the variation we would expect to
be associated with health status, but it does tap into a basic element of one's
current health and serves to control for that effect when we do not want it
to confound the relationships we study or we want to account for its selective effect on mortality outcomes.

SOCIAL AND ECONOMIC FACTORS

These variables are important in the sense that they are postulated to be
at the root of explanations of morbidity and mortality patterns. They relate
to, and should be considered in conjunction with, behavioral and health factors that we will discuss subsequently. Three broad sets of social and economic factors are socioeconomic status, family relations, and religious and
general social participation.

Socioeconomic status can incorporate knowledge, money, community
standing, and power (Kitagawa and Hauser 1973; Link and Phelan 1995;
Pearce 1996; Preston and Taubman 1994; Williams 1990). Poverty, as the
root cause of many diseases, was underscored early on. For example, Engels (1958/1845) noted such a connection among the Manchester factory
workers in the 1840s. Generally, the dimensions of high socioeconomic status provide the resources to avoid risk or to minimize the effects of disease
once it occurs. For example, high socioeconomic status reduces the risk of
chronic diseases and death through increased exercise, reduced smoking,
lower stress, and better diets; high socioeconomic status can also reduce the
risk of death from infectious diseases (like AIDS) through access to health
information and medical care (Adler et al. 1994). Thus, socioeconomic status acts by providing both knowledge about health risks and ways to avoid
them, and the means with which to manage risks and undergo treatment.
Such mechanisms are transportable to new situations and new diseases
(Link and Phelan 1995).

The general relationship between socioeconomic status and mortality is
well established; to understand it more fully, however, we need subtler

measures of socioeconomic status (Moss and Krieger 1995). The data set used here allows us to go beyond the one-dimensional measures of socioeconomic status that characterize much of the mortality literature and highlights the combined influences of education, family income, and occupation on mortality.

Family relations encompass marital status, family composition, social support, and social control. In general, married individuals have lower mortality risks than the unmarried because they exhibit more positive health behaviors and are linked to tighter-knit social support networks (Lillard and Waite 1995; Rogers 1995a). However, it is not just marriage in general that works in this positive fashion; the specific characteristics of spouses are important in understanding the mortality of individuals. For example, the educational background, income generation, health behavior, and health status of one's spouse can influence the mortality of the other spouse (Smith and Zick 1994). Social support also arises from other family members, other relatives and friends, and from participation in social activities—all factors that can affect health and mortality (Angel et al. 1997; House et al. 1988; Jarvis and Northcutt 1987; Rogers 1996). On the other hand, social relations can be stressful or damaging; for instance, caring for dependents may be financially and emotionally draining.

Religious and more general social participation can be associated with values and beliefs that can influence health and mortality, both through attitudes toward health behaviors and through the handling of stress and outlook on life. Measures of religious involvement and general social participation are not often included in mortality studies, yet we are aware of their importance (Jarvis and Northcutt 1987). The NHIS identifies the religious attendance and general social participation patterns of respondents. Although these variables are only crude indicators of religious and social participation, the analysis of them moves the mortality literature toward a more balanced inclusion of social factors.

All of the demographic, social, and economic causes mentioned above are treated in separate chapters, as well as integrated with other factors that are analyzed in particular chapters in this book.

BEHAVIORAL AND HEALTH FACTORS

Behavioral and health factors are those variables that are acquired in a person's lifetime that may lead more directly to poor or better survival outcomes. Here, we refer to several health behaviors, such as smoking, drinking, exercise, sleep, and body mass (e.g., leanness, obesity), and to patterns of health care, specified health conditions, and psychosocial factors. One principal health behavior is cigarette smoking, which is a major contributor to poor health and premature mortality and is considered the single most important preventable determinant of mortality in developed nations

(Centers for Disease Control 1993). The immense mortal effects of cigarette smoking in U.S. society will continue well into the next century, with literally millions of lives dependent upon current and projected smoking trends (Nam et al. 1996). Heavy alcohol use also increases the risk of death via accidents and violence and through certain organic diseases. However, moderate drinking has been shown to have a beneficial effect on health and survival from specific diseases, including heart diseases (Klatsky and Friedman 1995). Various studies have also demonstrated the linkage of body mass (height and weight) to mortality risks (Elo and Preston 1992; Lee et al. 1993). Some studies have shown other behaviors, such as exercise frequency and amount of sleep at night, to be related to mortality outcomes (Schoenborn 1986).

Several chapters in this book are devoted to a focus on the separate proximate factors, in conjunction with controls and fundamental causes, as they impact the probability of death.

OUTCOMES

Mortality outcomes constitute the main concern of this book. For the persons included in the NHIS samples at various dates, the MCD files identify those who were no longer alive by 1995. Knowing that individuals of given ages and sexes have died provides information that can be used to estimate risks of death, but our attempt to explain mortality patterns extends not only to elaborating the demographic, social, behavioral, and health factors associated with mortality risks, but also the nature of death. Here we can differentiate decedents according to the reported underlying cause of death—that cause which is believed to be the precipitating medical condition that led to death. From a large classification of such causes, we have extracted a condensed set of cause categories, emphasizing the cause groups that account for the major share of deaths in this country.

DATA ANALYSIS

Our broad analysis of factors related to adult mortality risks has been made possible by a recently released data set: the NHIS (from the National Center for Health Statistics), and its match to the NDI (also from the National Center for Health Statistics), resulting in the National Health Interview Survey Multiple Cause of Death linked file (NHIS-MCD). The NHIS includes annual information from about 120,000 people (encompassing over 40,000 households yearly) regarding such central items as age, race, sex, marital status, family size, income, education, and current occupation. It also includes supplemental questions that may vary from year to year, many of which are asked of the entire sample in a given sample year. These questions include items about religious attendance, income sources, social relations, health behaviors, and more. To date, individuals aged 18 and over from the NHIS surveys of 1986 to 1994 have been successfully matched with the NDI through 1995 (Horm 1993, 1996). That is, although of course most of the adults surveyed lived through the follow-up period, those who died have been identified. This source is ideal for more thoroughly understanding factors that lead some people to live and others to die in the U.S. population.

Early work on mortality employed fairly simple univariate statistics. Now, with new data sets and more sophisticated statistical techniques, it is possible to employ multivariate approaches. Consequently, we employ not only descriptive tables to tell our story but discrete hazard rate (i.e., event history) modeling as well. Throughout, we aim to present the data straightforwardly and therefore focus on new findings in each substantive chapter. But because of the importance of a full discussion of detailed sampling issues, methodological issues, and other statistical concerns, Chapter 2 deals with data and methods.

STRATEGY OF THE NARRATIVE

The book is organized in six parts. Following this Introduction and Chapter 2 on Data and Methods, we move (in Part II) to demographic and sociocultural characteristics associated with mortality. This encompasses chapters on sex effects, ethnicity, nativity, family relations, religious attendance, and social participation. Since the NHIS is a household-based survey of individuals, there are also unique opportunities to examine how the action of one family member affects other members within the family. Thus, we examine how family relations matter.

Part III focuses on socioeconomic effects, including basic socioeconomic status, occupational status, and health insurance. In these chapters, we expand previous research in several ways; for example, we show the importance of income, education, and other central measures of socioeconomic status, and demonstrate the significance of detailed socioeconomic measures for the understanding of U.S. adult mortality patterns.

The emphasis next shifts to health-related conditions and health status (Part IV). Chapters here deal with perceived health status, functional limitations, and mental health. Part V examines cigarette smoking, alcohol consumption, exercise, and other behaviors that influence the risk of mortality, including body mass, seat belt use, and sleeping patterns.

Finally, we try to bring together the several areas of the book, in the context of our conceptual framework, to elucidate the connections among the several factors as they relate to mortality chances. On the one hand, individual and social forces can provoke premature individual mortality, which can result in tragic consequences for the welfare of other family members and for the well-being of society. On the other hand, such forces can sway individuals to protect their health and thereby ensure their longer survival. This concluding section is intended to provide an integration of existing research, including our own, and point the way to future efforts to elaborate the mechanisms through which what occurs in our daily lives has an impact on the basic matters of life and death. We also examine our findings in light of past and potential future policy actions.

Overall, this book tells a story about social, behavioral, and health forces affecting U.S. adult mortality.

2

Data and Methods

This book provides a broad and detailed examination of adult mortality differences in the United States. Although the gist of the effort is to illuminate substantive differences in adult mortality, the results and conclusions are affected by the research methodologies involved. Thus, we devote this chapter to an explication of the data and methods used throughout the study. Such discussion should enlighten the reader regarding our research direction, inform the reader regarding the methodological and statistical issues we confronted and resolved, and enable future researchers to both replicate and extend our findings.

DATA

Dramatic changes have taken place in the sources of data used in research on U.S. adult mortality patterns. Although some studies continue to rely on vital statistics data compiled at the national level, many recent studies use survey-based data sets that are composed of (a) people who are exposed to the risk of death and then *die* over some follow-up time period, and (b) people who are exposed to the risk of death and *do not die* over the same follow-up period. Most simply, the decedents are compared to the survivors across various characteristics (such as sex, race/ethnicity, education, or cigarette smoking) to examine whether or not, and to what extent, they differ. Such prospective data sets have only recently come into existence at the national level, and have resulted in major breakthroughs in the ability of researchers to specify detailed mortality models (Hummer et al. 1998b).

Perhaps most ambitious was the National Center for Health Statistics (NCHS) effort to link the annual National Health Interview Survey (NHIS) to the Multiple Cause of Death (MCD) file compiled from the National Death Index (NDI). This linkage created a unique, powerful, but somewhat complicated source of mortality data that meets the above two criteria. The following subsections describe these data sets and their linkage for the purposes of analyzing U.S. adult mortality differentials.

NATIONAL HEALTH INTERVIEW SURVEY

In 1957, NCHS began conducting the NHIS, an annual household survey of individuals, to collect information on the health of U.S. individuals (Adams and Marano 1995). The NHIS, one of the oldest ongoing national surveys, is generally regarded as the main source of information for understanding health patterns in the population. In all, roughly 49,000 households yielding 125,000 people of all ages—children and adults—are included each year, with information gathered about each individual's health and sociodemographic characteristics (Adams and Marano 1995). The surveys are conducted in person by permanent staff interviewers of the Bureau of the Census. When possible, all adult household members participate in the interview. However, since the NHIS is a household survey of individuals, the household head or a responsible adult individual sometimes provides proxy answers for members who are not at home, and for those physically or mentally incapable of responding for themselves.

The annual NHIS is derived through a stratified, multistage probability design that allows for a continuous sampling of the civilian, noninstitutionalized population (Adams and Marano 1995). Each week, a probability sample of this population is interviewed, with the weekly samples additive over time. This type of design is especially important for calculating health or mortality estimates among small population subgroups in that they can be made from a longer period (even across multiple years) of data collection.

In the first stage of the design, the District of Columbia and the 50 U.S. states are divided into approximately 1,900 geographically defined primary sampling units (PSUs). A PSU is a county, a small group of contiguous counties, or a metropolitan statistical area. In some areas of the country, other divisions are employed, such as parishes in Louisiana, independent cities in Virginia, and minor civil divisions in some New England states. The PSUs are stratified by socioeconomic and demographic variables, and then selected with a probability proportional to their size within particular strata. The largest 52 of the PSUs are referred to as self-representing PSUs and are assured of selection into the sample. The other PSUs are clustered into 73 strata, with two sample PSUs chosen from each of the 73 in proportion to their population size. Thus, a total of 198 PSUs are selected in this first stage. To ensure ample cell sizes and to improve the statistical estimates for the African American population, geographic areas with PSUs that are predominantly African American are sampled at higher rates than other areas (Massey et al. 1989).

In the second stage, households are chosen within each PSU based on two types of units: area segments and permit area segments. Area segments are geographically defined based on the 1980 U.S. Census and contain an expected eight households; permit area segments cover geographical areas using updated lists of building permits and contain an expected four households. In all, the 7,500 segments yield about 59,000 sampled households, of which about 10,000 are expected, in any given year, to be vacant, demolished, or occupied by persons not in the target population (e.g., noncivilians or institutionalized persons). This NHIS sample design, based on results from the 1980 U.S. Census, was first used in 1985 and was consistently used through 1994 (Adams and Marano 1995). Fortuitously, this encompasses the complete period of our study, which uses NHIS data from 1986–1994.

The annual NHIS consists of two parts: (a) a basic health and demographic core questionnaire that remains largely the same from year to year and is completed for each household member; and (b) special topic (supplemental) questionnaires that vary from year to year and are completed for representative subsamples of the population. We use both the basic and supplemental portions of the NHIS in this monograph. For example, Chapter 3—which analyzes sex differences in mortality—employs the 1990 NHIS Health Promotion and Disease Prevention Supplement because of its rich inclusion of behavioral data. Chapter 4 on the other hand—which focuses on race/ethnic and nativity differentials in mortality—pools 6 years (1989–1994) of NHIS core data because the inclusion of relatively small race/ethnic groups requires a large sample of individuals at baseline for analysis. Potentially, Chapter 4 could also include the NHIS core data from 1986–1988; however the nativity variable was not available in the core data set during those years. In short, the selection of the specific NHIS data set(s) used for each chapter was made based on the substantive focus of the chapter, the availability of relevant variables in the NHIS, and sample sizes. Within each chapter, we briefly mention the specific NHIS data set(s) used. All of the NHIS data used throughout the monograph are public use data sets available from the National Technical Information Service (the national distribution center for NCHS data) or, for member institutions, from the Inter-university Consortium for Political and Social Research at the University of Michigan.

The NHIS consistently has very high response rates, ranging from 94 to 98% over the years (Adams and Marano 1995). About one-half of the non-responses comprises refusals, and the other half comprises households with no one home after repeated visits (Massey et al. 1989). These exceptionally high response rates are the result of mail contact prior to the interview, repeated interviewer trips to households, the fact that potential respondents are notified of the importance of the data collection effort and are assured of strict confidentiality, and extremely dedicated and talented U.S. Census Bureau interviewers. Estimates based on the NHIS, however, must reflect the fact that between 2 and 6% of selected individuals are not interviewed. Other characteristics—such as the oversampling of African Americans— must also be accounted for to produce accurate population estimates. This is accomplished through the weighting of the data set. The primary reason to weight the data is to make each NHIS sample—core and supplements— representative of the civilian noninstitutionalized population by age, sex, race, and residence (Adams and Marano 1995). Thus, our analyses throughout the monograph use weights provided by NCHS to account for the sampling characteristics and for nonresponse. More detail on the design and features of the NHIS from 1985–1994 is available in Massey et al. (1989).

MATCHING THE NHIS TO THE MULTIPLE CAUSE OF DEATH FILE

By themselves, the annual National Health Interview Surveys are of little use for the analysis of U.S. mortality patterns because they are cross-sectional surveys of living people whose future death patterns are unknown. Fortunately for mortality researchers, NCHS has recently linked the survey respondents of the NHIS to a national file of deaths that occur each year in the United States, called the Multiple Cause of Death file (MCD), through the NDI (Horm 1996; NCHS 1997b). That is, NCHS, through computer matching, has checked each survey respondent with the yearly NDI to best determine whether the sample person died during the year of the survey or in subsequent follow-up years. If a decedent is identified, the timing and cause of death information for that person are linked to their corresponding NHIS data. This linkage "permits the use of NHIS data for estimates of survival, mortality, and life expectancy while using the richness of the NHIS questionnaires, both core and supplements, as covariates" (NCHS 1997b: 4).

As of 1998, NCHS had linked individuals aged 18 and over in the NHIS files from 1986–1994 with the MCD file for the years 1986–1995 to create the NHIS-MCD linked file (NCHS 1997b). NCHS devised a program that uses a probabilistic scoring algorithm (Rogot et al. 1986) to best determine which individuals included in the NHIS subsequently died during follow-up

(NCHS 1997b). The approach assigns weights to each of 12 criteria—including social security number, first and last name, middle initial, father's surname, birth month and year, age, race, marital status, state of residence, state of birth, and combinations of these—and adds the weights to determine the quality of the potential matches (Horm 1996; NCHS 1997b). Agreement between the NHIS and NDI on any of the 12 criteria yields a potential match; thus, more than one death record may be matched to a given NHIS record using this procedure (NCHS 1997b). After scoring, the potential matches are classified into one of five classes based on the strength of the match. For example, Class One matches consist of exact or nearly exact agreement between the identifying information on the NHIS and NDI and are considered true matches (deceased individuals). On the other hand, Class Five matches contain disagreements on key items and are considered false matches, or survivors (NCHS 1997b). Ascertainment of the presumed survival status of individuals falling into Classes Two, Three, and Four—which are characterized by differing degrees of identification agreement between the NHIS and NDI—is based on NCHS recommendations according to the strength of the match within classes. It is also possible for researchers to use more liberal or conservative match classifications in comparison to NCHS recommendations. Liao et al. (1998), for example, found that the choice of match classification in the investigation of race/ethnic mortality differences was important only for Hispanics. Overall, though, they found that NCHS recommendations "appeared to provide the most consistent results" (Liao et al. 1998: 228)—and went on to analyze the data using the NCHS recommendations. Likewise, we have analyzed different match classifications and found that the NCHS recommendations provide highly sensible and reliable results (Hummer et al. 1999b). Throughout, then, this monograph uses the NCHS recommendations for determining the presumed death or survival of NHIS respondents.

Overall, Patterson and Bilgrad (1986) demonstrated that this matching methodology is highly accurate. The procedure used for the NHIS-MCD is also more advanced and flexible than has been incorporated in matches in previous studies, and has been refined and confirmed with the National Health and Nutrition Examination Survey Follow-up and the Longitudinal Study of Aging (NCHS 1997b). In fact, NCHS estimates that their recommendations correctly classify about 97% of deaths and an even higher proportion of survivors (NCHS 1997b). The linked data set also alleviates the problems of inconsistency between numerator and denominator often encountered when two diverse data sources are merged for mortality analyses. For example, race/ethnic reports are often inconsistent when death records are matched to census data (Hahn and Stroup 1994). In the case of the NHIS-MCD, race/ethnic reports stem from a single source—the household within which the individual lives.

DATA ISSUES AND LIMITATIONS

Despite all of the advantages of the linked NHIS-MCD file, there are some important data issues and limitations to consider. Some NHIS records, termed *ineligibles*, contain insufficient information to be matched to any death record. NCHS identifies ineligible individuals from the NHIS so that they can be dropped from subsequent analyses because ineligible individuals will never match death records, and so would appear to live forever (NCHS 1997b). In a related analysis, we found that the ineligible individuals were more likely to be women (most likely due to changing surnames over the life course), older, and of lower socioeconomic status than eligible individuals from the NHIS. With the exception that more ineligibles are women, the excluded individuals appear to exhibit a slightly higher risk profile for death compared to the remainder of the NHIS sample (Hummer et al. 1999a). Because of the relatively small size of the ineligible group (about 2% of the NHIS individuals in our analysis), the resulting bias from their exclusion, while unknown, is probably not large. Nevertheless, this is most likely one reason why death rate estimates and life expectancy calculations based on the NHIS-MCD data appear to be slightly more favorable compared to those made from vital statistics data (Hummer et al. 1999a).

The use of NHIS-MCD data also results in slightly lower death rate estimates than vital statistics data because the NHIS is based on the civilian, noninstitutionalized population of the United States. Thus, the NHIS initially excludes some of the least healthy people from consideration, most notably persons residing in nursing homes and prisons. In fact, of an estimated 33.5 million people in the United States aged 65 and over in 1995, about 4% (1.4 million) resided in nursing homes (Dey 1997). For the youngest individuals in the NHIS and the corresponding mortality analyses, the use of a noninstitutionalized population probably presents only a slight bias, although black males are more likely to be in the military and institutionalized than members of other race/ethnic groups. However, the bias may be greater at the oldest ages, where widowed, white women make up a substantial share of the nursing home population (Dey 1997). Moreover, because the NHIS is matched to the NDI for up to 9.5 years, it is possible that some respondents may become institutionalized at some point after the initial interview, but before death. Thus, our results cannot be generalized to the entire population, but assess the mortality experiences of civilian, noninstitutionalized persons at the time the surveys were conducted. Nevertheless, because our focus in this monograph is on mortality *differentials,* rather than absolute mortality levels per se, the exclusion of these specialized subpopulations should have relatively little influence on the study results.

As with any prospective study, our analyses may introduce biases because (with one exception, discussed in the statistical analysis section below) we do not have time-varying independent variables, a situation encountered in many other analyses of adult mortality. Indeed, it is important to recognize that the adult mortality process unfolds over many decades; clearly, then, one of the most difficult issues in modeling adult mortality is the influence of time (Hummer et al. 1998b). Because the NHIS data sets are cross-sectional, our models assume that the independent variables do not change between the time of the interview and the latest date through which the respondents are followed (through December 1995 or death). But some individuals may change over this period; for example, there may be income fluctuations, occupational changes, and changes in health and health behavior that are important for survival chances. Although this bias is important to keep in mind, it is at least partially offset by the relatively short time interval over the follow-up (which is, *at most,* about 9.5 years and sometimes as little as 1.5 years), the use of many variables that are largely time-invariant (e.g., education, sex, race/ethnicity) or relatively consistent year-to year (e.g., smoking and drinking behavior), and the clear advantages of the NHIS-MCD data set: the large sample sizes, linked death files, the substantial breadth of independent variables available for analysis, and detail on cause of death.

It is also the case that the NHIS excludes some important variables to consider for mortality analyses, while the measurement of other variables is imprecise. For example, the 1989–1994 versions of the NHIS asked whether individuals were born in the United States or elsewhere, but did not ascertain where immigrant individuals were born. Similarly, religious attendance was ascertained in 1987, but religious denominational membership and other aspects of religious behavior were not. Indeed, one could discuss a range of variables—biological, social, and psychological—that are not included in NHIS data and many similar survey-based data sets currently being employed in the mortality literature. The measurement of other variables in the NHIS may also be questioned. For example, it is difficult to obtain unbiased estimates of the influence of cigarette smoking, alcohol use, and weight-for-height on mortality when they are measured from a single point in time such as in the NHIS. Most simply, NHIS questionnaires were not designed with mortality follow-up as the main purpose of analysis; thus, the measures used throughout our analyses may not be as precise as we might prefer. The point of this discussion is not to be overly critical of the data set employed here; in fact, the NHIS-MCD may be the most inclusive data ever available to examine U.S. mortality patterns. Rather, it is important to keep in mind that the data employed here are imperfect: some important variables are completely missing, while others are available in cruder form than is desired.

Finally, it is also important to point out that our analysis focuses exclusively on survey-based responses of individuals. Therefore, on one end of the spectrum, we have no information on the genetic composition of individuals. Indeed, researchers in some studies are now adding the genetic information of survey respondents (using blood samples) to their questionnaire information, allowing for the analysis of biological and social determinants of mortality using single data sources (Vaupel 1998). On another end of the spectrum, we also do not have access to information on the neighborhood contexts in which the surveyed individuals live. Such information would allow for the multilevel analysis of contextual and individual level factors on mortality, also at the forefront of current mortality research (e.g., LeClere et al. 1997).

Despite these limitations, the NHIS-MCD is a prospective sample that is current, large, nationally representative, and includes some people who are exposed to the risk of death over the follow-up years but live, and some people who are exposed to the risk of death over the follow-up years but die. Moreover, the NHIS-MCD includes a wealth of demographic, social, economic, psychological, behavioral, and health information for both the individuals who live and for those who subsequently die, and it also provides information for females as well as males and young as well as old adults. Thus, this data set is exceptionally well suited for research questions involving current mortality differentials at the national level. Preston and Taubman (1994) described the NHIS as the "most authoritative source of national data on socioeconomic differences in health status" (p. 291). With the death matches to the NDI, we extend this high praise to vital status as well.

MEASUREMENT

Each chapter of this monograph includes measures specific to that chapter and are, thus, detailed in the appropriate place. In this section, we review the measurement schemes that are used repeatedly and consistently throughout.

MORTALITY MEASURES

Overall mortality provides a summary measure of all causes of death and is used frequently in the demographic and public health literatures and throughout this monograph. That is, our overall mortality measure contrasts those persons who die sometime during follow-up to those who survive through the entire period. The overall mortality measure also provides a point of departure for cause-specific analyses.

Underlying cause mortality is the cause-specific scheme used most frequently in the demographic and public health literatures. Nosologists at NCHS assign underlying cause of death by using an algorithm that examines each cause listed on the death certificate and by ascribing the underlying cause as the one which initiated the sequence of events leading to death. Other causes that are listed but which apparently did not trigger the sequence of events leading to death are designated as contributing causes. The coding is accomplished according to guidelines of the International Classification of Diseases (ICD), which contains a listing of three-digit codes corresponding to the various causes of death (U.S. Department of Health and Human Services 1990). ICD codes and guidelines are updated and revised about every 10 years; the NHIS-MCD file used here employs the ninth revision of the ICD.

We classify underlying causes of death into five to eight major cause categories in the different chapters, depending on the number of deaths available for each analysis and the focus of the chapter. The categories feature underlying causes of death that comprise major sub-sections of the ICD listings (for similar coding schemes, see Potter 1991; Rogers 1992; Sorlie et al. 1993). For example, Chapter 8, which examines the association between occupational status and mortality, employs six specific cause categories of death: circulatory diseases (ICD 390-459), cancers (ICD 140-239), respiratory diseases (ICD 460-519), diabetes (ICD 250), infectious and parasitic diseases (ICD 001-139), and social pathologies, which include accidents, suicides, homicides, and cirrhosis of the liver (ICD 571 and ICD E800-E999). In addition, a seventh residual cause category is specified. Circulatory diseases are the leading cause of death in the United States, and include heart and cerebrovascular diseases, as well as hypertension. Cancers are the second leading U.S. cause of death. Together, circulatory diseases and cancer account for over 60% of all U.S. deaths (Ventura et al. 1998). Some of the chapters focus on particular causes of death. For example, Chapter 12, which considers the association between mental health and mortality, includes suicide (ICD E950-E959) as a prime cause of death.

Note as well that we do not consider two other often-used measures of mortality: multiple cause of death and *life expectancy*. Multiple cause designations take account of all conditions (underlying and contributing) listed on the death certificate. The cause combinations are then organized into different schemes for analytic purposes (Nam 1990). Various works (e.g., Nam et al. 1994; Wrigley and Nam 1987) have shown that the interpretation of mortality differentials between groups may vary depending on whether an underlying cause or multiple cause scheme is used. Nevertheless, we focus here on the more basic overall and underlying cause measures to paint a broad picture of U.S. mortality differentials. Future work, of course, may expand into the multiple cause arena to take advantage of all of the available information in the MCD file.

Life expectancy is a measure of mortality often used in the demographic literature and presents expected remaining years of life at specified ages for individuals in a population, given current age-specific mortality rates. Life expectancy is a particularly useful measure for demographic characteristics of populations such as sex and race/ethnicity; in other words, for population characteristics that are least apt to change. Using the NHIS-MCD data, we have calculated life expectancy at age 55 (e55) for each sex and race (Rogers et al. 1997) and at age 20 (e20) by religious attendance (Hummer et al. 1999a). We find that estimates of life expectancy based on the NHIS-MCD tend to be somewhat higher than those of vital statistics data, most likely because (a) the NHIS-MCD stems from a noninstitutionalized sample of adults; (b) some deaths—perhaps 3 to 5%—are missed in the NDI (NCHS 1997b); and (c) some participants in the NHIS cannot be followed (ineligibles) because of a lack of identifying information. Further, life expectancy figures are most often presented without controlling for other covariates and, thus, are not adjusted for other influential variables related to mortality risk. Therefore, for the analyses throughout this monograph, we focus on *differential overall and cause-specific mortality,* as measured by odds ratios of death and with controls for various mortality covariates. The actual models we employ are discussed in the statistical methodology section below.

COVARIATES OF MORTALITY

A variety of factors are associated with the risk of mortality for individuals. This monograph depicts factors ranging from age, race, and sex, to cigarette smoking, religious participation, and mental health. While the different chapters highlight the specific measures that are the focus for that chapter, several measures are consistently used throughout the monograph. *Age,* for example, is measured throughout in single years ranging from 18 to 99. Due to confidentiality concerns, children (younger than 18 years of age) who are included in the NHIS are not matched with the NDI and must be excluded from the mortality analyses. Thus, our analyses are contingent upon individuals surviving until the age of 18. While age is perhaps the most critical variable for the analysis of mortality, we do not include a separate chapter on age effects here because the NHIS-MCD data set does not include the large number of oldest-old individuals that are necessary for stable estimates of mortality at these ages (see, for example, Kestenbaum 1997). Indeed, the very oldest ages are also where U.S. mortality patterns are the most uncertain (Kestenbaum 1997; Manton and Vaupel 1995). Nevertheless, we include a control for age in every mortality model we present throughout the monograph.

Other covariates included in most chapters include sex, race, education, family income, marital status, and self-reported health. *Sex,* of course, is included as a dichotomous variable, with males compared to females. While we examine race and ethnicity in detail in Chapter 4, most chapters include a dichotomous control for *race* by contrasting African Americans with persons of other races. Most chapters include three categories for both education and marital status. The *education* measure contrasts those persons with 0–11 years and 12 years of education with those persons with 13 or more years of education. *Marital status* contrasts persons who are separated/divorced and widowed with those who are currently married. We measure *family income* on an equivalence scale, which takes account of the family size of the respondent (Buhmann et al. 1988). Here, income equivalence (W) is equal to family income (I) divided by family size (S), raised to an equivalence elasticity of .38 (Van der Gaag and Smolensky 1982), which adjusts for differences in consumption across families of different sizes:

$$W = I/S^{.38}$$

This measure exhibited a stronger association with mortality than competitors, such as income in dollars or logged dollars (see Chapter 7). We measure income equivalence continuously in units of $10,000.

Self-reported health is a frequently used five-level measure ranging from poor to excellent. Despite being self-reported, it reflects a person's general health condition well and has found to be a strong predictor of subsequent mortality in many studies (Idler and Benyamini 1997; McGee et al. 1999; Mossey and Shapiro 1982). Other covariates (e.g., behavioral, other health variables) are used less consistently through the monograph and, thus, their measurement schemes are detailed in the appropriate chapters.

MISSING DATA

Yet another outstanding feature of the NHIS-MCD data set is that for most variables there are very small percentages of missing data. For example, the 1989 NHIS shows no missing data for age and sex; less than 1% missing for race, marital status, and self-reported health; and less than 2% missing for education (NCHS 1991b). Thus, cases with missing data are generally dropped from the analyses.

One notable exception is detailed family income, which generally has a nonresponse rate of 10 to 15% in the various years of the NHIS. Rather than exclude this substantial number of cases, we imputed values for detailed family income based on regression models of age, sex, marital status, and education, and stratified by whether the person's categorized family income was less than $20,000 or $20,000 or more, which was usually missing for only about 2% of the cases. This imputation allowed us to preserve a great majority of the cases for analysis. Further, we observed no difference in conclusions based on whether we included or excluded the imputed cases for income; our decision to include the imputed cases resided mainly in our desire to maintain the nationally representative character of the data and large sample sizes for analyses.

STATISTICAL ANALYSES

DESCRIPTIVE ANALYSES

Within each chapter, we present a basic descriptive table of data that shows, for most covariates, the percentage distribution of cases specific to survival status. For example, the descriptive tabulations consistently show that women are somewhat more likely to be represented in the survivor group than men (usually about 55% compared to 45%, respectively) and somewhat less likely to be represented in the decedents than men (usually about 45% compared to 55%). This is because adult women outnumber men in the U.S. population and have lower death rates. For continuously measured covariates, such as age, the mean values specific to survival status are shown. Thus, for example, our descriptive tabulations consistently show a much lower mean age for the survivor population in comparison to the decedent population. All of the descriptive tabulations are weighted to represent the civilian, noninstitutionalized population of survivors and decedents.

DISCRETE TIME HAZARDS MODELING

Most of the analyses in the book are built around regression models of mortality risk that take into account different sets of covariates as explanatory variables. To examine mortality within such a multivariate framework, we use discrete-time hazard models (Allison 1984). These models are appropriate for data that include a *risk set*—a set of individuals who are at risk of dying during each follow-up interval—and a *hazard*—the event of interest (death) that may occur during a particular interval to a particular individual in the risk set. Discrete-time hazard models also provide consistent estimators of the true standard errors of the regression coefficients (Allison 1984; Teachman et al. 1994).

Because NHIS interviews are conducted throughout the year, respondents are considered at risk of dying for one-half of the interview year and for the entire year for each subsequent year of follow-up through the end of 1995. Therefore, the individual person-records in these data are transformed into a *person-year* file where individuals contribute the number of person-years they lived before death or before the end of the follow-up period (Allison 1984). For survivors of the 1986 NHIS to the end of follow-up, each person contributes 9.5 person-years to the file. For those who die during the follow-up period, the number of person-years depends on the timing of death. For example, persons interviewed in 1986 and who died in 1988 contribute just 2.5 person-years. The transformation of individual records to person-year files is commonplace in mortality studies—particularly when individuals are interviewed and then followed over time (Rogers et al. 1996b).

While our data generally do not include time-varying covariates (as discussed above), the age of individuals in the person-year file is adjusted for each year that the individual is followed. For example, if a person was originally interviewed in 1986 and was 24 years old, the first person-year record for that individual would list their age as 24, their values for the other covariates, and their survival status for that year. If they survived 1986, the person-year record for that individual for 1987 would list them as 25 years old, would list the same values for the other covariates, and would list their survival status for 1987. In this fashion, age and survival status are appropriately adjusted for each person-year record, while the values for the other covariates necessarily remain unchanged.

Once a person-year data set is developed, the estimation of discrete-time hazard models is accomplished through the logistic regression specification in common statistical packages (Allison 1984). For overall mortality (died during follow-up versus survival) models, we use dichotomous logistic regression to compare individuals who died sometime during the follow-up period (coded one) to those who survived the follow-up (coded zero). The logistic regression specification estimates the amount of change in the dependent variable given a change in the independent variables, contingent on the specific value of the independent variables being examined (Aldrich and Nelson 1984). For the cause of death analyses, we employ multinomial logistic regression methods. This type of analysis compares those who survive to those who die from one of a number of different causes, say cancer, or circulatory disease, or respiratory disease, or accidents. Generally, we make comparisons between survival and a particular cause of death. But we also compare the odds of dying from one cause to those of dying from another (e.g., how much greater are the odds of dying from cancer compared to those of dying from respiratory disease?). The multinomial logistic regression model is a direct extension of the dichotomous logistic regression model (Hanushek and Jackson 1977; Maddala 1983). In the multinomial case, the dependent variable is the log of the conditional odds of the probability of each cause of death relative to surviving.

Other recent mortality studies have used continuous-time hazard models, where time is measured from date of the interview to date of death and not in yearly intervals (e.g., LeClere et al. 1997). Generally, the results provided by these two approaches will be very similar. Allison (1984: 22), for example, notes that the discrete-time method will virtually always give results that are similar to continuous-time models, and the choice between the two methods "should generally be made on the basis of computational cost and convenience." We compared the results given by discrete-time and continuous-time methods for many of our models and present one such comparison in a simple model shown in Table 2.1. The discrete-time hazard model results are shown in the left columns, while the continuous-time hazard model results are shown in the right columns. In these models, the risk of mortality is regressed on age, measured in single years, and a dichotomous measure of sex, with women specified as the reference category. Indeed, as we consistently found, the two methods yield nearly identical results. In each, the risk of mortality increases about 8% with each additional year of age, and men exhibit a 72 to 73% higher mortality risk over the follow-up period compared to women. Because the estimation of the discrete-time models were more convenient for our purposes and because many readers in the social science and public health areas are very familiar and comfortable with logistic regression results and in the interpretation of odds ratios—as specified by the discrete-time hazard model—we chose to use the discrete-time hazard models throughout.

Further, we report the results of all of the discrete-time models in the form of odds ratios of death (see Hosmer and Lemeshow 1989). Odds ratios are the exponentiated form of the regression coefficients that the discrete-time hazard models produce. Throughout this monograph, individuals who survive each person-year are coded zero, while those who die during the year are coded one. Thus, odds ratios above 1.00 indicate a higher risk of death for that particular category of the independent variable, while those below 1.00 signify a reduced risk of mortality. Again, referring to the simple model in Table 2.1, older persons and males exhibit higher odds of death compared to younger persons and females. The reference categories for each categorical covariate are listed in the tables, with "ref" in the tables indicating the comparison odds ratio (or 1.00) for each particular variable.

TABLE 2.1   A Comparison of Results Produced by a Discrete-Time Hazard Mortality Model with Those Produced by a Continuous-Time (Cox Proportional) Hazard Mortality Model, U.S. Adults, 1990–1995

	Discrete-time model results		Continuous-time model results	
	Coefficient	Odds ratio	Coefficient	Hazard ratio
Age (continuous)	.08*	1.08*	.08*	1.08*
Sex				
Male	.55*	1.73*	.54*	1.72*
Female	ref	ref	ref	ref

Source: NCHS 1993c, 1997b.
$+ p \leq .10;\ * p \leq .05.$

Within each chapter we present a series of models, focusing on the odds ratio of mortality for the covariate being focused upon. Thus, for example, we portray race/ethnic differences in mortality adjusted for only age and sex, then further adjusted for socioeconomic factors such as education and family income, and then further adjusted for other factors. This strategy is commonplace in the mortality literature and allows for the interpretation of mortality differentials within the multivariate context.

STATISTICAL INFERENCE IN
COMPLEX SAMPLE SURVEYS

The NHIS is not a strict random sample of the U.S. civilian, noninstitutionalized population; rather, the annual NHIS is derived through a stratified, multistage probability design. These design effects are used to increase sample sizes for some relatively small population groups and to reduce field costs, as cases are sampled from selected geographic areas. However, such methods may also produce a loss of statistical power in the data because of the intracluster correlation of responses. In fact, the effects of sampling design on statistical inferences—particularly on the estimation of standard errors for regression coefficients—are often overlooked by researchers. The more popular statistical packages—SAS, SPSS, and BMDP—generally assume that data are drawn from strictly random samples and, therefore, do not correctly incorporate the design effects into the calculations of the standard errors. We use the statistical package SUDAAN 7.0 (Shah et al. 1996), which incorporates information about the design of the sample to correctly estimate the coefficients and standard errors for our models (Forthofer 1992). Notably, the regression (discrete-time hazard) coefficients produced by SUDAAN are identical to those produced by other packages such as SAS; however, standard errors estimated in SUDAAN tend to be larger than those produced by standard packages and yield more conservative estimates of statistical significance. We report significance levels for all coefficients at the .05 and .10 levels.

HEALTH SELECTIVITY

Some individuals who are NHIS respondents are quite unhealthy and are, thus, likely to die shortly after the time of the survey. Other individuals, on the other hand, are very healthy at the time of the survey and are much more likely to survive the duration of the follow-up period. Further, *if* the health status of individuals is related to the mortality differential being investigated (say, for instance, mortality differences by religious attendance), the effects of the variable being estimated (e.g., religious attendance) may be biased because it, in part, reflects health status. Thus, when health status may be confounding the relationship between the independent variable in question and the risk of mortality, we statistically control for the health status of individuals at the time of the survey. This is usually accomplished through the use of the self-reported health status variable, as well as through the use of other health controls (see, for example, Chapter 6 on the relationship between religious attendance and mortality, where three measures of health status at baseline are controlled). Further, recall that the data set we employ excludes some of the most unhealthy people from the analysis at the baseline time because it is a sample of the *noninstitutionalized* population. We return to the issue of health selectivity separately in several of the individual chapters.

CONCLUSION

This chapter has presented the NHIS-MCD data set to be used throughout the book, and explained some of the basic measures and statistical methods that are used. The NHIS-MCD linked data set, while containing some disadvantages, is one of the largest, most timely, and comprehensive data sets ever compiled for investigating differential mortality in the United States. We rely on discrete-time hazards modeling, with coefficients presented in the form of odds ratios, as our prime statistical methodology. The analysis chapters employ a consistent format and methodology (as detailed in this chapter), facilitating concordance between chapters and ease of interpretation throughout. The key methodological difference between chapters involves the choice of particular NHIS data set(s) and specific variables employed. Thus, the individual chapters detail the data set selections and the specific measures used.

DEMOGRAPHIC AND SOCIOCULTURAL CHARACTERISTICS

3

THE SEX DIFFERENTIAL IN MORTALITY

For most of the 20th century, the sex gap in U.S. life expectancy at birth widened, moving from 1.8 years in 1920 to a peak of almost 8 years in the mid-1970s (Knudsen and McNown 1993). In the last 20 years, the sex mortality gap has slowly narrowed; U.S. women currently enjoy a 6.0 year advantage in life expectancy compared to men (Peters et al. 1998). While a very small portion of this female advantage is attributable to survival advantages during infancy and childhood, the large majority is due to causes of death operating during adulthood. Most importantly, this includes heart disease, but also accidents and violence, cancer, and respiratory diseases (Nathanson 1984). Recent data indicate that close to 40% of the U.S. sex mortality differential is due to ischemic heart disease alone, although this percentage has been declining (Knudsen and McNown 1993; Trovato and Lalu 1998).

This chapter explores the current sex differential in U.S. mortality by examining the influences of demographic, social, economic, and behavioral factors on overall and cause-specific mortality. In addition, we examine whether the magnitude of the sex mortality gap differs across categories of education, income, employment, and marital status—a possibility that has been proposed in recent literature, but which remains largely unexplored (Nathanson 1995; Nathanson and Lopez 1987; Vallin 1995).

PREVIOUS LITERATURE ON THE SEX MORTALITY GAP

Two broad explanations have been offered for understanding the female mortality advantage vis-à-vis men in the United States. First, biological factors may be responsible for some portion of the difference. In a classic study that compared Roman Catholic Brothers and Sisters, Madigan (1957) found that the sex mortality difference between these two groups was similar to the general population. This finding was interpreted to suggest that biological differences between the sexes must be important, because the social environments of the Brothers and Sisters were thought to be quite similar. These results were later questioned, since there was selectivity in age at entry into the monestaries and convents. Further, the study did not fully control for sex differences in health behavior or health conditions.

Much later work in demography and public health focused on the explanatory influence of behavioral factors for understanding the sex mortality gap. However, Verbrugge (1989), noting the inability of behaviorally based statistical models to fully account for sex differences in mortality, also suggested that the answer may lie in biological factors (also see Wingard et al. 1983). More recent evidence indicates that women may be protected from a limited number of infectious and degenerative diseases because of the presence of reproductive physiology, protective hormones, and certain X-linked genes (Gage 1994; Waldron 1983). This is probably most important in the case of heart disease mortality, where the production of estrogen in premenopausal women and estrogen replacement therapy in postmenopausal women appear to reduce the risk of death from this leading cause (Grodstein et al. 1997; Horiuchi 1997). Moreover, differences in the distribution of body fat appear to be associated with women's lower mortality due to heart disease (Waldron 1995). Furthermore, different types of cancer have been linked to reproductive physiology differences between the sexes (Waldron 1983).

It is also clear that the influence of biological factors on sex mortality differences varies across social and cultural environments. For example, the physical toll of childbearing—an important biologically based contributor to female mortality historically and in some modern developing nations—poses relatively little mortality risk to women in modern industrial societies (Waldron 1983). In a similar sense, estrogen replacement therapy is a medical innovation that seems to lower women's mortality risk (Grodstein et al. 1997), but is relevant only in modern industrialized nations. While we cannot directly measure the impact of biological factors or their interactions with social and cultural factors in our data set, strong evidence suggests that the U.S. sex mortality difference is at least partially rooted in biological differences between the sexes (Carey 1997; Waldron 1995).

Sex mortality differentials, however, have been found to vary substantially over time and place, and by social class and marital status, suggesting that biological theories of causation may address only part of the puzzle (Lopez 1983; Nathanson 1984; Nathanson and Lopez 1987; Waldron 1983). Behavioral explanations suggest that male-female differences in mortality risks are due to the contrasting behavior patterns exhibited by men and women. Most often cited are male excesses in cigarette smoking, alcohol use, occupational hazards, and dangerous behavior, such as high speed driving and the excessive use of violence in stressful situations. Retherford (1975), for example, analyzed the impact of cigarette smoking on increased U.S. sex mortality differences between 1910 and 1962 and found that smoking accounted for 75% of the increase. While male and female patterns of smoking have become more similar in recent decades, historical and continued differences in cigarette smoking patterns, especially at high levels of consumption, continue to favor women (Rogers and Powell-Griner 1991; Rogers et al. 1995; Waldron 1986). Additional evidence, however, indicates that other behavioral differences between women and men may have limited impact on the sex mortality differential. Wingard (1982), for example, found that physical activity, weight status, and several psychosocial risk factors favored male as opposed to female survival. Thus, while behavioral explanations—and especially cigarette smoking—are surely important for continued evaluation, to date they have not been able to account for the entire sex gap in U.S. mortality.

In more recent years, a conceptual framework focusing on the differing social structural positions of men and women and their impact on the mortality gap between the sexes has been advanced. In the case of heart disease, Nathanson and Lopez (1987) argue that gender differences in smoking and other behavioral risk factors have become increasingly concentrated among the lower classes. Correspondingly, risk factor differences are less pronounced among the middle and upper classes, and may result in a much smaller sex mortality gap in those structural positions (also see Vallin 1995). Indeed, Nathanson and Lopez (1987) suggest that "sex mortality differentials may converge at upper socioeconomic status levels, due primarily to the presence at these levels of structural and cultural supports for relatively healthy male behavior" (p. 133). Strengthening this argument is the fact that U.S. smoking rates are relatively similar among white collar men, blue collar women, and white collar women, but substantially higher among blue collar men (Nathanson and Lopez 1987). A similar sex mortality pattern may also be evident by marital status; that is, the sex mortality gap has been found to be smaller among married individuals and larger among unmarried individuals (Gove 1973; Rogers 1995a). Thus, the sex mortality gap is not static across social groups and reflects the sex-specific socialization patterns and norms within U.S. subpopulations (Nathanson 1984; Nathanson and Lopez 1987). However, surprisingly little empirical research—particularly at the population level—has investigated the sex mortality gap within specific social and economic groups.

It is also the case that the generally more privileged social and economic position of males vis-à-vis females in U.S. society works to keep the sex mortality gap from being even larger than it is. That is, much scientific literature has documented the educational, income, and occupational advantages of men in U.S. society, but few studies of sex mortality differences take such basic compositional differences into account. Compared to women, a higher percentage of adult men are also married—which is yet another compositional difference that favors male survival prospects (Lillard and Waite 1995; Rogers 1995a). Thus, although recent decades have witnessed substantial gains by women in labor force participation, income, and education, the gendered structure of stratification in U.S. society continues to favor men. In attempting to explain sex differences in mortality, however, few studies have considered such male advantages, most likely because statistical adjustment for such factors may only work to widen the observed gaps.

DATA

This chapter uses the 1990 Health Promotion and Disease Prevention (HPDP) supplement of the National Health Interview Survey (NHIS). The survival status of persons in this data set is ascertained through matches with the Multiple Cause of Death (MCD) file through the end of 1995 (NCHS 1993c, 1997b). The NHIS-HPDP contains a nationally representative sample of 41,104 adults aged 18 and over. Linkage with the MCD file results in 237,929 person years for this analysis, along with 2,388 deaths. The dependent variable for most of the analysis is overall mortality versus survival, but we further specify underlying cause mortality for a portion of the analysis. The cause groups include circulatory diseases (International Classification of Diseases [ICD] 390-459), cancers (ICD 140-239), respiratory diseases (ICD 466-496), social pathologies—which include suicide, accidents, homicide, and cirrhosis of the liver (ICD 571 and ICD E800-E999)—and a residual fifth group of causes, which includes infectious diseases, diabetes, and more.

The analysis focuses around the sex variable; we code women as the reference group in the statistical models because of their generally lower mortality in comparison to men. The NHIS-HPDP contains numerous covariates thought to be related to sex differentials in mortality that we build into the analysis. Our demographic measures include age, ranging from 18 to 99, and a dichotomous measure of race, contrasting African Americans and others. Social and economic variables include education, employment status, family income, and marital status. In this chapter, education is specified as four groups: 0–11 years, 12 years, 13–15 years, and 16 and more years. Employment status is coded as three groups and specifies individuals who are unemployed, those not in the labor force, and those who are employed, while income is measured continuously in units of $10,000 on an equivalence scale, as detailed in Chapter 2. Marital status is coded as four categories: never married, widowed, divorced or separated, and currently married. We expect that the inclusion of the social and economic factors in the mortality models will widen the sex mortality differential because, overall, U.S. women are in disadvantaged social and economic positions compared to men. Further, we expect that the magnitude of the sex mortality gap will vary across the categories of these social and economic variables, as suggested in the review of previous studies above.

Behavioral factors include cigarette smoking, alcohol use, exercise, and body mass. Cigarette smoking includes four groups: never smokers, former smokers, current smokers who consume less than 20 cigarettes per day (current light), and current smokers who consume 20 or more cigarettes per day (current heavy). Similarly, alcohol use includes never drinkers, former drinkers, light drinkers (less than 3 drinks per day on days drank), and heavy drinkers (three or more drinks per day on days drank). The exercise variable contrasts individuals who report exercising or playing sports regularly compared to those who report that they do not. The body mass variable specifies three groups according to self-reported weight and height. Women and men in the bottom and top 10% of the body mass index distribution are compared to those in the middle 80% of the distribution. Each of these behavioral factors is analyzed in more depth in Chapters 13 through 16. We expect that the sex mortality gap will close substantially with inclusion of the behavioral factors in the models; indeed, cigarette smoking differences between men and women is often speculated to be the key behavioral factors affecting differential mortality by sex (e.g., Retherford 1975; Rogers and Powell-Griner 1991).

RESULTS

DESCRIPTIVE STATISTICS

The descriptive data in Table 3.1 for both sexes illustrates that the United States is characterized by a larger female noninstitutionalized adult population, but that more adult men died over the follow-up period. By sex, there are large differences in the distribution of some of the social and economic covariates. About twice as many women as men are out of the paid labor force, an employment status that has been demonstrated to be associated with higher U.S. mortality (Sorlie et al. 1995). Women also live, on average, in families with slightly lower mean incomes than men and are less likely to have a college degree. Furthermore, women are more likely than men to be separated or divorced, and are far more likely to be widowed. Thus, U.S. women display disadvantaged social and economic characteris-

TABLE 3.1   Descriptive Statistics for Demographic, Social, Economic, and Behavioral
Factors Related to Sex Differences in U.S. Adult Mortality, 1990–1995

	Both sexes		Women		Men	
	Survived	Died	Survived	Died	Survived	Died
Demographic factors						
Sex						
Male	47.5	55.0	0.0	0.0	100.0	100.0
Female	52.5	45.0	100.0	100.0	0.0	0.0
Age (mean)	46.0	70.3	46.9	72.7	45.1	68.3
Race						
African American	11.1	12.3	11.8	11.9	10.3	12.6
Not African American	88.9	87.7	88.2	88.1	89.7	87.4
Social and economic factors						
Employment status						
Unemployed	3.1	1.8	2.8	0.6	3.4	2.7
Not in labor force	30.6	75.5	39.7	84.0	20.6	68.5
Employed	66.3	22.8	57.4	15.4	76.0	28.8
Income equivalence	2.1	1.6	2.0	1.5	2.2	1.7
(mean in $10,000s)						
Education						
Less than 12 years	20.6	45.1	20.9	44.1	20.3	45.9
12 years	38.6	32.8	41.0	36.3	36.0	30.0
13–15 years	20.6	11.9	20.8	11.3	20.5	12.3
16+ years	20.1	10.2	17.3	8.2	23.2	11.8
Marital status						
Never married	18.6	7.2	15.9	5.9	21.6	8.2
Divorced/separated	9.7	9.3	11.3	9.3	7.9	9.3
Widowed	6.6	26.1	10.8	45.0	2.1	10.7
Married	65.1	57.4	62.0	39.8	68.5	71.8
Behavioral factors						
Cigarette smoking						
Current heavy (20+/day)	14.4	16.5	11.5	12.0	17.5	20.1
Current light (<20/day)	11.1	10.3	11.3	10.9	10.9	9.8
Former	24.3	36.8	19.4	25.3	29.9	46.2
Never	50.2	36.3	57.8	51.8	41.7	23.8
Alcohol use						
Current heavy (3+/day)	30.7	21.9	23.7	13.7	38.5	28.6
Current light (<3/day)	30.2	21.8	27.3	16.3	33.3	26.3
Former	9.4	20.4	7.6	15.4	11.3	24.5
Never	29.5	35.6	41.3	54.4	16.5	20.2
Exercise						
No regular exercise	58.9	75.1	61.9	80.3	55.6	70.9
Regular exercise	41.1	24.9	38.1	19.7	44.4	29.1
Body mass						
Bottom 10%	10.0	12.4	10.0	11.8	10.0	12.9
Top 10%	10.0	11.2	10.0	11.5	10.0	10.9
Middle 80%	80.0	76.4	80.0	76.7	80.0	76.2
Person-years and deaths	237,929	2,388	124,903	1,074	113,026	1,314

Sources: Derived from NCHS 1993c, 1997b.

tics compared to men—a situation that should favor the survival prospects of men.

In contrast, the distribution of most of the behavioral factors favors women. While about equal percentages of men and women are current light smokers, men are more likely to be heavy smokers. Notably, men are also far more likely to be former smokers, in large part due to the earlier and more pronounced development of normative smoking behavior among U.S. men in comparison to women during past decades (Rogers et al. 1995). Men are also more likely than women to be heavy or former drinkers, while women are far more likely to be never drinkers. However, not all behavioral factors favor women; men are more likely to report that they exercise regularly. Given, however, the powerful influence of cigarette smoking on U.S. mortality patterns (further reinforced in Chapter 13), the behavioral differences exhibited here should favor women's survival. We now turn to the multivariate examination of sex mortality differences.

THE SEX DIFFERENCE IN OVERALL MORTALITY

Table 3.2 displays the sex difference in overall (all-cause) mortality for the entire age range of adults while considering the simultaneous influence of demographic, social, and economic factors. Model 1, which controls for only basic demographic factors, shows that men exhibit 73% higher odds of mortality than women during the follow-up period. However, further control for individual social and economic factors in Models 2 through 5 illustrates that, with the inclusion of any one of the variables, the sex mortality differential widens in comparison to Model 1. The most likely reason for the widening is because women tend to be in more disadvantaged social and economic positions compared to men, as illustrated in Table 3.1. Controlling for the complete set of demographic, social, and economic factors in Model 6 increases the odds ratio of male-to-female mortality to 2.0. In other words, the odds of male mortality during the follow-up period are twice those of female mortality, with the control of demographic, social, and economic characteristics. Thus, the disadvantaged social and economic situation of U.S. women prevents the sex mortality gap from being even wider than it already is. While some literature (e.g., United Nations 1991) has offered speculation that women's social and economic gains vis-à-vis men might lead to narrowed sex mortality differences, the findings here support the notion that the improving status of women, all else being equal, may work to widen the U.S. sex mortality gap (e.g., Nathanson 1995).

Table 3.3 focuses on the influence of behavioral factors. Model 1 simply repeats the basic demographic model, again illustrating the baseline 1.73 difference in mortality odds between the sexes. The inclusion of cigarette smoking in Model 2 helps to close the sex mortality gap. In fact, controlling

TABLE 3.2   Odds Ratios for Sex Differences in Mortality, Focusing on the Influence of Social and Economic Covariates, U.S. Adults, 1990–1995

	Model 1	Model 2	Model 3	Model 4	Model 5	Model 6
Demographic factors						
Sex						
Male	1.73*	1.84*	1.82*	1.78*	1.84*	2.00*
Female	ref	ref	ref	ref	ref	ref
Age (continuous)	1.09*	1.07*	1.08*	1.08*	1.08*	1.07*
Race						
African American	1.48*	1.46*	1.30*	1.36*	1.41*	1.25*
Other	ref	ref	ref	ref	ref	ref
Social and economic factors						
Employment status						
Unemployed		1.99*				1.78*
Not in labor force		1.95*				1.78*
Employed		ref				ref
Income equivalence (continuous)			0.82*			0.92*
Education						
Less than 12 years				1.94*		1.55*
12 years				1.56*		1.37*
13–15 years				1.32*		1.19+
16+ years				ref		ref
Marital status						
Never married					1.33*	1.24*
Divorced/separated					1.38*	1.36*
Widowed					1.21*	1.17*
Married					ref	ref
−2*Log-likelihood	22,310.9	22,178.7	22,216.8	22,120.4	22,279.3	21,970.9

Sources: Derived from NCHS 1993c, 1997b.
+ $p \le .10$; * $p \le .05$.

for cigarette smoking results in a sex mortality gap that is substantially smaller than that exhibited in the baseline model. Controlling for the other behavioral factors has a more modest impact on the sex mortality gap. The inclusion of the exercise variable in Model 4, in fact, slightly increases the gap in comparison to the baseline demographic model since, compared to females, males are more likely to regularly exercise. The simultaneous inclusion of smoking, alcohol use, exercise, and body mass (Model 6) demonstrates that this set of behavioral factors accounts for some, but not nearly all, of the current sex mortality gap in the United States. What most research in this area has not considered, however, is that the disadvantageous social and economic position of women in U.S. society keeps the sex mor-

TABLE 3.3   Odds Ratios for Sex Differences in Mortality, Focusing on the Influence of Behavioral Factors, U.S. Adults, 1990–1995

	Model 1	Model 2	Model 3	Model 4	Model 5	Model 6	Model 7
Demographic factors							
Sex							
Male	1.73*	1.53*	1.69*	1.77*	1.72*	1.57*	1.75*
Female	ref	ref	ref	ref	ref	ref	ref
Age (continuous)	1.09*	1.09*	1.08*	1.08*	1.08*	1.09*	1.08*
Race							
African American	1.48*	1.51*	1.44*	1.42*	1.46*	1.39*	1.26*
Other	ref	ref	ref	ref	ref	ref	ref
Behavioral factors							
Cigarette smoking							
Current heavy (20+/day)		2.56*				2.43*	2.28*
Current light (<20/day)		2.22*				2.23*	2.08*
Former		1.39*				1.44*	1.42*
Never		ref				ref	ref
Alcohol use							
Current heavy (3+/day)			1.15*			0.97	1.01
Current light (<3/day)			0.81*			0.74*	0.82*
Former			1.35*			1.16*	1.14*
Never			ref			ref	ref
Exercise							
No regular exercise				1.57*		1.44*	1.40*
Regular exercise				ref		ref	ref
Body mass							
Bottom 10%					1.51*	1.37*	1.32*
Top 10%					1.27*	1.26*	1.22*
Middle 80%					ref	ref	ref
Social and economic factors							
Employment status							
Unemployed							1.77*
Not in labor force							1.76*
Employed							ref
Income equivalence (continuous)							0.95*
Education							
Less than 12 years							1.27*
12 years							1.18*
13–15 years							1.09
16+years							ref

(*continues*)

TABLE 3.3 (*continued*)

	Model 1	Model 2	Model 3	Model 4	Model 5	Model 6	Model 7
Marital status							
Never married							1.29*
Divorced/separated							1.20*
Widowed							1.16*
Married							ref
−2*Log-likelihood	22,310.9	21,713.8	21,762.8	21,890.9	22,095.0	21,291.8	21,077.8

Sources: Derived from NCHS 1993c, 1997b.
$+ p \leq .10; * p \leq .05.$

tality gap from being even larger. Thus, Model 7 additionally includes the social and economic factors that were included in Table 3.2. The inclusion of all of these covariates results in a sex mortality gap nearly equal to the baseline demographic model (compare Model 7 to Model 1). Thus, our analysis suggests that the higher male risks associated with these behavioral factors are about equal—in terms of their impact on the sex mortality gap— to the social and economic disadvantages experienced by women.

SEX DIFFERENCES IN
CAUSE-SPECIFIC MORTALITY

Considering the inability of the overall mortality models presented in Tables 3.2 and 3.3 to statistically eliminate the sex mortality gap, Table 3.4 examines sex mortality differentials across five cause-of-death categories. For each cause, three models are presented. Model 1 for each cause includes only demographic factors; Model 2 for each cause additionally includes social and economic factors; Model 3 for each cause additionally includes behavioral factors.

Comparing the baseline sex mortality differential across causes (Model 1 for each) illustrates that the magnitude of the gap varies, with the largest being a 2.76 differential in odds exhibited for social pathologies. This large gap is particularly unfortunate, given that a substantial proportion of social pathological deaths occur at young ages and are due to homicide, suicide, and automobile accidents (Trovato and Lalu 1998). In fact, we found the largest age-specific sex mortality differential to be evident among 18–44 year olds, where men exhibited 2.45 times the odds of death than women over the follow-up period (data not shown).

Each cause category of death, though, is characterized by higher male mortality. Perhaps most important, the odds of death due to circulatory diseases for men over the follow-up period are nearly 1.8 times those of women. This cause group accounts for over 40% of U.S. adult deaths and, thus, is the major contributor to overall sex mortality differences (e.g. Knudsen and McNown 1993; Trovato and Lalu 1998). Model 2 for circulatory diseases shows that, similar to overall mortality, controlling for social and economic factors magnifies the mortality difference between men and women. In turn, controlling for behavioral factors in Model 3 works to narrow the difference, although men still exhibit about twice the odds of circulatory disease mortality compared to women when controlling for the complete set of mortality covariates included here. Keep in mind that while control for cigarette smoking works to narrow the male-female gap in circulatory disease mortality, control for exercise—also a powerful risk factor for circulatory disease mortality (see Chapter 15)—has the opposite effect (e.g., Waldron 1995). The unexplained excess circulatory disease male mortality in Model 3 may, in part, be due to the incomplete measurement of social and behavioral risk factors. For example, our measure of cigarette smoking, while powerful, cannot take into account the complete life history of individual smoking patterns. Other factors thought to be relevant for circulatory disease mortality risks and which also might favor women— such as personality type and specific dietary patterns (Waldron 1995)—are also not available in this data set. Given, however, the mounting biological evidence linking, most importantly, sex hormones and the distribution of body fat to differential sex patterns of heart disease mortality, the unexplained wide gap for circulatory diseases evident in our Model 3 is not surprising.

Cancer and respiratory disease mortality also exhibit wide sex differences. Controlling for only demographic factors, men exhibit about twice the odds of respiratory disease mortality and about 1.6 times the odds of cancer mortality. For these two causes, the addition of behavioral factors in Model 3 substantially reduces the sex mortality gap. The cancer mortality differential, in fact, is nearly eliminated when comparing Model 2 to Model 3. For these two causes, cigarette smoking has been demonstrated to be the key behavioral risk factor (Hummer et al. 1998a; Nam et al. 1994; Peto et al. 1995). Thus, it is not surprising that a substantial narrowing of the mortality gaps occur when smoking is added to the models. With large reductions in smoking in recent decades exhibited especially by men, the short-term future sex gap in mortality from these two causes could decline even further. Nevertheless, more U.S. men than women still smoke cigarettes; further, men continue to be heavier smokers than women (Rogers et al. 1995). Unless these patterns change, men can still expect to experience significantly higher death rates from these causes well into the 21st century (Nam et al. 1996; also see Carter and Lee 1992).

TABLE 3.4 Odds Ratios for Sex Differences in Cause-Specific Mortality, Controlling for Demographic, Social, Economic, and Behavioral Factors, U.S. Adults, 1990–1995

	Circulatory			Cancer			Respiratory			Social pathologies			Residual		
	Model 1	Model 2	Model 3	Model 1	Model 2	Model 3	Model 1	Model 2	Model 3	Model 1	Model 2	Model 3	Model 1	Model 2	Model 3
Demographic factors															
Sex															
Male	1.77*	2.09*	1.98*	1.61*	1.59*	1.20*	2.01*	2.46*	1.67*	2.76*	3.15*	3.64*	1.52*	1.96*	1.74*
Female	ref	ref	ref	ref	ref	ref	ref	ref	ref	ref	ref	ref	ref	ref	ref
Age (continuous)	1.10*	1.08*	1.09*	1.08*	1.08*	1.08*	1.11*	1.09*	1.10*	1.02*	1.01*	1.02*	1.09*	1.06*	1.06*
Race															
African American	1.34*	1.11	1.12	1.40*	1.38*	1.38*	0.54+	0.43*	0.49+	1.14	0.85	0.86	2.84*	2.17*	2.18*
Other	ref	ref	ref	ref	ref	ref	ref	ref	ref	ref	ref	ref	ref	ref	ref
Social and economic factors															
Employment status															
Unemployed		2.01*	2.04*		1.08	1.04		1.85	1.80		1.69	1.59		3.18*	3.34*
Not in labor force		2.08*	2.05*		1.28*	1.22+		1.71*	1.58+		1.18	1.19		3.14*	3.36*
Employed		ref	ref		ref	ref		ref	ref		ref	ref		ref	ref
Income equivalence (cont)		0.89*	0.93+		1.01	1.02		0.84+	0.89		0.88	0.91		0.86*	0.92
Education															
Less than 12 years		1.76*	1.44*		1.39*	1.14		1.73+	1.27		1.83*	1.63+		1.19	0.99
12 years		1.45*	1.31*		1.45*	1.22		1.74+	1.36		1.03	0.90		1.09	0.93
13–15 years		1.29+	1.25		1.16	1.04		1.83+	1.46		1.02	0.97		0.86	0.75
16+ years		ref	ref		ref	ref		ref	ref		ref	ref		ref	ref

Marital status															
Never married		1.12	1.16		0.80	0.82		0.76	0.77		1.46	1.40		2.02*	2.09*
Divorced/separated		0.97	0.88		1.42*	1.14		2.73*	2.21*		1.57+	1.43		1.73*	1.67*
Widowed		1.24*	1.20*		0.73*	0.74*		1.25	1.18		1.69+	1.75+		1.56*	1.61*
Married		ref	ref		ref	ref		ref	ref		ref	ref		ref	ref
Behavioral factors															
Cigarette smoking															
Current heavy (20+/day)			2.20*			2.94*			5.25*			1.27			1.80*
Current light (<20/day)			2.24*			2.27*			3.39*			1.35			1.78*
Former			1.30*			1.77*			3.54*			0.49*			1.29+
Never			ref			ref			ref			ref			ref
Alcohol use															
Current heavy (3+/day)			0.86			1.21			0.82			1.20			1.09
Current light (<3/day)			0.66*			1.07			0.66+			0.84			0.96
Former			1.03			1.49*			1.19			0.77			1.00
Never			ref			ref			ref			ref			ref
Exercise															
No regular exercise			1.43*			1.27*			1.83*			1.09			1.76*
Regular exercise			ref			ref			ref			ref			ref
Body mass															
Bottom 10%			1.02			1.33*			2.01*			1.09			1.77*
Top 10%			1.41*			1.08			0.49+			1.12			1.55*
Middle 80%			ref			ref			ref			ref			ref
−2*Log-likelihood	10,628.7	10,445.2	9,970.5	8,258.3	8,191.9	7,896.5	2,473.6	2,426.9	2,283.2	2,549.0	2,515.1	2,431.2	4,607.1	4,458.6	4,231.1

Sources: Derived from NCHS 1993c, 1997b.

$+ p \leq .10$; $* p \leq .05$.

SEX MORTALITY DIFFERENTIALS ACROSS
SOCIAL AND ECONOMIC FACTORS

Our overall and cause-specific mortality models suggested that the male-female gap might be even greater if the social and economic positions of men and women were more equal in U.S. society. Some have also suggested that sex mortality gaps are not static among social and economic groups; that is, male and female mortality might be highly similar in more advantaged structural positions (Nathanson and Lopez 1987). One implication, if such a hypothesis holds, is that social positions have different implications for male and female mortality. Second, similar or identical mortality experiences by sex within social and economic groups would dampen the argument that sex mortality differentials are primarily rooted in biological determinants (e.g., Carey 1997). However, few studies have compared sex mortality differences within social and economic positions of the U.S. population.

Thus, Tables 3.5 through 3.8 display the results from all-cause mortality models run within categories of employment status, family income category, educational level, and marital status, respectively. Because family income was measured on a continuous equivalence scale in earlier models, we categorize this variable into quartiles to best show sex mortality differences across the different levels of income. For each of these tables, we display only the odds ratio for male to female mortality. Note also that the three models specified for each category of the social and economic factors controls for the covariates listed at the bottom of each table.

Together, these tables demonstrate that males exhibited higher mortality than females over the follow-up period within all of the social and economic positions that we specified. Nevertheless, rather wide variation in the sex mortality gap is evident when comparing across the social and economic positions. For employment status (Table 3.5) , the odds of male mortality is over five times that of female mortality for unemployed persons. While the percentage of unemployed people in the population is relatively small (in this data set, about 3% for both men and women; see Table 3.1), this category poses an exceptionally higher comparative risk for men. In contrast, employed males and males not in the labor force exhibit just under twice the odds of mortality compared to their female counterparts. Married individuals (Table 3.6) are also characterized by a smaller sex mortality gap, while divorced and separated individuals are characterized by somewhat higher gaps. Consistent with the findings for employment status, the mortality gap is sizable for each of the marital status groups and remains large even with control for demographic, social, economic, and behavioral covariates.

For family income categories and educational levels (Tables 3.7 and 3.8, respectively), the most advantaged social positions are characterized by no-

TABLE 3.5 Odds Ratios for Sex Differences in Mortality for Adults Who are Employed, Unemployed, and Not in the Labor Force, Controlling for Demographic, Social, Economic, and Behavioral Factors, U.S. Adults, 1990–1995[a]

	Employed			Unemployed			Not in labor force		
	Model 1	Model 2	Model 3	Model 1	Model 2	Model 3	Model 1	Model 2	Model 3
Sex									
Male	1.94*	1.99*	1.70*	5.18*	5.72*	5.07*	1.79*	1.97*	1.73*
Female	ref	ref	ref	ref	ref	ref	ref	ref	ref
−2*Log-likelihood	6,528.3	6,483.4	6,264.3	476.1	468.6	454.2	15,149.1	14,979.8	14,298.6

Source: Derived from NCHS 1993c, 1997b.
[a] Model 1 controls for demographic factors. Model 2 controls for demographic, social, and economic factors. Model 3 controls for demographic, social, economic, and behavioral factors. (See Tables 3.2, 3.3, and 3.4 in this chapter for a more complete illustration of this modeling.)
$+ p \leq .10$; $* p \leq .05$.

TABLE 3.6 Odds Ratios for Sex Differences in Mortality Specific to Four Marital Statuses, Controlling for Demographic, Social, Economic, and Behavioral Factors, U.S. Adults, 1990–1995[a]

	Married			Never Married			Divorced/separated			Widowed		
	Model 1	Model 2	Model 3	Model 1	Model 2	Model 3	Model 1	Model 2	Model 3	Model 1	Model 2	Model 3
Sex												
Male	1.74*	1.90*	1.67*	1.98*	2.09*	2.09*	2.21*	2.39*	1.92*	1.81*	1.88*	1.57*
Female	ref	ref	ref	ref	ref	ref	ref	ref	ref	ref	ref	ref
−2*Log-likelihood	13,164.6	13,017.8	12,519.6	1,878.1	1,843.9	1,773.6	2,195.7	2,115.5	1,996.9	4,991.7	4,925.2	4,683.8

Source: Derived from NCHS 1993c, 1997b.

[a] Model 1 controls for demographic factors. Model 2 controls for demographic, social, and economic factors. Model 3 controls for demographic, social, economic, and behavioral factors. (See Tables 3.2, 3.3, and 3.4 in this chapter for a more complete illustration of this modeling.)

+ $p \leq .10$; * $p \leq .05$.

TABLE 3.7 Odds Ratios for Sex Differences in Mortality Specific to Four Levels of Family Income, Controlling for Demographic, Social, Economic, and Behavioral Factors, U.S. Adults, 1990–1995[a]

	Lowest quartile			Second quartile			Third quartile			Highest quartile		
	Model 1	Model 2	Model 3	Model 1	Model 2	Model 3	Model 1	Model 2	Model 3	Model 1	Model 2	Model 3
Sex												
Male	1.92*	2.15*	1.97*	1.84*	2.02*	1.71*	1.97*	1.97*	1.75*	1.32*	1.52*	1.33*
Female	ref	ref	ref	ref	ref	ref	ref	ref	ref	ref	ref	ref
−2*Log-likelihood	7,422.6	7,294.6	6,963.4	7,689.6	7,612.4	7,263.6	3,955.2	3,926.7	3,772.1	3,091.2	3,077.9	2,993.3

Source: Derived from NCHS 1993c, 1997b.
[a] Model 1 controls for demographic factors. Model 2 controls for demographic, social, and economic factors. Model 3 controls for demographic, social, economic, and behavioral factors. (See Tables 3.2, 3.3, and 3.4 in this chapter for a more complete illustration of this modeling.)
+ $p \leq .10$; * $p \leq .05$.

TABLE 3.8 Odds Ratios for Sex Differences in Mortality Specific to Four Levels of Educational Attainment, Controlling for Demographic, Social, Economic, and Behavioral Factors, U.S. Adults, 1990–1995[a]

| | 0–11 Years | | | 12 Years | | | 13–15 Years | | | 16+ Years | | |
	Model 1	Model 2	Model 3	Model 1	Model 2	Model 3	Model 1	Model 2	Model 3	Model 1	Model 2	Model 3
Sex												
Male	1.89*	2.11*	1.90*	1.67*	1.89*	1.64*	1.83*	2.12*	1.90*	1.47*	1.68*	1.50*
Female	ref	ref	ref	ref	ref	ref	ref	ref	ref	ref	ref	ref
−2*Log-likelihood	9,080.4	9,007.8	8,557.6	7,567.9	7,517.6	7,264.1	2,865.4	2,840.2	2,730.6	2,567.2	2,556.7	2,448.2

Sources: Derived from NCHS 1993c, 1997b.

[a] Model 1 controls for demographic factors. Model 2 controls for demographic, social, and economic factors. Model 3 controls for demographic, social, economic, and behavioral factors. (See Tables 3.2, 3.3, and 3.4 in this chapter for a more complete illustration of this modeling.)

$+ p \leq .10$; $* p \leq .05$.

tably smaller sex mortality gaps. For example, men living in high-income families exhibit only 32% higher odds of mortality compared to women in high-income families, controlling for demographic factors. Even within the highest income quartile and among college graduates, however, the sex mortality gap persists after control for the measured social, economic, and behavioral factors. Because measures of family income for individuals beyond the age of 65 may not reflect the accurate socioeconomic status of elderly adults, we further modeled the sex mortality differential among the highest family income quartile *only for those individuals 18 through 64 years of age.* For these high-income young adults, the odds of mortality for men exceed women by just 20%, controlling for age and race (results not shown). This further supports the notion that the U.S. sex mortality gap is variable across subpopulations, with our estimates suggesting that the lowest gap exists among the most economically advantaged segment of the population. In contrast, large sex mortality gaps exist when considering the most socially and economically disadvantaged segments of the adult population.

CONCLUSION

Sex differentials in mortality have long intrigued scientists in many academic disciplines. This topic continues to be of concern in the U.S. demographic literature because (a) the overall sex mortality difference has changed rather remarkably over the course of the century; (b) the overall differential, although narrowing in recent years, remains substantial, with a current life expectancy at birth advantage of 6.0 years for women; and (c) a full understanding of the explanatory factors has remained elusive. This chapter has examined the current sex mortality differential using individual level data from a large supplement of the 1990 NHIS matched to mortality follow-up data through the end of 1995.

Our findings indicated that U.S. adult men exhibited 1.7 times the odds of mortality in the 5-year follow-up period compared to adult women. Controlling for the complete set of social, economic, and behavioral factors in the analysis left the overall odds ratio of mortality basically unchanged (e.g., Verbrugge 1989; Wingard 1982). However, this does not mean that the covariates had no influence on the sex mortality differential. In contrast, controlling for social and economic factors actually widened the sex mortality gap while, on the other hand, controlling for behavioral factors narrowed the overall difference, in large part due to the more hazardous cigarette smoking patterns exhibited by men. In fact, our estimates suggest that cigarette smoking accounts for about 25% of the current overall sex mortality difference, and a much larger percentage when cancer mortality and respiratory disease mortality are separately considered. Thus, contin-

ued aggressive efforts to combat cigarette smoking will not only be instrumental for reducing overall U.S. adult mortality, but also could substantially reduce the sex difference in mortality as well (e.g., Nam et al. 1996).
It will be important for future analysts to consider an even wider range of
social, economic, and behavioral factors to further understand the sex
mortality gap. Such factors include those that may favor men, such as
wealth, but perhaps many more that may favor women, such as religious
involvement, the presence of social support networks, the propensity to
seek medical care, and a host of difficult-to-measure high-risk behavioral factors (e.g., occupational hazards, driving habits, drug use, use of
weapons, use of cigars and/or smokeless tobacco, and specific dietary intake). To date, even the most wide-ranging data sets in this area of study
have lacked the ability to tap such a comprehensive set of possible explanatory factors.

Our separate cause-specific models further illustrated that the magnitude of the sex mortality gap varies by cause, although all causes examined
favor women. Perhaps most unfortunate is the nearly threefold differential exhibited for social pathologies—a differential which actually widened
with control for the social and behavioral factors in our statistical models.
Our data set could not account for many of the social and behavioral
factors associated with deaths due to social pathologies, which may include drug abuse, gang membership, the use of force in problem-solving,
loneliness and depression, and unsafe driving practices. Nevertheless,
the cause-of-death results suggest that powerful efforts to curb dangerous and violent behavior disproportionally exhibited by (and harmful
to) young males must be made if the substantial gap in mortality due to
social pathologies is to be closed (e.g., Sells and Blum 1996). Given the
young ages at which many of these deaths occur, including during childhood (Singh and Yu 1996b), these efforts must be geared to even young
children.

Among older adults, recent research has highlighted the persistent contribution of circulatory diseases for the U.S. sex mortality difference
(Knudsen and McNown 1993; Trovato and Lalu 1998). Our results demonstrated that men exhibited about 75% higher odds of death over the follow-
up period for circulatory disease mortality, and that the inclusion of social
and economic covariates widened the observed gap. Somewhat surprisingly, controlling for behavioral factors (including cigarette smoking) only
slightly narrows the circulatory disease mortality difference; one reason is
that men are more likely than women to regularly exercise, which is a significant risk factor for this cause (see Chapter 15). Our review of the literature earlier in this chapter suggested that biological factors may be especially important in protecting women from circulatory disease mortality,
particularly at young adult ages. While we could not directly address this
hypothesis, our findings provide indirect support for this assertion because

the social and behavioral-based statistical models did not effectively account for the circulatory disease mortality difference.

Perhaps the most promising result we uncovered is that sex mortality differentials for the most highly educated and, particularly, the most economically advantaged segments of the population are much smaller than those exhibited by the more disadvantaged segments of the population. These findings provide convincing evidence for the structural hypothesis advanced by Nathanson and Lopez (1987) and, most importantly, suggest that men *can* achieve a lower level of mortality much more similar to that of women. Further, such findings provide evidence that despite the relevance of biological factors discussed above, sex mortality differentials also seem to be strongly rooted in the social structure of U.S. society. Consequently, future work should further investigate why advantaged social and economic conditions are especially favorable for male survival and how such advantages can be diffused to men in disadvantaged social and economic positions.

On the negative side, some subgroups of men exhibit substantially higher risks of death than women; two such groups include those who are unemployed and those who are separated or divorced. While the unemployed category of adults is fairly small, our findings demonstrate that this is an especially hazardous position for males. Thus, another area for future research could explore the differences between male and female unemployment for health and mortality prospects, as well as the effects of male unemployment for the health and mortality of all members of those particular families and households.

4

RACE/ETHNICITY, NATIVITY,

AND ADULT MORTALITY

Similar to the vast interest in sex mortality differentials, demographic and health researchers over many decades have documented mortality differentials across U.S. race/ethnic groups. Most often investigated are differences between African and Caucasian Americans (e.g., Otten et al. 1990; Rogers 1992; Sorlie et al. 1992a), but studies of Asian American and Hispanic mortality are becoming more common as well (e.g., Hoyert and Kung 1997; Liao et al. 1997, 1998; Sorlie et al. 1993). The U.S. foreign-born population has also been shown to exhibit *more favorable* levels of health and mortality than their U.S.-born counterparts, a pattern that has puzzled the demographic and public health communities for decades (Rumbaut and Weeks 1989; Scribner 1996; Singh and Yu 1996a). With few exceptions (e.g., Elo and Preston 1997; Fang et al. 1997; Hummer et al. 1999b; Kestenbaum 1986; Sorlie et al. 1993), however, most of this work has focused on infant health and mortality. Relatively little work has considered the influence of nativity on adult mortality, particularly at the national level.

The increase in the foreign-born and minority populations makes the need for such analyses more pressing. In 1996, 24.6 million persons, or 9.3% of the U.S. population, were foreign-born. This is the largest foreign-born population in U.S. history, as well as the largest share of the population since 1930, when the foreign-born comprised 11.6% of the total population (Hansen and Faber 1997; Jasso and Rosenzweig 1990; U.S. Bureau of the Census 1993). While one-half of the foreign-born had their origins in the Western Hemisphere in 1996, with a quarter of the total from Mexico, nearly 25% originally came from Asia. In addition, over 10% originated in the Caribbean, which has been a traditional source of the foreign-born black population. Notably, one-half of the current foreign-born population came to the United States in the last 15 years (Hansen and Faber 1997). These migration trends have fueled the rapid growth in the last two decades of the Asian and Pacific Islander population, which grew 108%, and the Hispanic population, which grew 53%, during the 1980s (DeVita 1996; Kitano and Daniels 1995; U.S. Bureau of the Census 1992). The foreign-born African American population also nearly doubled between 1980 and 1990, numbering about 1.6 million people in 1990, which is more than 5% of the total African American population (U.S. Bureau of the Census 1992). It is clear, then, that the study of race/ethnic mortality differentials must take into account the varied nativity composition of the groups. Thus, this chapter documents and examines differences in adult mortality between seven numerically major U.S. race/ethnic groups, while taking into account the influence of nativity and the length of time lived in the United States for the foreign-born (e.g., Hummer et al. 1999b). In addition, we examine race/ethnic mortality differentials by age and cause of death, also within the context of nativity.

INTRODUCTION

Current life expectancy at birth for African Americans is about 7 years shorter than that of Caucasian Americans, a demographic fact that has drawn considerable attention from the research and policy communities. Most scholars agree that a substantial portion of the difference between the two groups is a result of the harsh socioeconomic circumstances in which many African Americans live (National Research Council 1989; Rogers 1992). Some studies, however, suggest that a substantial mortality gap between these groups persists beyond socioeconomic differences, particularly among young adults (e.g., Elo and Preston 1996; Otten et al. 1990; Sorlie et al. 1992a). This may be due to unmeasured socioeconomic factors such as wealth or the effects of discrimination on health and mortality (Hummer 1996; Williams et al. 1994). The African-Caucasian American mortality differential also varies across specific age groups (Elo and Preston 1997; Nam 1995) and by cause of death (Elo and Preston 1997; Rogers 1992). Little work, however, has explored African American mortality compared to a wide range of other race/ethnic groups or within the context of nativity. Indeed, the foreign-born African American population nearly doubled between 1980 and 1990.

The life expectancy gap between African and Asian Americans is even wider than between African and Caucasian Americans. The Asian and Pacific Islander population, in itself a heterogeneous mixture of ethnic groups, appears to have the lowest mortality of any U.S. subpopulation and, together with non-Hispanic whites, the most advantaged socioeconomic composition (Elo and Preston 1997; Hoyert and Kung 1997; Rogers et al. 1996b). Relatively few adult mortality studies at the national level, however, have examined the Asian American population. Some have used data sources that ascertained race/ethnic numerator (death) and denominator (survivor) information from different sources (e.g., Day 1993; Yu et al. 1985), that may lead to biases in mortality estimates (Sorlie et al. 1992b). Indeed, national-level mortality data from a single source for Asian Americans continue to be sparse (Hoyert and Kung 1997). Fortunately, the NHIS-MCD data file employed here provides national level mortality data with race/ethnic information from a single source—the household within which the individual lives.

Even though some recent literature continues to examine Hispanics as a single group (e.g., Elo and Preston 1997; Liao et al. 1997, 1998), most adult mortality studies specify Hispanic subpopulations separately (e.g., Rosenwaike 1987, 1991; Sorlie et al. 1993). This is because the diverse national origins, migratory histories, assimilation processes, and geographical locations of these populations have produced important socioeconomic, cultural, and health differences across them (Bean and Tienda 1987; Vega and Amaro 1994). The most recent descriptive findings from the U.S. Vital Statistics system suggest that Puerto Ricans suffer from the highest age-adjusted rates of mortality compared to the other Hispanic groups, while Cubans, Mexican Americans, and Other Hispanics display an age-adjusted rate of mortality lower than Caucasian Americans (Anderson et al. 1997). These patterns also differ by age and cause of death. In general, Hispanics are characterized by high mortality among young adults due to homicide, HIV/AIDS, and chronic liver disease, but lower heart disease and cancer mortality among older adults vis-à-vis Caucasian Americans (Anderson et al. 1997; Liao et al. 1998; Rosenwaike 1987). Few studies, however, have been able to examine detailed age and cause-of-death mortality patterns among the different Hispanic groups, particularly with a data set that contains a consistent race/ethnic reporting source (see Sorlie et al., 1993, for an exception).

Because they are the largest Hispanic subgroup, most in-depth studies in this area have focused on Mexican Americans. Socioeconomically, Mexican Americans are disadvantaged similar to African Americans, so it is often assumed that their mortality patterns are also similar. That is, individuals from both groups are more likely to be unemployed, poor, and without a high school degree than Caucasian Americans, and both groups have experienced a long history of discrimination (Bean and Tienda 1987; National Research Council 1989). However, life expectancy at birth for Mexican Americans is similar to, if not higher than, that of Caucasian Americans (Bradshaw and Liese 1991; Rogers et al. 1996b; Sorlie et al. 1993; Wei et al. 1996). The term epidemiologic paradox has been used to describe this unexpected result (Markides and Coreil 1986). Some other Hispanics—those originating from Central and South America, for example—seem to be similar in this way to Mexican Americans (Rosenwaike 1987; Sorlie et al. 1993), although a great deal of the literature on the epidemiologic paradox focuses exclusively on Mexican Americans.

In recent years, researchers have hypothesized that nativity may help account for the favorable health and mortality patterns of Mexican Americans (Cobas et al. 1996; Scribner 1996; Scribner and Dwyer 1989). First, consider that high levels of migration from Mexico to the U.S. in the last 30 years has resulted in a substantial percentage of Mexican American adults who are foreign-born (U.S. Bureau of the Census 1992). Second, international migration tends to select healthy, eager individuals; in other words, frail, unmotivated individuals are not likely to migrate (Rosenwaike 1991). Third, U.S. residents exhibit higher levels of smoking and drinking than Mexicans, and, in some ways, may also have poorer dietary practices (Scribner 1996). Thus, the nativity hypothesis suggests that the Mexican immigrants' superior health behaviors, family support systems, and health status upon entry to the United States compensate for the high-risk socioeconomic status of Mexican Americans in general. It has also been suggested that the U.S. acculturation process wears away some of the advantages of Mexican nativity; that is, the health advantages of immigration are most apparent shortly after entry to the United States and weaken over time (Guendelman and English 1995; Scribner 1996).

By extension, the nativity hypothesis also suggests that within each race/ethnic group, foreign-born persons may exhibit lower mortality risks than their U.S.-born counterparts. For example, studies of the African and Asian American foreign-born populations demonstrate that they also display more positive health characteristics and health behaviors than their native-born counterparts (Cabral et al. 1990; Kleinman et al. 1991; Rumbaut and Weeks 1989, 1996; Singh and Yu 1996a). However, relatively few studies of adult mortality have considered the mortality of foreign-born groups other than Mexican Americans, and none that we are aware of have considered the length of time spent in the United States (for a work similar in this regard, see Hummer et al. 1999b).

DATA

The data set used for this chapter consists of the combined 1989–1994 versions of the core National Health Interview Survey (NHIS) linked to the Multiple Cause of Death (MCD) file for the years 1989–1995 (NCHS 1991b, 1992b, 1993d, 1994d, 1995d, 1996c, 1997b). For the analysis in this chapter, it was necessary to use the core NHIS (rather than its smaller, but more detailed supplements) because of the relatively small size of some of the race/ethnic and nativity groups considered here. Unfortunately, the use of the core NHIS data limits the scope of available variables; for example, there are no measures of health behavior available in the core NHIS. Combining six years of core NHIS data yields a sample size of over 400,000 and thus makes possible the analysis of mortality patterns among relatively small race/ethnic and nativity groups.

We exclude Native Americans due to their nearly complete U.S.-born composition; further, we exclude a small number of other individuals because of missing race/ethnic identification. Linkage of the NHIS with the MCD file indicated that 19,086 of the surveyed individuals died between 1989 and 1995. The linked NHIS-MCD data set is thought to be among the most accurate available for measuring race/ethnic differences in adult mortality, in large part because it relies on single, self-reports of race/ethnic identification both for survivors of the follow-up period and for persons who die during follow-up (Liao et al. 1998; Rogers et al. 1996b). In addition, the core NHIS includes information on the nativity of sampled individuals and length of time spent in the United States for foreign-born individuals, variables that are not often available in other data sets used for mortality analyses.

Race/ethnicity and **nativity** are the key independent variables in this chapter. We demarcate Caucasian Americans, African Americans, Mexican Americans, Puerto Ricans, Cuban Americans, Other Hispanics, and Asian and Pacific Islanders. While more detailed than most similar analyses, this race/ethnic measurement scheme is far from ideal; one major limitation is that the Asian and Pacific Islander population is examined as a whole here. In fact, the Asian and Pacific Islander population is composed of many diverse subgroups. For example, the 1994 NHIS includes 842 Chinese, 840 Filipino, 482 Asian Indian, 400 Vietnamese, 393 Japanese, and 377 Korean individuals; these six subgroups make up 87% of the Asian and Pacific Islander sample in the 1994 NHIS (NCHS 1996d). A similar limitation is that persons originating from Central and South America and other persons of Spanish descent are grouped together into our Other Hispanic category. Note that we consider race/ethnic groupings to be essentially social phenomena. In terms of their implications for mortality patterns, race/ethnic groups appear to vary socially, culturally, and historically rather than biologically (Hummer 1996; Jones et al. 1991; Kaufman and Cooper 1995; Williams et al. 1994).

Beginning only in 1989, the core NHIS asked respondents about their place of birth and the length of time they had lived in the United States. Using this information, we created a three-category nativity variable indicating whether the individual was born in the United States, born elsewhere and had lived in the United States less than 15 years (short-term immigrant), or born elsewhere and lived in the United States 15 or more years (long term-immigrant). This distinction is important because one-half of the current foreign-born population came to the United States in the last 15 years (Hansen and Faber 1997). Further note that the NHIS considers island-born Puerto Ricans and those persons originating from Guam and the U.S. Virgin Islands to be foreign-born (NCHS 1991b). Thus, most importantly, island-born Puerto Ricans are grouped here in the foreign-born category, although it is important to recognize their status as U.S. citizens by birth.

Most of the chapter examines overall mortality as the dependent variable; we also examine cause categories of death in a portion of the analysis as well. The causes of death are grouped into four categories: circulatory diseases (International Classification of Diseases [ICD] 390-459), cancers (ICD 140-239), social pathologies—which include suicide, accidents, homicide, and cirrhosis of the liver (ICD 571 and ICD E800-E999)—and a residual fourth group. This scheme is similar to those employed in our other chapters and related studies of adult mortality (e.g., Potter 1991; Rogers 1992; Rogers et al. 1996b), but includes somewhat less detail because of the limited number of deaths among some of the numerically smaller race/ethnic groups.

RESULTS

DESCRIPTIVE STATISTICS

The top portion of Table 4.1 provides descriptive statistics for race/ethnicity and nativity by survival status. For race/ethnicity, a comparison of the two columns shows that death during the follow-up period is comparatively more likely to occur among African Americans and Caucasian Americans and less likely among the other race/ethnic groups. For example, Mexican Americans constitute 4.2% of the adults who survive and only 2.0% of those who die during follow-up. Part of the comparatively high mortality among Caucasian Americans can be attributed to their older age distribution, which is not considered in this descriptive table. By nativity, U.S.-born adults and long-term foreign-born residents exhibit disproportionately high percentages of deaths, while short-term foreign-born residents exhibit a comparatively low percentage of death. Again, however, note that there are age structure differences between nativity groups that must be kept in mind when examining these descriptive data. The bottom portion of Table 4.1 presents descriptive statistics for the demographic and social factors. In keeping with most prior research on adult mortality, individuals are less likely to survive the follow-up period if they are older, male, less educated, lower income, not in the labor force, or previously married.

Table 4.2 provides the percentage distribution or mean for each variable

TABLE 4.1 Descriptive Statistics for Demographic, Social, and Economic Factors Related to Race/Ethnic and Nativity Differences in Mortality, U.S. Adults, 1989–1995

	Survived (%)	Died (%)
Race/Ethnicity		
African American	11.1	11.9
Asian American	2.7	1.1
Mexican American	4.2	2.0
Puerto Rican	0.9	0.5
Cuban American	0.5	0.5
Other Hispanic	2.1	1.0
Caucasian American	78.5	83.0
Nativity		
Foreign born, <15 years in United States	5.1	1.6
Foreign born, +15 years in United States	5.2	5.8
U.S. born	89.7	92.6
Demographic factors		
Age (mean)	45.8	70.7
Sex		
Male	47.5	54.4
Female	52.5	45.6
Social and economic factors		
Education		
Less than 12 years	20.6	44.5
12 years	38.4	32.2
13+ years	41.0	23.3
Income equivalence (mean in $10,000s)	1.9	1.4
Employment status		
Unemployed	3.2	1.2
Not in labor force	31.2	78.1
Employed	65.7	20.6
Marital status		
Never married	19.1	8.0
Divorced/separated	9.4	8.8
Widowed	6.7	27.6
Married	64.8	55.6
Person-years and deaths	2,160,511	19,086

Sources: Derived from NCHS 1991b, 1992b, 1993d, 1994d, 1995d, 1996c, 1997b.

separately by race/ethnicity. Of central interest is nativity. While about 95% of Caucasian and African American adults are U.S.-born, individuals in the other groups are far more likely to be foreign-born. For example, only 19.4% of Asian Americans and 27.5% of Cuban Americans, respectively, are U.S.-born. As might be expected given recent immigration patterns, African American, Mexican American, Other Hispanic, and Asian American foreign-born individuals tend to be of more recent entry, while

TABLE 4.2 Descriptive Statistics for Demographic, Social, and Economic Variables by Race/Ethnicity, U.S. Adults, 1989–1995

	African American	Asian American	Mexican American	Puerto Rican	Cuban American	Other Hispanic	Caucasian American
Nativity							
Foreign born, <15 years	3.8	55.7	27.6	18.1	21.8	37.9	1.3
Foreign born, 15+ years	2.3	24.9	18.9	38.6	50.7	23.4	3.1
U.S. born	94.0	19.4	53.5	43.2	27.5	38.7	95.6
Demographic factors							
Age (mean)	43.3	41.2	38.3	39.6	48.4	40.4	47.2
Sex							
Male	44.7	47.8	50.4	44.0	47.3	45.7	47.9
Female	55.3	52.2	49.6	56.0	52.7	54.3	52.1
Social and economic factors							
Education							
<12 years	29.8	15.6	51.8	40.2	31.2	29.6	17.5
12 years	39.6	25.9	29.4	34.0	29.7	32.3	39.4
13+ years	30.6	58.5	18.8	25.8	39.2	38.2	43.1
Income equivalence (mean in $10,000s)	1.3	2.0	1.3	1.4	1.6	1.7	2.0
Employment status							
Unemployed	5.5	2.5	4.8	3.6	3.6	3.8	2.7
Not in labor force	33.6	30.4	30.3	39.7	34.1	29.2	31.3
Employed	60.9	67.1	64.9	56.7	62.3	67.0	66.0
Marital status							
Never married	31.5	26.2	23.2	27.5	18.5	25.1	16.5
Divorced/separated	15.7	4.5	8.6	14.8	12.6	11.8	8.6
Widowed	8.1	3.9	3.0	3.9	8.0	4.1	7.1
Married	44.8	65.3	65.2	53.8	60.9	59.0	67.8

Sources: Derived from NCHS 1991b, 1992b, 1993d, 1994d, 1995d, 1996c, 1997b.

Caucasian American, Puerto Rican, and Cuban foreign-born persons are less likely to be of recent entry.

The race/ethnic groups also exhibit considerable variation for each of the social factors. Asian Americans and Caucasian Americans, respectively, are by far the most highly educated groups and exhibit the highest incomes, on average. Together with Mexican Americans, they are also most likely to be married. In contrast, African Americans, Mexican Americans, and Puerto Ricans exhibit the lowest average incomes, while Mexican Americans and Puerto Ricans are least likely to possess a high school degree. Cubans and Other Hispanics tend to exhibit intermediate levels on the socioeconomic factors. Thus, these descriptive figures show clear social advantages for Asian and Caucasian Americans, clear disadvantages for African Americans, Mexican Americans, and Puerto Ricans, and a widely varied distribution of nativity across the seven race/ethnic groups. We now turn to the multivariate analysis, which examines race/ethnic mortality patterns while simultaneously considering demographic and social factors, including nativity.

RACE/ETHNICITY, NATIVITY, AND MORTALITY ACROSS ALL ADULT AGES

Table 4.3 considers the associations between race/ethnicity, nativity, and mortality across the entire adult age range. Controlling only for age and sex, Model 1 shows that, compared to Caucasians, African Americans exhibit the highest odds of mortality, while Asian Americans exhibit 31% lower odds of mortality. The four Hispanic groups display rather varied risks of mortality. Puerto Rican mortality is comparatively highest, but not as high as African Americans; this finding is consistent with age-adjusted mortality figures published by the NCHS Vital Statistics system (Anderson et al. 1997). On the other hand, Mexican and Cuban Americans display odds of mortality about equal to those of Caucasians, while Other Hispanics display lower odds of mortality than Caucasians. The epidemiologic paradox—the fact that some U.S. minority groups display lower odds of mortality than their social circumstances and discriminatory histories would lead one to expect—is clearly evident here for Mexican Americans, Cubans, and Other Hispanics. Overall, then, there is considerable variation in the odds of mortality across race/ethnicity (also see Figure 4.1). Even wider variation would be evident if Asian Americans were specified as the reference group; indeed, African Americans exhibited over twice the odds of adult mortality over the follow-up period compared to Asian Americans ($e^{[\ln(1.41)-\ln(0.69)]} = 2.04$).

Model 2 shows that both groups of foreign-born individuals display lower odds of mortality than individuals born in the United States. How-

TABLE 4.3   Adjusted Odds Ratios for the Associations between Race/Ethnicity, Nativity, and Mortality, U.S. Adults, 1989–1995

	Model 1	Model 2	Model 3	Model 4
Race/ethnicity				
African American	1.41*		1.41*	1.17*
Asian American	0.69*		0.78*	0.81*
Mexican American	1.03		1.12*	0.95
Puerto Rican	1.33*		1.59*	1.28*
Cuban American	1.01		1.21+	1.12
Other Hispanic	0.83*		0.92	0.87+
Caucasian American	ref		ref	ref
Nativity				
Foreign born, <15 years		0.82*	0.87*	0.82*
Foreign born, 15+ years		0.77*	0.77*	0.78*
U.S. born		ref	ref	ref
Demographic factors				
Age (continuous)	1.09*	1.09*	1.09*	1.07*
Sex				
Male	1.70*	1.69*	1.70*	1.95*
Female	ref	ref	ref	ref
Social and economic factors				
Education				
<12 years				1.29*
12 years				1.14*
13+ years				ref
Income equivalence (continuous)				0.92*
Employment status				
Unemployed				1.44*
Not in labor force				1.96*
Employed				ref
Marital status				
Never married				1.48*
Divorced/separated				1.47*
Widowed				1.20*
Married				ref
-2*Log-likelihood	181,531.3	181,262.3	181,021.3	176,879.2

Sources: Derived from NCHS 1991b, 1992b, 1993d, 1994d, 1995d, 1996c, 1997b.
   $+ \, p \leq .10$; *$p \leq .05$.

ever, there are only slight differences in the odds ratios of death by length of time in the United States, which offers little support to the suggestion that the survival advantages of migration lessen with time. Of course, the mortality patterns of second and third generation immigrants may be different than the first generation immigrants due to acculturation; however, we cannot directly test that proposition here. When the race/ethnic and nativity variables are both included in Model 3, the general similarity in mortality between Caucasians, Mexican Americans, and Cubans exhibited in Model 1 now favors Caucasians. That is, Mexican and Cuban Americans are much more likely to be foreign-born than Caucasians, helping to account for the overall similar mortality prospects between these groups (e.g., Hummer et al. 1999b). Similarly, Puerto Rican mortality is even higher vis-à-vis Caucasians when nativity is controlled. A parallel pattern is also evident when we compare Asian Americans and Other Hispanics to Caucasians; although both groups continue to exhibit lower odds of mortality than Caucasians after nativity is controlled, the advantage is narrowed in comparison to Model 1. As a whole, race/ethnic mortality differences are influenced by nativity: race/ethnic groups with high percentages of foreign-born individuals benefit in that their mortality prospects are lower than would otherwise be the case. On the other hand, the African-Caucasian American mortality gap is unaffected by the inclusion of the nativity variables, most likely because the percentage of foreign-born persons for both groups is relatively small.

Model 4 additionally includes social and economic factors and demonstrates several important findings. First, the excess mortality of African Americans in comparison to Caucasians is substantially narrowed, but not eliminated, with their introduction. Others (e.g., Elo and Preston 1996; Rogers et al. 1996b; Sorlie et al. 1992a) have also shown a moderate mortality difference between these groups after controlling for similar variables. While differences in the social and economic factors included here are clearly critical, then, for understanding the racial gap in mortality, there are also other factors not measured here that are instrumental in creating this gap. Second, the excess mortality of Puerto Ricans, Mexican Americans, and Cubans in comparison to Caucasians seen in Model 3 is reduced or eliminated with the introduction of social and economic factors in Model 4. This finding provides evidence that social disadvantages elevate mortality levels among these Hispanic groups, although the protective effect of nativity (compare Model 1 to Model 3) works to offset these disadvantages. Third, the mortality advantage Asian Americans exhibit relative to Caucasians remains stable with the introduction of social factors, most likely because Asian and Caucasian Americans both display advantageous social characteristics (also see Figure 4.1). Finally, the nativity differentials in mortality remain consistent with the introduction of social and economic factors. Thus, the relatively high mortality of U.S.-born adults, in comparison to their foreign-born counterparts, is independent of the distribution of the social and economic factors considered here. We cannot account here for the health selection of foreign-born individuals at time of U.S. entry, which has been hypothesized to be, at least in part, responsible for their favorable outcomes. A second reason for the remaining mortality difference

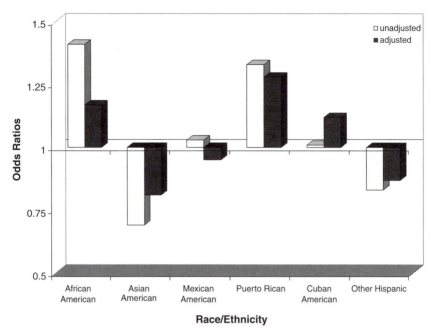

FIGURE 4.1   Odds ratios of dying by race/ethnicity for U.S. Adults, 1989–1995. Note: Referent is Caucasian American.

between the foreign- and native-born populations may be health behavior. Foreign-born individuals have been shown to exhibit lower rates of smoking, alcohol use, and drug use than U.S.-born individuals and may have healthier diets, all factors that help to maintain better health and lower mortality (Cabral et al. 1990; Rumbaut and Weeks 1989; Scribner 1996).

To better understand race/ethnic and nativity patterns of mortality, Table 4.4 examines combined race/ethnic and nativity groups, with native-born Caucasians specified as the reference group. Note also that the long-term and short-term groups of foreign-born persons have been combined in this table because the mortality experiences of these two groups were similar for the overall population (Table 4.3) and for each of the race/ethnic groups (from preliminary models, not shown here). Interestingly, Model 1 shows that foreign-born African American and Other Hispanic individuals exhibit the lowest odds of mortality compared to Caucasians. In fact, foreign-born African Americans exhibit 41% lower odds of mortality during the follow-up period than native-born Caucasians and about 59% lower odds of mortality when compared to native-born African Americans ($e^{[\ln(.58)-\ln(1.43)]}$). The relatively small percentage of foreign-born African Americans, however, largely negates the influence of this low mortality pattern on overall African American mortality. On the other hand, the low mortality of foreign-born Other Hispanics is instrumental in their overall

TABLE 4.4 Adjusted Odds Ratios for the Association between Race/Ethnicity/Nativity and Mortality, U.S. Adults, 1989–1995

	Model 1	Model 2
Race/Ethnicity/Nativity		
African American, foreign born	0.58*	0.54*
African American, native born	1.43*	1.19*
Asian American, foreign born	0.68*	0.68*
Asian American, native born	0.67*	0.70*
Mexican American, foreign born	0.97	0.81*
Mexican American, native born	1.05	0.91
Puerto Rican, foreign (island) born	1.24+	0.98
Puerto Rican, native (mainland) born	1.63*	1.41+
Cuban American, foreign born	0.91	0.85
Cuban American, native born	1.49+	1.40
Other Hispanic, foreign born	0.59*	0.55*
Other Hispanic, native born	1.14	1.08
Caucasian American, foreign born	0.82*	0.82*
Caucasian American, native born	ref	ref
Demographic factors		
Age (continuous)	1.09*	1.07*
Sex		
Male	1.70*	1.95*
Female	ref	ref
Social and economic factors		
Education		
<12 years		1.29*
12 years		1.14*
13+ years		ref
Income equivalence (continuous in $10,000s)		0.92*
Employment status		
Unemployed		1.43*
Not in labor force		1.96*
Employed		ref
Marital status		
Never married		1.48*
Divorced/separated		1.46*
Widowed		1.20*
Married		ref
−2*Log-likelihood	181,433.3	177,267.0

Sources: Derived from NCHS 1991b, 1992b, 1993d, 1994d, 1995d, 1996c, 1997b.
+ $p \le .10$; *$p \le .05$.

low mortality because Other Hispanics are predominantly (61%) foreign-born. Some other foreign-born groups—including Asian and Caucasian Americans—also display lower mortality than native-born Caucasians. Of equal interest, mortality for foreign-born Mexican Americans is roughly equal to that of native-born Caucasians, even though foreign-born Mexican Americans on the whole are socially and economically disadvantaged. In fact, controlling for social and economic characteristics in Model 2 evinces a change in the mortality of foreign-born Mexican Americans vis-à-vis native-born Caucasians; net of these characteristics, foreign-born Mexican Americans exhibit about 19% lower odds of mortality than native-born Caucasians.

Model 2 also shows that, net of social and economic factors, each group of foreign-born individuals displays mortality equal to or lower than native-born Caucasian Americans, a pattern that is highly suggestive of healthy migration selectivity for each of the race/ethnic groups. Within each of the seven race/ethnic groups, Model 2 also shows that foreign-born mortality is lower than mortality among the native-born—although the difference is quite small for Asian Americans. We now turn to the analysis of race/ethnic patterns of mortality by age and cause-of-death groups, again with a focus on the influence of nativity.

SEPARATE MODELS BY AGE GROUP AND CAUSE OF DEATH

Tables 4.5 and 4.6 show race/ethnic and nativity patterns of mortality specific to age group and cause-of-death, respectively. Note that the race/ethnic and nativity variables are specified separately in these tables. Table 4.5 displays three different sets of models specific to young adults, middle-aged adults, and older adults. The results show that the associations between race/ethnicity and mortality and between nativity and mortality vary considerably by age. It is perhaps most widely documented that the African American-Caucasian American mortality gap is widest among young adults and narrows with age, with some analysts suggesting that a crossover occurs at about age 87 or 88 (Kestenbaum 1997; Nam 1995). We cannot effectively address the crossover hypothesis because of the limited sample size of the oldest adults in our data set; however, these data show a much narrower racial differential among middle-aged and, especially, older adults than among younger adults. Even more striking patterns—with crossovers—are evident when the four Hispanic groups are compared to Caucasians. Controlling for demographic characteristics and nativity, each of the four Hispanic groups displays higher odds of mortality than Caucasians among the 18–44 group. In fact, young adult mortality among Puerto Ricans is the highest among any of the race/ethnic groups (e.g., Anderson et al. 1997), a disadvantage that is reduced, but not eliminated, with controls for social and economic factors. Among adults aged 45–64, only Puerto Ricans (among the Hispanic groups) exhibit higher mortality than Caucasians, with most of the excess mortality attributable to their disadvantaged social and economic characteristics. Within the 65 and older group, all four Hispanic groups exhibit odds of mortality equal to or lower than Caucasians, with the mortality advantages vis-à-vis Caucasians relatively stable even after control for social and economic factors.

The mortality difference between Asian Americans and Caucasians also varies by age, with virtually no difference among the two youngest age groups (controlling for nativity), and considerably lower mortality among Asian Americans in the oldest age category. Because the two groups exhibit relatively similar social and economic characteristics, their mortality differences are unaffected by controlling for such characteristics. Overall, Caucasian mortality is comparatively highest vis-à-vis each of the other race/ethnic groups at the oldest ages and comparatively lowest among young adults.

By nativity, middle-aged and older foreign-born adults display lower odds of mortality than native-born adults, with little change in the associations when social and economic factors are controlled (see Models 2 and 3 for both the age 45–64 and age 65+ groups). Among young adults, mortality differences by nativity are smaller in magnitude and not statistically significant. The influence of nativity on the race/ethnic mortality differentials (comparing Model 2 to Model 1 within each age group) is also clear for each age group, and most prominent for middle-aged adults. That is, nativity works to lower the odds of mortality for each race/ethnic group vis-à-vis Caucasians in nearly every case. For example, compared to Caucasians, Asian Americans display 23% lower odds of mortality over the follow-up period among adults aged 45–64 (Model 1 among ages 45–64); when nativity is controlled, the Asian mortality advantage is erased (Model 2 among ages 45–64). Note, too, that both the race/ethnic and nativity associations with mortality among middle-aged and older adults persist net of one another; that is, both race/ethnicity *and* nativity impact U.S. adult mortality prospects.

Table 4.6, which displays cause of death patterns by race/ethnicity and nativity, shows that mortality differences between race/ethnic groups vary considerably across causes (also see Figure 4.2). In contrast, the influence of nativity is rather consistent across causes: foreign-born individuals have generally lower odds of death for each cause, although the foreign-born advantage for social pathologies is not statistically significant. The most pronounced foreign-born advantage is for cancer, with the odds of death about 35% lower among short-term immigrants and 25% lower among long-term immigrants. Because cigarette smoking accounts for a substantial share of cancer deaths in the United States, health behavior differences between the foreign- and native-born groups may be crucial. The multifactorial nature of each of these causes of death, however, makes it necessary to be extremely cautious in interpreting the importance of cigarette smoking, dietary practices, or any other specific factor in the creation of the mortality differences by nativity. Comparing Models 2 and 3 for each cause of death,

TABLE 4.5 Adjusted Odds Ratios for the Associations between Race/Ethnicity, Nativity, and Age for Three Different Age Groups, U.S. Adults, 1989–1995

	Ages 18–44			Ages 45–64			Ages 65+		
	Model 1	Model 2	Model 3	Model 1	Model 2	Model 3	Model 1	Model 2	Model 3
Race/Ethnicity									
African American	2.20*	2.21*	1.45*	1.72*	1.72*	1.24*	1.22*	1.21*	1.07*
Asian American	0.95	1.01	0.93	0.77*	1.05	1.12	0.61*	0.69*	0.70*
Mexican American	1.65*	1.71*	1.32*	0.99	1.11	0.83+	0.87+	0.95	0.87+
Puerto Rican	3.29*	3.48*	2.31*	1.47*	1.91*	1.26	0.73+	0.89	0.79
Cuban American	1.79+	1.91+	1.66	1.02	1.33	1.18	0.95	1.15	1.09
Other Hispanic	1.28	1.36+	1.14	0.80	1.01	0.91	0.76*	0.84+	0.82*
Caucasian American	ref	ref	ref	ref	ref	ref	ref	ref	ref
Nativity									
Foreign born, <15 years		0.91	0.87		0.68*	0.60*		0.80*	0.80*
Foreign born, 15+ years		0.91	0.90		0.67*	0.70*		0.79*	0.79*
U.S. born		ref	ref		ref	ref	ref	ref	
Demographic factors									
Age (continuous)	1.05*	1.05*	1.08*	1.10*	1.10*	1.07*	1.09*	1.09*	1.08*

Sex									
Male	2.06*	2.07*	2.45*	1.57*	1.57*	2.01*	1.71*	1.71*	1.87*
Female	ref	ref	ref	ref	ref	ref	ref	ref	ref
Social and economic factors									
Education									
<12 years			1.63*			1.43*			1.24*
12 years			1.26*			1.12*			1.11*
13+ years			ref			ref			ref
Income equivalence (continuous in $10,000s)			0.88*			0.89*			0.95*
Employment status									
Unemployed			1.65*			1.18			1.37*
Not in labor force			2.36*			2.37*			1.56*
Employed			ref			ref			ref
Marital status									
Never married			2.19*			1.65*			1.14*
Divorced/separated			1.76*			1.46*			1.41*
Widowed			2.09*			1.45*			1.15*
Married			ref			ref			ref
−2*Log-likelihood	22,017.2	21,952.8	21,236.9	42,996.5	42,874.8	41,426.9	116,223.0	115,892.8	113,767.4

Sources: Derived from NCHS 1991b, 1992b, 1993d, 1994d, 1995d, 1996c, 1997b.

$+ p \leq .10; * p \leq .05.$

TABLE 4.6 Adjusted Odds Ratios for the Associations between Race/Ethnicity, Nativity, and Cause-Specific Mortality, U.S. Adults, 1989–1995

	Circulatory			Cancer			Social pathologies			Other causes		
	Model 1	Model 2	Model 3	Model 1	Model 2	Model 3	Model 1	Model 2	Model 3	Model 1	Model 2	Model 3
Race/ethnicity												
African American	1.41*	1.40*	1.17*	1.24*	1.23*	1.13*	1.28*	1.28*	0.97*	1.66*	1.65*	1.32*
Asian American	0.79*	0.83	0.86	0.61*	0.79	0.81	0.50*	0.48*	0.44*	0.69*	0.89	0.93
Mexican American	0.94	1.02	0.87	0.71*	0.77*	0.69*	1.50*	1.56*	1.27+	1.27*	1.46*	1.24*
Puerto Rican	1.08	1.24	1.02	0.94	1.11	0.96	2.28*	2.46*	1.87*	1.69*	2.30*	1.74*
Cuban American	0.99	1.11	1.03	1.10	1.39+	1.31	0.48	0.52	0.46	1.11	1.52*	1.41+
Other Hispanic	0.64*	0.69*	0.65*	0.71*	0.85	0.82	1.39+	1.48*	1.33	1.01	1.18	1.11
Caucasian American	ref	ref	ref	ref	ref	ref	ref	ref	ref	ref	ref	ref
Nativity												
Foreign born<15 years		1.05	1.01		0.63*	0.63*		0.90	0.86		0.71*	0.66*
Foreign born, 15+ years		0.80*	0.81*		0.75*	0.76*		0.93	0.95		0.67*	0.69*
U.S. born		ref	ref		ref	ref		ref	ref		ref	ref
Demographic factors												
Age (continuous)	1.11*	1.11*	1.09*	1.08*	1.08*	1.07*	1.02*	1.02*	1.01*	1.09*	1.09*	1.07*
Sex												
Male	1.76*	1.76*	2.01*	1.58*	1.57*	1.62*	2.51*	2.49*	3.02*	1.62*	1.62*	2.00*
Female	ref	ref	ref	ref	ref	ref	ref	ref	ref	ref	ref	ref

Social and economic factors												
Education												
<12 years			1.35*			1.31*			1.29*			1.15*
12 years			1.11*			1.22*			1.20*			1.06
13+ years			ref			ref			ref			ref
Income equivalence (continuous in $10,000s)			0.92*			0.98			0.89*			0.88*
Employment status												
Unemployed			1.68*			1.00			1.59*			1.55*
Not in labor force			1.89*			1.59*			1.78*			2.82*
Employed			ref			ref			ref			ref
Marital status												
Never married			1.30*			0.93			1.71*			1.94*
Divorced/separated			1.37*			1.41*			1.84*			1.64*
Widowed			1.22*			0.86*			1.61*			1.34*
Married			ref			ref			ref			ref
−2*Log-likelihood	83,306.4	83,135.5	81,282.5	66,022.5	65,804.7	64,916.6	21,697.5	21,572.9	21,082.2	55,144.8	54,985.2	53,286.9

Sources: Derived from NCHS 1991b, 1992b, 1993d, 1994d, 1995d, 1996c, 1997b.

$+ p \leq .10$; $* p \leq .05$.

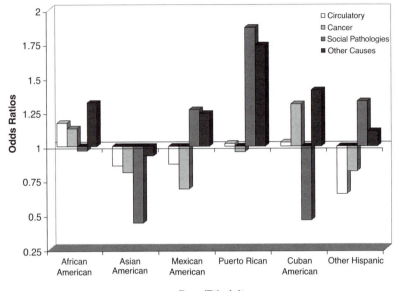

FIGURE 4.2   Adjusted odds ratios of cause-specific mortality by race/ethnicity, U.S. Adults, 1989–1995. Note: Referent is Caucasian American.

however, shows that the social and economic factors considered here have very little impact on the mortality differences between the foreign-born and native-born populations.

Consistent with the influence of nativity on race/ethnic mortality differences among different age groups, it is also clear that nativity plays an important part in the race/ethnic mortality differences across causes of death. For Asian Americans, Mexican Americans, Puerto Ricans, Cubans, and Other Hispanics, controlling for nativity (Model 2 for each cause of death) in nearly every case raises the risk of death for these groups vis-à-vis Caucasian Americans. For example, Asian Americans exhibit 39% lower odds of cancer mortality compared to Caucasians when nativity is not included in the model (Model 1 for cancer); with the addition of nativity, Asian Americans exhibit just 21% lower odds of cancer mortality compared to Caucasians. In contrast, and also as seen in the age-specific models in Table 4.5, the African American versus Caucasian American differences in mortality for each cause are unaffected by the inclusion of nativity.

Overall, African Americans have higher mortality than non-Hispanic whites for all causes. Because circulatory disease and cancer account for nearly two-thirds of all U.S. deaths, the moderately higher African American mortality for these causes results in huge losses in life expectancy compared to Caucasians. Note that the excess circulatory disease, cancer, and other cause mortality among African Americans is substantially reduced, but not eliminated, when social and economic factors are controlled.

The high risks for social pathologies among Mexican Americans, Puerto Ricans, Other Hispanics, and African Americans compared to Caucasians and, especially, Asian Americans could result from a combination of factors, including relatively high rates of alcohol and drug use among young males. For example, Mexican American males who drink on average consume about four drinks of liquor daily (Rogers 1991b). However, the reduced odds ratio in Model 3 for each of these groups vis-à-vis Caucasian Americans demonstrates that social disadvantages are, at least in part, also responsible. Prior studies have also reported relatively low risks of cancer and heart disease mortality among Hispanics and Asian Americans, compared to Caucasians (Rogers et al. 1996b; Sorlie et al. 1993). We also find this to be the case, corresponding to the favorable mortality patterns for older Hispanics and Asian Americans seen in Table 4.5. Indeed, Mexican Americans exhibit 13% lower odds of circulatory disease mortality and 31% lower odds of cancer mortality than Caucasians, respectively, when other variables are controlled. Notably, circulatory disease and cancer mortality is no higher among Puerto Ricans compared to Caucasian Americans. These causes of death are both strongly linked to health behaviors, such as smoking and dietary practices, for which Hispanics and Asian Americans generally appear to exhibit healthier patterns than do Caucasian or African Americans (e.g., Rumbaut and Weeks 1996; Vega and Amaro 1994).

Compared to Caucasians, Asian Americans display lower mortality for most causes, but exceptionally low mortality due to social pathologies. In fact, they exhibit about one-half the odds of death from social pathologies over the follow-up period compared to Caucasians, with the differentials even wider when compared to Mexican Americans, Puerto Ricans, Other Hispanics, or African Americans. Others have reported that Asian Americans demonstrate a low propensity to die due to homicides and motor vehicle accidents (Fingerhut et al. 1994). Furthermore, Fingerhut et al. (1994) report very low rates of alcohol use among Asian Americans. And compared to other race/ethnic groups, Asian Americans are far less likely to use marijuana, cocaine, and other illegal drugs (Zane and Kim 1994). The low odds ratio exhibited by Cubans for social pathologies is of similar interest, although the extremely small number of deaths warrants caution for this particular finding.

CONCLUSION

This chapter explored the association between race/ethnicity and U.S. adult mortality, with special emphasis on the influence of nativity. African Americans suffer from the highest odds of mortality across nearly all adult ages (eclipsed only by Puerto Ricans among young adults), although their heightened risk vis-à-vis Caucasian Americans is especially pronounced for younger adults. The mortality risk for each of the young adult Hispanic groups is also higher than Caucasians. In contrast, the Hispanic subgroups exhibited mortality equal to, or lower than, Caucasians among the 65 and older age group, which demonstrates a mortality crossover phenomenon with non-Hispanic whites.

Asian American mortality is generally lower than that of Caucasians, yet the advantage differs by age and cause, with the most favorable Asian American mortality patterns exhibited among the elderly and for social pathological deaths and cancer. The generally low mortality exhibited by Asian Americans reported here is consistent with others who suggest that Asian American mortality is among the lowest in the world (Hahn 1995). This is a reversal from earlier in the century; in 1920, Caucasian Americans displayed significantly lower mortality than Asian Americans (Barringer et al. 1993). It will be interesting to monitor the mortality patterns of Asian Americans as this group continues to experience tremendous growth, particularly through immigration. The analysis of Asian and Pacific Islander population subgroups—in particular Chinese, Filipino, Hawaiian, Korean, Vietnamese, Japanese, Asian Indian, Samoan, and Guamanian Americans—will also become possible with continued growth in the Asian and Pacific Islander population and with the recent specification of Asian American subgroups in the NHIS. Indeed, limited evidence suggests some rather wide variation in Asian American adult mortality by specific subgroup, with Hawaiians and Samoans demonstrating much higher rates of age-adjusted mortality compared to the other groups (Hoyert and Kung 1997). Clearly, the analysis of differentials within the Asian and Pacific Islander group will be of immense interest.

In contrast to Asian Americans, African Americans suffer from the highest mortality risks compared to the other groups across nearly all of the age and cause-of-death categories, and the social factors included here account for a large portion of this disadvantage. Social disadvantages also help to explain some of the higher mortality risks of Mexican Americans and Puerto Ricans vis-à-vis Caucasian and Asian Americans, particularly among the youngest adults. While the significance of social factors for understanding mortality differentials is not new, it may be important to recognize their relevance at a time when U.S. policy seems to be de-emphasizing basic social programs geared toward minority groups, new immigrants, and the poor. For example, the reduction and/or elimination of affirmative action programs may further marginalize the most disadvantaged groups in U.S. society, maintain or widen current social inequalities, and have detrimental consequences for the health and welfare of minority group members. Similar questions surround welfare reform, the failure of national health insurance proposals, and cutbacks in programs like Medicaid. Consequently, it will be increasingly important to monitor the health and mortality outcomes of African Americans, Mexican Americans, and Puerto Ricans as the United States experiences these profound shifts in social policy. Given the importance of social factors for mortality outcomes, and the lack of momentum for dealing with basic social inequalities at the national level, the prospects of closing the race/ethnic mortality gaps we reported here—particularly between African Americans and other race/ethnic groups—are not promising in the near future.

We re-emphasize, though, that race/ethnic mortality patterns should not be interpreted outside of the context of nativity. One exception is that African American-Caucasian American mortality differences are relatively unaffected by nativity, only because of the small foreign-born proportion of these populations; nevertheless the recent growth and low mortality of the foreign-born African American population makes it important that nativity continues to be considered here as well. Moreover, Asian American, Mexican American, Cuban American, and Other Hispanic mortality vis-à-vis Caucasians is lower than what might otherwise be the case because of the influence of nativity. That is, controlling for nativity increased the risk of mortality for each of these minority groups compared to Caucasians. This suggests that the generally low mortality of the foreign-born, in combination with the high percentage of foreign-born residents among the Asian American and Hispanic populations, help to maintain the largely favorable mortality profile of these groups. While often not thought about in debates about immigration policy, such patterns suggest that continued streams of what appears to be healthy and select migrants may be important in maintaining a healthy profile for several U.S. race/ethnic groups.

When looking strictly at nativity, foreign-born adults exhibit lower mortality than native-born adults for nearly all causes of death, with the advantage most pronounced among middle-aged and older individuals. Within race/ethnic group, the foreign-born advantage is also most pronounced among African Americans and Other Hispanics, although a great deal of the literature in this area focuses on the association between immigration and health among Mexican and Asian Americans (e.g., Markides and Coreil 1986; Rumbaut and Weeks 1996; Scribner 1996). Indeed, foreign-born African Americans demonstrated the lowest mortality risks of any group considered here. The amount of time spent in the United States by the foreign-born, however, exhibited little impact on mortality patterns; that is, the foreign-born advantage was nearly identical for short- and long-term immigrants. In general, then, foreign-born nativity is associated with lower mortality across nearly all ages and causes of death, with the magnitude of the advantage varying by race/ethnicity.

5

FAMILY COMPOSITION
AND MORTALITY

Although most mortality research focuses on risk factors for individuals, mortality prospects are also determined by other persons who are close by (Link and Phelan 1995; Pearce 1996): spouses, children, parents, and other relatives. Neglecting such social relations overlooks vast parts of individuals' lives. A family's social, emotional, instrumental, and financial support can influence the risk of death of individual family members. Thus, this chapter illuminates the relations between family composition and mortality among adults in the United States.

A death in the family can be devastating. The death of the family's breadwinner may mean that other family members must change their roles and may be forced into the labor force. The death of one family member may result in the family moving, selling their home, or further changing their family composition to adjust for the lost member. Further, a family member's death may mean the loss of health insurance coverage for the entire family (for more detail about health insurance and mortality, see Chapter 9).

One hundred years ago, marital disruption was more likely to be due to the death of a spouse than to divorce. Now, because mortality rates have dropped to such relatively low levels, marital disruption is more likely to be a result of divorce (Bumpass et al. 1991). But, as we will demonstrate, the risk of mortality is not the same for all family members or for people who reside in different families. Thus, family arrangements and rearrangements are due in part to mortality: for example, the death of a husband transforms a married woman into a widow, and the death of either parent transforms a three-person family into a single parent with child.

There are no studies that we know of that examine the association between family arrangements and mortality; instead, there is a substantial marital status/mortality literature. The existing explanations for the marital advantage in longevity—explanations stressing integration, marital protection, and marital selectivity—are not mutually exclusive, and each may help to explain why married people in general live longer than others. Selectivity theory contends that the mortality difference between married and unmarried individuals is due to selection of healthy individuals for marriage (Kisker and Goldman 1987; Lillard and Panis 1996). Single individuals who are ill, the theory contends, are less likely to marry. Thus, their illness, along with a lack of social ties, contributes to social isolation, less social support, little social control, and a higher risk of mortality.

Marriage may protect individuals by focusing attention on health, reducing risks, and increasing compliance with medical regimens. Generally, compared to unmarried individuals, married persons eat better, take better care of themselves, and live a more stable, secure, and scheduled lifestyle (Gove 1973; Trovato and Lauris 1989). Status integration assesses the degree of social isolation that a person experiences (Durkheim 1951/1897; Ross 1995). By virtue of their spouses, married individuals are usually more integrated into society than unmarried ones. Social integration encourages social control and social support. Social support provides emotional reassurance. People who feel that they are loved, valued, and cared for have a sense of belonging (Antonucci 1990; Cobb 1976).

Bumpass et al. (1991) conclude that marital status categories no longer satisfactorily capture people's living situation. Indeed, Ross maintains that "marital status is a crude indicator of certain underlying concepts—social attachment, integration, and support, and the economic well-being of the household" (1995, p. 139). To more fully understand the relations between marriage and mortality requires a broader investigation that includes family arrangements, family roles, and health and financial considerations.

Family composition more adequately captures the complex relation of family members to mortality. For example, there are large and important differences between a family with a married couple only, with a married couple and child(ren), with parents, and with other relatives. Such differences must be distinguished and examined.

Moreover, *family relations* are often overlooked, but nonetheless important. There are large and critical differences between being married and a household head, being a young adult residing with parents, and being a young unmarried adult with a child and living with parents. Thus, it is not just the family configuration that matters, but also the position that individual family members assume: household head, parent, child, or sibling.

Family size can affect mortality in multiple ways. More individuals provide the opportunity for rich and complex ties and networks. Married couples comprise a family of at least two, while unmarried individuals often live alone. Larger families increase the opportunity to provide members additional social, emotional, instrumental, and financial support. At the same time, larger families can create additional emotional stress and financial strain. We incorporate family size in this chapter through the family composition variable and through the income equivalence scale.

Family composition is related to family income. Married couples, especially those with dual incomes, enjoy economic advantages not afforded unmarried people. Further, a large family provides a large reserve labor, or more earners. And female-headed families are more vulnerable to poverty than other family types. In fact, in 1990, just 5.7% of married-couple families lived in poverty, compared with 33.4% of female-headed families with no husband present (U.S. Bureau of the Census 1991). Economic hardship can lead to depression, anxiety, and ultimately, death (Ross and Mirosky 1989).

While adjustment for economic resources provides partial explanation for the relation between family composition and mortality, other economic factors may be at play. Some family living arrangements are formed based not on consumption patterns, but on dire economic need. Economic necessity is the key reason adult children sometimes reside with their parents (Speare and Avery 1993). Severe economic need can be partly assessed through welfare program participation. Programs like Aid to Families with Dependent Children (AFDC) provide support for single-parent families. By examining the effects of welfare receipt within the family it is possible to identify families in dire economic need, and to determine how much welfare payments reduce the risk of mortality.

Some individuals require and receive instrumental support (Antonucci 1990). This support may affect relations within the family. For example, ill children may depend on their parents for their entire lives, which can increase emotional and financial strain (Atchley 1991). One-quarter of elderly in ill health live with an adult child, often an adult daughter. Thus, the family often assumes the primary caregiving function for family members who are physically or mentally ill. This chapter examines the relations between family composition and mortality, with particular attention to the moderating effects of family relations and financial and instrumental support.

DATA AND METHODS

Since the National Health Interview Survey (NHIS) is a household-based survey of individuals, there are unique opportunities to examine how the action of one family member affects other members within the family.

We use the 1987 NHIS person file for our analyses of family composition and mortality because it is a full sample with mortality follow-up through 1995 (NCHS 1988). We could have merged several years of NHIS data, but such linkages would have increased the complexity of an already difficult coding scheme. Recall that the NDI includes only those individuals aged 18 and over, so children who live in the sampled households are included to determine the family structure, but are not included in the mortality analyses. Furthermore, we use the 1990 NHIS Family Resource Supplement for a portion of the analyses because it includes information on welfare receipt (NCHS 1995d).

To construct family composition, we incorporate information about marital status, type of family (primary or secondary), relationship to the reference person, and family size. Most NHIS samples do not include more than 16 individuals within one family. But as many as 16 individuals in the family, along with the other relationship information, translates into multiple relationships.

NHIS provides detailed marital statuses. A negligible number of people are of unknown marital status, which we exclude from the analyses. We include as married those with and without a spouse in the household; only 2% of marriages do not have a spouse in the residential household, because that person resides elsewhere. Thus, we distinguish between those who are married and those who are not married.

NHIS provides information on the type of family and on the relationship to the reference person. There are two types of families: primary and secondary. A primary family includes two or more individuals related by blood, marriage, or adoption who are living together. A secondary family would be another unrelated family living within the same household. There is only a tiny fraction of individuals living in secondary families in this data set; because of their small number, we drop them from the analyses.

NHIS lists the following relationships to the reference person: reference person or spouse, child, grandchild, parent, or other relative of the reference person. There are thousands of possible family configurations. We balance the needs to present detailed categories, to present a diversity of family arrangements, to examine welfare receipt within the family, to accurately assess the mortal risks associated with various family arrangements, and to maintain reasonably large cell sizes for analyses. Note that we are not examining total family size, but individuals who *currently* live in the household.

For those who are married, we distinguish married with spouse only, with 1, 2, 3, or 4 or more children, and with other relatives (all other combinations, including grandchildren, parents, and more distant relatives). When we define a household with a married couple and 1, 2, 3, or 4 or more children, we do not include any other relatives; if a household with a married couple and children includes other relatives, such as an uncle, we define that household as living with other relatives.

For those who are not married, we distinguish among those who have established independent households, those who are not the household head and are living with non-relatives, and those who are still living at home with their married parents. Since the sample includes individuals aged 18 and over, some households will have young adults living with married parents. We categorize those who are living with their parents and no one else, those with parents and other adult siblings, and those living with parents and with their own child. Those who are household heads may live by themselves. Such individuals do not live with other relatives but may reside with nonrelatives. Unmarried household heads may also live with children or with other relatives. Or, individuals may live in an unmarried parent's home.

Coding family relationships from a household file is complex. Although the NHIS is a household survey, the records are arranged by family member, with as many as 16 records (one for each family member). Our first step was to read each individual record. Figure 5.1, Panel A, depicts a hypothetical set of nine individual records from three different households. The first four individuals reside in a family comprised of a married couple and their two children. The first record in each household lists the reference person. Thus, each household record is related to the first record, the reference person. The second step, depicted in Panel B, combines all of the individual records into one household record, with detailed information about each family member. We created 16 separate data sets from the person file, one for each possible family member, with detail on the family relationships, and then merged these 16 files into 1 long family file, with codes relating each person to others in the family. Thus, the first four records in the person file (Panel A) become one record in the family file (Panel B), with detailed information about each family member. For example, in the first family record, the reference person is married, with a spouse and two children.

The last step is to code the family relations of each member and write the records back to an individual person file (see Panel C). Once the individual person records are merged into the household file, there are still 16 required data passes to correctly code each person with his or her other relations. Rather than cycle through the data set 16 times, especially when most of the common family relations will be selected with fewer passes, we coded family relations not for everyone in the family but for the first six individuals. The first six individuals capture 99% of the sample, and the other family members are generally under the age of 18, and often provide few additional cases (there is one family with 16 members). Providing codes for the first six family members will introduce some biases, especially for the largest families with more diverse relations, and may be more likely to bias

A. Read individual records

Record number	Household number	Person number	Marital status	Family relation
1	1	1	Married	Referent
2	1	2	Married	Spouse
3	1	3	Unmarried	Child
4	1	4	Unmarried	Child
5	2	1	Unmarried	Referent
6	2	2	Unmarried	Child
7	3	1	Married	Referent
8	3	2	Married	Spouse
9	3	3	Unmarried	Parent

|
|
V

B. Convert individual records to household records

Household	Famrel1	Famrel2	Famrel3	Famrel4
1	Self	Spouse	Child	Child
2	Self	Child		
3	Self	Spouse	Parent	

|
|
V

C. Transfer household information to individual records

Record number	Household number	Family relation code
1	1	Married, with spouse and two children
2	1	Married, with spouse and two children
3	1	Adult child living with one sibling and two married parents
4	1	Adult child living with one sibling and two married parents
5	2	Single parent living with one child
6	2	Adult child living in single parent household
7	3	Married, living with spouse and one parent
8	3	Married, living with spouse and one parent
9	3	Parent living with married children (ref)

FIGURE 5.1   Creating detailed household information from combined individual records and writing that information back to the individual.

some ethnic groups that have more diverse family arrangements. Most relations, however, are captured through this process.

Rather than focus on the family arrangement and how it affects individual members, we are concerned with the exact relation of a particular family member to others in the family. Conceptually, it becomes difficult to create individual records from family records since each person is related to others in the family in different ways. For example, the first family portrayed includes four members. The *family* represents a married couple and two children. But the individual relations vary: the first member is married, living with a spouse and two children; the second member is also married and living with a spouse and two children; but the third member, the child, is living with married parents and one sibling. In Panel C, we have created four records for the first family. Since we can only analyze those individuals over the age of 18, we code the family relations, but some members may be dropped from subsequent analyses. For example, the first family listed in Panel B can produce the four individual records listed in Panel C, or three records if one of the children is under the age of 18, or just two records if both of the children are under the age of 18. Cycling through the data set to code other respondents becomes easier after the first pass, since the family relationships are complementary. For example, once we know that there are two individuals in the household and that the first person is a parent living with a child, then we know that the other person is a child living with a parent.

We have incorporated household information, which is already an integral part of the survey, with individual records. Thus, we can include information at both the individual and family level. Such advantages introduce new methodological issues. One potential problem is that the assumption of independence of the observations is called into question. Because we have family information, large families will contribute family characteristics multiple times. For example, an adult child living with three siblings and a parent will contribute four times (one for each adult child). This question of independence is not crucial, since it parallels the relations of marital status, where married individuals are interrelated. Thus, we adhere to the position that family relations are similar to marital status and therefore no special statistical adjustments of independence are needed. Moreover, many of the family relationships are unique and do not represent dependency. On the other hand, future research could test for dependence of observations by randomly sampling individuals within a particular family type to determine if the results remain consistent.

Defining family relationships with the 1987 NHIS is difficult because of the structure of the data. The NHIS has asked all family members to state their association to the referent person. Thus, family composition can be constructed for the referent person, since each person is linked to that one person. Other family relations can be constructed, but with less precision. For example, an in-law may be related to the referent person, but may be more closely related to others in the household. Such other codes are complicated, since we only know partial information. Fortunately, NCHS had the insight to change their family relation coding with the 1996 NHIS re-design, which should enable future research of family composition to be methodologically easier and can allow for more detailed coding of family relations.

When examining relations between family arrangements and mortality, we adjust for age, sex, race, income equivalence, and health status (for more detailed discussion of income equivalence and health status, refer to

Chapters 7 and 10, respectively). The relations between family composition and mortality vary by sex. Moreover, compared to younger adults, older adults (those over age 65), live in different family arrangements, are more likely to be out of the labor force, and are more likely to rely on Social Security, pensions, and assets rather than earnings. Thus, we stratify several analyses by sex and by broad age groups—young and old adults.

Welfare receipt includes whether an individual received:

> Money from the State or Local welfare agency under the Aid to Families with Dependent Children Program (AFDC, ADC) or other assistance programs such as 1) general assistance, 2) emergency assistance, 3) Refugee Assistance, or Indian Assistance (on reservations or Indian lands) (NCHS 1991c: BB17-5).

RESULTS

Table 5.1 shows that the most common family arrangements are to be married and living with spouse only, 24%, with spouse and one or two children, 28%, with a spouse and 3 or more children, 8%, and to be unmarried and live alone, 14%. Almost 10% of the sample includes adults living with one or both of their parents.

The multivariate models in Table 5.2 progress from examining the association between family living arrangements and mortality, controlling just age, sex, and race (Model 1), to later models that also control for income and health status. For each model, the referent category is married individuals who are living with two children. Mortality differences are apparent for different family arrangements. For example, compared to those who are married and living with two children, those who are married and living with spouse only are 21% more likely to die, and those who are married and living with four or more children are 39% more likely to die (Panel A, Model 1).

Married individuals living with other relatives find an additional risk of death. For example, compared to married couples living with two children, married spouses living with other relatives are 57% more likely to die. Living with other relatives—say aunts, uncles, nieces, nephews, and cousins—may not provide the close ties that a spouse, children, or parents provide. Moreover, living with distant relatives suggests living arrangements based in part on need—financial, instrumental, or emotional—a risk factor for mortality.

Part B shows individuals who are not married but are living with a married couple. Note that a married individual living with three children experiences low mortality, but one of adult children living with married parents and two siblings experiences high mortality. For instance, compared to a married person living with a spouse and two children, one adult living with

TABLE 5.1   Percentages of U.S. Adults Residing in Various Family Relations for
Those Who Survived 1987–1995[a]

Family composition	Percentages
A. Married, household head or spouse, live with	
Spouse only	24.4
1 child	13.6
2 children	14.1
3 children	5.9
4 or more children	2.4
Other relatives	6.3
B. Not married, living with married couple, not household head	
Adult child living with married parents	2.2
Adult child living with married parents and 1 sibling	2.2
Adult children living with married parents and 2 or more siblings.	2.0
Adult living with own child and married parents	1.0
C. Not married, household head, live with	
Self only, no other relative	14.4
1 child	2.7
2 children	1.6
3 children	0.7
4 or more children	0.3
Other relatives	2.4
D. Not married, not household head, live with	
Adult child living with unmarried parent	1.3
Adult child living with unmarried parent and 1 or more siblings	1.2
Other relatives	1.3

Sources: Derived from NCHS 1995d and 1997b.
[a]Unweighted person years: 695971.

married parents and two or more siblings is three times more likely to die. High mortality is also evident for a single parent living with child and married parents.

Part C of Table 5.2 shows risks of death for individuals who are the household head and are unmarried. Individuals who are not married and who do not live with other family members experience relatively high mortality. Compared to married couples living with two children, nonmarried individuals living alone are 58% more likely to die. Some individuals may live alone because they have no other choice and were not selected for marriage (see Kisker and Goldman 1987). Such individuals may have personality, physical/mental health, or financial problems that hinder their marriage prospects and increase their chances of death. Some individuals who live alone were previously married. Individuals who are divorced or separated may have personality, health, or financial problems that increase their

TABLE 5.2   Odds Ratios of Family Composition and U.S. Adult Mortality, 1987–1995[a]

Family composition	Model 1	Model 2	Model 3
A. Married, household head or spouse, live with			
Spouse only	1.21*	1.23*	1.15*
1 child	1.21*	1.25*	1.17*
2 children	ref	ref	ref
3 children	0.96	0.92	0.94
4 or more children	1.39*	1.23	1.27
Other relatives	1.57*	1.51*	1.31
B. Not married, living with married couple, not household head			
Adult child living with married parents	1.48+	1.38	1.29
Adult child living with married parents and 1 sibling	1.94*	1.84*	1.86*
Adult child living with married parents and 2+ siblings	3.08*	2.74*	2.76*
Adult living with own child and married parents	2.36*	2.08*	2.05*
C. Not married, household head, live with			
Self only, no other relatives	1.58*	1.46*	1.48*
1 child	1.58*	1.47*	1.39*
2 children	1.82*	1.58*	1.48*
3 children	2.01*	1.65+	1.61+
4 or more children	3.16*	2.38*	2.22*
Other relatives	1.49	1.39	1.35
D. Not married, not household head, live with			
Adult child living with unmarried parent	2.72*	2.36*	2.29*
Adult child living with unmarried parent and 1+ siblings	2.90*	2.48*	2.27*
Other relatives	1.95	1.72	1.76
Demographic			
Age	1.11*	1.10*	1.09*
Sex	1.88*	1.92*	1.90*
Race	1.44*	1.29*	1.18*
Income equivalence		0.82*	0.92*
Health status			1.43*
−2*Log-likelihood	63,853.45	63,601.22	62,552.87

Sources: Derived from NCHS 1995d and 1997b.
[a] Unweighted person years: 695971, with 6832 deaths.
$+ p \leq .10, *p \leq .05$.

chances of divorce and death. Widowed individuals may have lost not only their spouse but also part of their financial support.

There is a consistent mortality gradient for unmarried individuals who have children living with them. Compared to married individuals who live with their spouses and two children, unmarried individuals who live with one child have 58% higher mortality, with two children the mortality is

82% greater, with three children it is twice as high, and with four or more children it is three times greater. Thus, whereas children are seen as providing social integration for married couples, they provide a higher risk of death for unmarried individuals. Most likely, the emotional and financial burden of raising a child single-handedly becomes more onerous with a greater number of children.

Unmarried adults who are not household heads and who live with others experience high mortality (Part D). For example, compared to a married couple living with two children, an adult child living with an unmarried parent is 2.7 times more likely to die. This higher mortality may be due to the family configuration, but could also be due to health and financial needs.

Table 5.2 shows that some of the burdens of family arrangements are financial. If these financial costs are controlled, then the risk of mortality should be reduced. Model 2, which adjusts for family income, supports this supposition. In every instance, the odds ratios decline between Models 1 and 2 for those who are not married, which implies that part of the high mortality experienced by individuals in various family configurations is economically based. The high mortality risk for couples living with four or more children is also reduced with the introduction of income equivalence. Large families may miss some of the benefits of social integration because of the losses due to increased financial strain. For example, compared to married couples with two children, an unmarried parent with four or more children is 3.2 times more likely to die without income controls, but 2.4 times more likely to die when income is considered in the analysis.

Health status also affects the relations between family composition and mortality. The mortality risk for many family configurations drops for many individuals, including individuals who are married and living with spouse only, and married and living with only one child. These relations hint that childless couples may experience health problems that prevent them from producing children, and that couples with one child may also experience health problems that either prevent or discourage them from producing additional children. Of course, other factors may be at play; we certainly recognize that a married couple with no children or with one child could still have grown children who have moved out of the household, or may have children from a previous marriage or relationship who live with the ex-spouse or ex-partner.

Table 5.3 shows the relations between family composition and mortality separately for males and females, and controlling for age, race, income equivalence, and health status. Generally the risks are similar, but males are more likely to experience greater risks of death from most family arrangements, especially those in which adult children are living with married parents. Compared to a married male living with his spouse and two

TABLE 5.3   Odds Ratios of Family Composition and U.S. Adult Mortality, by Sex, 1987–1995[a]

Family composition	Male	Female
A. Married, household head or spouse, live with		
Spouse only	1.23*	1.01
1 child	1.16	1.18
2 children	ref	ref
3 children	1.02	0.75
4 or more children	1.26	1.29
Other relatives	1.32	1.24
B. Not married, living with married couple, not household head		
Adult child living with married parents	1.10	1.81
Adult child living with married parents and 1 sibling	1.89*	1.65
Adult child living with married parents and 2+ siblings	3.38*	0.83
Adult child living with own child and married parents	2.21+	1.84
C. Not married, household head, live with		
Self only, no other relatives	1.63*	1.26+
1 child	1.27	1.30+
2 children	1.20	1.46+
3 or more children	2.22	1.70*
Other relatives	1.42	1.27
D. Not married, not household head, live with		
Adult child living with unmarried parent	2.12*	2.58*
Adult child living with unmarried parent and 1+ siblings	2.39*	1.72
Other relatives	1.97	1.33
Demographic		
Age	1.09*	1.10*
Race	1.27*	1.11
Income equivalence	0.89*	0.95+
Health status	1.42*	1.44*
−2*Log-likelihood	32,683.86	29,834.64

Sources: Derived from NCHS 1995d and 1997b.

[a] Unweighted person years: 320,477, with 3661 deaths for males. Unweighted person years: 375,494, with 3171 deaths for females.

$+ p \leq .10, *p \leq .05$.

children, a male living with his parents and two or more siblings is over three times more likely to die. Thus, compared to females, males suffer much higher mortality in family arrangements that suggest emotional, physical, or financial dependence.

There are age differences in family composition and mortality (see Table 5.4). The first outstanding feature of this table is that older adults do not commonly live in several types of households. Thus, for example, Panel B

TABLE 5.4   Odds Ratios of Family Composition and U.S. Adult Mortality, by Age, 1987–1995[a]

Family composition	18–64	65+[b]
A. Married, household head or spouse, live with		
Spouse only	1.18+	0.83
1 child	1.24*	0.86
2 children	ref	ref
3 children	0.92	1.11
4 or more children	1.35+	0.82
Other relatives	1.36	0.69
B. Living with married couple, not household head		
Adult child living with married parents	1.22	
Adult child living with married parents and 1 sibling	1.95*	
Adult child living with married parents and 2 or more siblings	2.78*	
Adult living with own child and married parents	2.01*	
C. Not married, household head, live with		
Self only, no other relatives	1.92*	0.97
1 child	1.28	1.02
2 children	1.56+	1.06
3 children	1.46	1.62
4 or more children	2.55*	
Other relatives	2.12*	0.93
D. Not married, not household head, live with		
Adult child living with unmarried parent	2.46*	1.28
Adult children living with unmarried parent and 1 or more siblings	2.61*	0.51
Other relatives	1.78	
Demographic		
Age	1.09*	1.10*
Sex	2.01*	1.81*
Race	1.35*	1.00
Income equivalence	0.90*	0.93*
Health status	1.58*	1.37*
−2*Log-likelihood	22,569.56	39,880.88

Sources: Derived from NCHS 1995d and 1997b.

[a] Unweighted person years: 566,010, with 1876 for 18–64. Unweighted person years: 129,961, with 4,956 deaths for 65 and over.

[b] Empty cells for those 65 and over indicate very few individuals comprise that particular family arrangement; they were combined with other relatives.

$+ p \leq .10$, $*p \leq .05$.

does not present comparisons for older adults living with their married parents. On the other hand, it is more likely and more life promoting for older adults to live with their spouses only, or with a spouse and one child. Most likely, younger married adults are establishing their families, whereas older adults are more likely to expect all or most of their children to have moved out of the house.

Living alone is risky for young, but not older adults. For example, compared to those who are married and living with two children, young adults who live alone are twice as likely to die, but older adults who live alone have even odds of dying. Thus, it is not only family living arrangements, but also age composition and life-course factors that affect subsequent mortality.

One advantage of examining family composition is that it is possible to determine the effects of family factors on individual mortality, controlling for demographic factors, income equivalence, and health status. Table 5.5 displays mortality by family composition and by welfare participation for 1990–1995. Model 1 includes family composition, Model 2 introduces welfare receipt of the individual, and Model 3 introduces welfare receipt for 1, 2, and 3 or more family members. We have shaded those areas where 15% or more of the families receive welfare: those are also the areas that should experience the greatest change in mortal risk.

Compared to those who are married and living with two children, those household heads who are not married and living with three children are 35% more likely to die without consideration of welfare support (Model 1, Part C), but just 26% more likely when welfare support is considered (Model 2). Forty percent of single parents living with three children receive welfare support (data not shown). Welfare support reduces but does not eliminate the excess risk of death for individuals in family configurations that are in economic need.

The numbers of family members receiving welfare support also affect mortality. Some families may have three or more members receiving welfare support. Once welfare support of family members is considered, the mortality for unmarried individuals living with three or with four or more children substantially declines (see Model 3, Part C). Furthermore, Model 3 reveals a welfare gradient: compared to those who do not receive welfare, those individuals who live in families in which one member receives welfare are no more likely to die, those individuals who live in families in which two members receive welfare are 30% more likely to die, and those individuals who live in families in which three or more members receive welfare are 70% more likely to die. Those individuals who live in families with multiple welfare recipients experience high mortality and demonstrate high financial need that is not fully met with welfare disbursements.

CONCLUSION

The family is an important social institution. Link and Phelan (1995) make a plea for researchers to uncover the factors that place individuals "at risk of risks." We assert that the family is a central place to ferret out these

TABLE 5.5   Odds Ratios of Family Composition and U.S. Adult Mortality, with an Emphasis on Individual and Family Member Welfare Participation, 1990–1995[a]

Family composition	Model 1	Model 2	Model 3
A. Married, household head or spouse, live with			
Spouse only	1.08	1.09	1.09
1 child	1.19+	1.20+	1.20+
2 children	ref	ref	ref
3 children	1.10	1.10	1.08
4 or more children	1.05	1.03	1.00
Other relatives	1.05	1.16	1.21
B. Living with married couple, not household head			
Adult child living with married parents	2.86*	2.89*	2.91*
Adult child living with married parents and 1 sibling	2.20*	2.22*	2.23*
Adult child living with married parents and 21 siblings	3.79*	3.81*	3.82*
Adult child living with own child and married parents	3.34*	3.26*	3.23*
C. Not married, household head, live with			
Self only, no other relatives	1.40*	1.40*	1.41*
1 child	1.38*	1.37*	1.38*
2 children	1.22*	1.19	1.17
3 children	1.35	1.26	1.20
4 or more children	1.33	1.23	1.10
Other relatives	1.04	1.01	1.11
D. Not married, not household head, live with			
Adult child living with unmarried parent	2.09*	2.09*	2.13*
Adult child living with unmarried parent and 1+ siblings	2.17*	2.13*	2.13*
Other relatives	1.88	1.88	1.86
Demographic			
Age	1.10*	1.10*	1.10*
Sex (1 = male)	1.84*	1.84*	1.84*
Race (1 = black)	1.17+	1.16+	1.16+
Income equivalence	0.93*	0.93*	0.93*
Health status	1.47*	1.14*	1.47*
Welfare receipt		1.24*	
Number of family welfare recipients			
No welfare recipients			ref
1 member			0.95
2 members			1.30
3 or more members			1.71*
−2*Log-likelihood	41,285.42	41,280.97	41,273.69

Sources: Derived from NCHS, 1995d and 1997b.
[a] Unweighted person years: 702,900, with 4136 deaths. Shaded areas represent families in which 15% or more receive welfare.
+ $p \leq .10$, * $p \leq .05$.

risks. Family composition differentially affects mortality. Married individuals living with their spouses and two children experience lower mortality than most other configurations, and individuals in larger families often experience relatively high mortality.

Status integration, selectivity, and marital protection theories assert that, compared with unmarried individuals, married individuals generally have more social bonds, are healthier, and exhibit favorable health behavior. Although we suggest that all family relations benefit from social integration, it is most apparent for married couples, and married couples with children. On average, marriage appears to provide increased social support, positive social control, and to encourage health promotion and disease prevention. Although social factors are important in the relations between family composition and mortality, so too are economic influences.

A married couple has the opportunity for dual earners. If one spouse works, the other spouse can provide other services, and acts as reserve labor. Even retired couples can both receive pensions and/or Social Security, in addition to other economic returns. Although marriage can provide some protection from premature mortality, high incomes within marriage can further increase that protection and can provide the necessary means for a healthy and secure lifestyle (see also K. Smith and Waitzman 1994).

Part of the high mortality experienced by unmarried individuals who live with their parents and/or who live with their children is due to their lower income. Thus, some of the integrative aspects are either stronger for smaller families, or are partly lost due to the additional financial strains often characterized by large families, especially those headed by single parents. For some family configurations, the incomes are so low that they are supplemented with welfare support. Welfare may support one or more individuals in the family. Our results indicate that individuals in families that receive welfare experience higher morality, even controlling for income equivalence. We suggest that this higher mortality is due to the disadvantaged situation that welfare recipients find themselves in that is helped but not ameliorated by welfare receipt. To more fully understand the mechanisms that operate between welfare receipt, family composition, and mortality would require more detailed comparisons of similar families that differ only on whether they receive welfare. Young adult children who live with their parents experience high mortality, but are unlikely to qualify for welfare support. Perhaps new social policies could be enacted to assist young adults so that they can establish independent households.

Adam Smith (1937/1776) talked of the invisible hand of the marketplace influencing market forces. We see the helping hand of a relative affecting social forces. Such helping hands are often quite visible at the family level, but are invisible or unacknowledged at the larger societal level. Plainly, the large percentage of individuals with mental, addictive, physical, and functional disorders, and financial difficulties who survive in the community would be reduced without the helping hand of relatives.

In many instances, rather than the family living arrangements affecting mortality, the family rearranges itself to protect family members against mortality. Compared to married couples with two children, single parents with four or more children are two to three times as likely to die. Such individuals might substantially reduce their own mortality if they were not caring for their children; they could send the children to the other parent or give the children up for adoption. But by risking their own lives by taking care of their children, they ensure a brighter, longer future for their children. Thus, the family forms and reforms as if to ensure longer lives of everyone in the family, rather than to increase the survival probability of one member.

It is difficult to parse out the benefits of social integration from the accommodations some family members make to support their kin. Some individuals who have lost their spouse, their job, their house, or their physical independence may be institutionalized if they are not accepted into the home of another relative. These types of events are difficult to measure, since the comparison should not be with either the past or current living situation, but with the hypothetical situation that might have occurred had the relative not opened his or her home. For example, adults who live with their children but in their married parents' house experience high mortality; but how much higher would their mortality be if their parents did not take them in and provide the needed emotional, social, instrumental, and financial support?

Many recent studies have begun to examine contextual factors, especially how the effects of county, tract, or block level characteristics affect individual mortality risk. Part of the justification for including contextual or neighborhood effects is that social institutions—church, school, government, and work—directly affect individuals and their mortality. We assert that the family has been overlooked in contextual studies, but is of central importance. The family provides support that is much more proximate, important, and relevant to the individual than more distal factors.

Longitudinal data can further elaborate some of our results. For example, it would be informative to see how the forming, reforming, and dissolution of families affects mortality for family members. It would also be useful to know how a change in income may initiate a chain of events that results in changes in one or more households.

This chapter has demonstrated the importance of examining family relations and mortality. This examination is broader than the inclusion of marital status; instead family studies of mortality should include information on spouses, children, parents, and other relatives. This study more clearly reveals the relations between family composition and mortality in the United States.

6

Religious Attendance, Social Participation, and Adult Mortality

This chapter broadens the examination of demographic and sociocultural influences by investigating the associations between religious attendance, general social participation, and U.S. adult mortality. In large part because of the pioneering work of Durkheim (1951), the influence of religion and other forms of social participation on suicide has become an important part of mortality discourse, particularly in sociology. In the demographic literature, however, few studies have examined the relationship between religious involvement, other forms of social participation, and mortality at the national level (for exceptions, see Bryant and Rakowski 1992; Hummer et al. 1999a; Rogers 1996). In large part, this is because data on religious and other forms of social participation are often unavailable or of poor quality. In fact, with the exception of marital status, the U.S. Vital Statistics System does not collect any information on social or religious participation at all. This chapter shows that religious and general social participation are, indeed, associated with adult mortality and that both selection variables (who is socially and religiously active) and intervening variables (how religious and general social participation influence the lives of individuals) play important parts in the explanation.

LINKING RELIGIOUS AND GENERAL SOCIAL PARTICIPATION TO MORTALITY

Few national studies have explored the relationships that we are addressing here, that is, the association between religious participation, general social participation, and U.S. adult mortality. While many studies of adult mortality have focused on marital status, we are concerned here with other aspects of social participation, including peoples' ties with a religious community and participation in other social activities.

Many studies have, in fact, investigated the association between religious denominational membership and mortality. In general, people belonging to behaviorally strict and wealthy denominations are found to have lower mortality risks than people who belong to other or no religious groups (Dwyer et al. 1990; Goldstein 1996; Kark et al. 1996; Lyon et al. 1977; Lyon et al. 1976; Phillips et al. 1980). Much of this line of research focuses on Mormons, Seventh Day Adventists, and Jews. Evidence also suggests that more strict adherents of some religious groups, such as Mormons, tend to exhibit lower mortality than those more loosely tied to the same groups (Gardner and Lyon 1982a, 1982b).

Other studies have investigated the association between various measures of religious participation and health outcomes (e.g., Ellison 1991; Gartner et al. 1991; Gottlieb and Green 1984; Idler 1987, 1995; Levin and Markides 1986; Levin and Vanderpool 1989; Musick 1996). Most of these studies uncover a positive association between religious participation and health, regardless of the specific measurement of the key independent and dependent variables (also see Jarvis and Northcott 1987; Levin 1994a). Yet another line of research examines the effects of various measures of religion on the timing of death. Recent evidence indicates that elderly religious individuals are less likely to die in the period before the most significant celebrations of their respective traditions (Idler and Kasl 1992; also see Phillips and Smith 1990).

Just a few studies, however, have focused on the linkage between religious participation and mortality, and most of these have focused on specific U.S. communities. Comstock and Partridge (1972), for example, documented a measurable beneficial association between church attendance and mortality from several causes among adults in Washington County, Maryland. Nevertheless, Comstock and Tonascia (1977) later suggested that such an association was spurious because of the socioeconomic selectivity of church attendance. Using the Alameda County Study data, Wingard (1982) demonstrated that church membership was related to lower mortality for both women and men, but that the association disappeared with controls for socioeconomic and behavioral factors. A more recent analysis of the Alameda County data suggest that religious attendance at baseline is associated with lower mortality over a 28-year follow-up period, even net of social and behavioral variables (Strawbridge et al. 1997).

In addition, both the Alameda County Study and the Tecumseh Community Health Study found that a social network index, one component of which was church membership, was negatively associated with mortality, net of other factors (Berkman and Syme 1979; House et al. 1982; Seeman et al. 1987). Seeman et al. (1987) went so far as to say that some social ties, but particularly church membership, may be more important than marital status in predicting mortality. Furthermore, Zuckerman et al. (1984) analyzed a sample of poor, elderly residents in Connecticut and found that their index of religiousness was a highly significant predictor of lower mortality among people who were in poor health; the effect was not evident for healthy individuals.

Other studies, of nationally representative data, have included a religion variable in analyses focused on the family, other social activities, and mortality. For example, Rogers (1996), in an analysis of adults 55 and older, employed a variable indicating whether or not individuals had attended church or services in the past 2 weeks. He found that those who had done so exhibited about 30% lower mortality in a subsequent 7-year follow-up period than those who had not, net of a number of demographic, social, and health characteristics. In a similar analysis of African Americans 55 and older, Bryant and Rakowski (1992) also found that church attendance in the past 2 weeks was strongly associated with lower subsequent mortality, net of demographic, social, and health characteristics. Both studies, however, focused only on older adults and included only a dichotomous measure of religious attendance. Beyond religious participation, Rogers (1996) also suggests that other forms of social participation—with friends, with relatives outside the household, and in the community—are associated with reduced risks of death (e.g., Berkman and Syme 1979; House et al. 1982; Moen et al. 1992).

Thus, there is some evidence from both community and national-level studies that religious and other forms of social participation are associated with reduced risks of adult mortality. However, few studies, particularly at the national level, have considered these factors as important social indicators that contribute to the survival chances of individuals. Given the studies identified above, we expect that those individuals who are more religiously and socially active will exhibit lower risks of adult mortality. In this section, we speculate on some of the reasons why these relationships might exist and what variables will tap this logic. We begin with a brief discussion of the religious and general social participation variables.

RELIGIOUS ATTENDANCE

Our data set limits the focus on religious participation to religious attendance and includes the following question: "How often do you go to church, temple, or other religious services?" Respondents were allowed to choose the number of times per week, month, or year, in addition to a "never" option (Chyba and Washington 1993). We recognize that there are other, perhaps very important, dimensions of religious participation that we cannot consider in this analysis. For example, our data set contains no information on individuals' religious affiliation, frequency of prayer or meditation, belief in a god or the afterlife, or intensity of religious beliefs. Nevertheless, religious attendance has been the most commonly used and robust indicator of religious participation in many studies, including those related to health outcomes (Williams 1994). Because the reasons for religious attendance vary from habit to social desirability to spiritual reasons, we consider religious attendance to be a general indicator of a person's involvement in a religious community. Religious communities, while usually centered around spiritual matters, constitute a network of people who provide social resources, behavioral norms, and instrumental support to one another (Ellison and George 1994; Jarvis and Northcott 1987; Musick 1996). Moreover, involvement in a religious community may be psychologically rewarding and stress reducing, particularly in times of personal difficulty. Thus, there are multiple reasons why one might expect religious attendance to be associated with improved health and reduced mortality risks.

GENERAL SOCIAL PARTICIPATION

Our data set includes one question on general social participation. That is, "What is your frequency of participation in social activities?" Again, respondents were allowed to choose the number of times per week, month, or year, in addition to a "never" option (Chyba and Washington 1993). We also recognize that there are various types of social activity that individuals become involved in, various ways that individuals define social activity, and various costs and benefits that individuals accrue from participating in social activities. Thus, we concentrate not on the frequency of participation but on the fact that some individuals report that they do not participate in social activities at all. We assume that such individuals may not receive the same social support, have the same friendships, and be exposed to the same behavioral norms as their more socially active counterparts (e.g., House et al. 1988; Rogers 1996).

SELECTION FACTORS

People who do not attend religious services or who do not participate in social activities may abstain because their health limits their activities (Jarvis and Northcott 1987; Levin and Markides 1986). Our analysis addresses this issue in two ways. First, our data are a sample of the noninstitutionalized U.S. population, thus eliminating from consideration some of the most unhealthy and activity-limited people (for example, individuals who reside in nursing homes, mental health facilities, and prisons). Second, we statistically control for the baseline health status and activity limitation status of individuals in our data set through the use of self-reported measures of health and activity limitation.

Another type of potential selectivity involves social and economic factors. For example, individuals who are more educated, who have higher incomes, or who are married may be more likely to attend religious services and participate in other social activities (e.g., Comstock and Tonascia 1977). Thus, an observed association between, say, religious attendance and lower mortality may in fact be due to social and economic characteristics that select people into more active lifestyles. Our data set allows for education, income, employment status, and marital status controls; consequently, we can directly assess the impact of social selectivity on the religious and social participation linkages with mortality.

MEDIATING FACTORS

Other factors are best viewed as mediating the relationship between religious attendance, general social participation, and mortality (Jarvis and Northcott 1987). For example, the association between religious attendance and lower mortality may be due to differential health behavior exhibited between religious attendance groups. That is, through norms and denominational prescriptions, people who attend religious services more often are less likely to smoke cigarettes and engage in other unhealthy behavior than people who attend services less regularly (Gottlieb and Green 1984; Levin 1994a, 1994b). These behavioral factors are associated with adult mortality, particularly for certain causes of death. For example, cigarette smoking is a well-known risk factor for cancer, respiratory disease, and heart disease (Hummer et al. 1998a; Nam et al. 1994; Ravenholt 1984). We include a measure of smoking status here, with the understanding that religious involvement may influence other health behavioral factors (e.g., alcohol and drug use, driving practices, exercise) that also have important implications for survival chances.

Finally, general social participation and religious attendance may be related to other unmeasured factors that also work to reduce the risk of mortality. That is, recent theoretical work suggests that the association between religious factors and health is multifactorial in origin and that statistical models may not account for the complete set of religious effects (Levin 1994a: 10). For example, religious participation may generate increased self-esteem and a more coherent worldview, and may mitigate the impact of stressful life events such as illness and grief (Ellison 1994; Kark et al. 1996; Levin and Vanderpool 1987). Churches and temples may provide food and clothing, financial and housing assistance, and counseling to individuals, particularly attending members (Antonucci 1990). Informally, individual church members often provide support for one another through prayer and friendship (Bryant and Rakowski 1992; Taylor and Chatters

1986). Ellison and George (1994), in fact, report that frequent religious participation is related not only to an increased number of social ties and interactions, but also to more positive evaluations of those ties (also see Bradley 1995).

DATA

This chapter utilizes the Cancer Risk Factor Supplement of the 1987 National Health Interview Survey (NHIS) matched to the Multiple Cause of Death (MCD) file through the end of 1995 (NCHS 1989c, 1997b). The 1987 Cancer Risk Factor Supplement is the only recent NHIS survey that includes both a measure of religious attendance and an indicator of general social participation. Also included were behavioral questions such as cigarette smoking and the usual demographic, health, and household questions that are available on the NHIS core questionnaire. In all, 22,080 persons were interviewed in this supplement, the purpose of which was to collect in-depth information on cancer-related behaviors and exposures for a representative sample of the noninstitutionalized U.S. adult population (NCHS 1989c). Of the 22,080 respondents, 2,056 were identified as having died between 1987 and the end of 1995; our person-year file for this chapter contains 189,685 records.

The main independent variables considered here are religious attendance and general social participation. Following suggestions from earlier literature (e.g., Levin and Schiller 1987; Williams 1994), we create four categories of religious attendance: those who never attend services, those who attend less than once a week, those who attend weekly, and those who attend more than once a week. Those individuals who attend more than once a week are designated as the reference group. About 2% of the respondents did not answer this question; these individuals are subsequently dropped from the analysis. We dichotomize the general social participation variable, designating those people who participate in social activities as the reference group. Again, about 2% of the sample did not answer the question involving participation in social activity, and these individuals have also been dropped from the analysis.

We consider several sets of mortality covariates. Demographic factors include age, sex, and race; social factors include income equivalence, education, employment status, and marital status; and our health selection variables include a continuous measure of self-reported health ranging from one (excellent) to five (poor), and a dichotomous indicator of activity limitation. We designate people as activity limited if they are unable to perform, or are limited in performing, their major activity (such as paid employment or housework), or are limited in any way from performing other unspecified activities for health reasons (NCHS 1989c). This is a very inclusive measure of activity limitation, specifically constructed to eliminate, in the most comprehensive manner possible, any notion of health selectivity. Finally, we include cigarette smoking as a key behavioral factor related to mortality. For this measure, we specify four groups—never, former, current light, and current heavy smokers.

Most of the analysis in this chapter employs a dichotomous measure of survival status as the key dependent variable; that is, whether individuals interviewed in 1987 died or survived between the time of the interview in 1987 and the end of the follow-up period in 1995. We also use a five category cause of death scheme, which includes circulatory diseases (International Classification of Diseases [ICD] 390-459), cancers (ICD 140–239), respiratory diseases (ICD 466–496), social pathologies (which include suicides, accidents, homicides, and cirrhosis of the liver, ICD 571 and ICD 800–999), and a residual fifth category.

RESULTS

Table 6.1 provides descriptive statistics for all variables included in the analysis by survival status. For categorical variables, percentage distributions are shown; for continuous variables, mean values are reported. Note first that nearly 37% of the survivors (and about the same percentage of persons who died in the follow-up period) report that they attended church or service weekly or more than once a week. Thus, our data are highly consistent with other national surveys that report that about 40% of U.S. adults attend services during any given week (U.S. Bureau of the Census 1996: 70). Our data also show that nearly one-third of the survivors and about 40% of the persons who died over the follow-up period reported that they never attend services. A full comparison of the two columns for the religious attendance variable shows that death is especially more likely to occur among those who never attend services and less likely to occur among those who attend less than one time per week. Keep in mind, however, that this is simply a bivariate tabulation.

The general social participation variable indicates that socially active individuals are more likely to survive the follow-up period. For example, 63.9% of persons who survive the follow-up period report that they were involved in at least one social activity at baseline, while only 47.3% of persons who died reported involvement in at least one social activity. Among the other variables, death in the follow-up period is more likely among people who are older, male, black, lower income, less educated, not in the labor force, and widowed. In addition, individuals who are activity-limited, who are in poor health, and who are former smokers are more likely to die during follow-up than individuals in other categories of these variables. We now turn to the multivariate analysis to determine whether religious atten-

TABLE 6.1   Descriptive Statistics of Religious Attendance, General
Social Participation, and Other Mortality Covariates by Survival Status,
U.S. Adults, 1987–1995

	Survived	Died
Religious attendance		
Never attend	31.7	41.0
Attend <1 time/week	31.5	22.0
Attend weekly	28.2	30.0
Attend >1 time/week	8.6	7.0
General social participation		
No social activities	36.1	52.7
One or more activities	63.9	47.3
Demographic factors		
Age (mean)	46.6	70.5
Sex		
Male	47.3	53.0
Female	52.7	47.0
Race		
African American	10.9	12.8
Other	89.1	87.2
Health factors		
Activity limitations		
Limited	15.1	45.5
Not limited	84.9	54.5
Self-reported health (mean)	2.2	3.1
Social and economic factors		
Income equivalence (mean in $10,000s)	1.9	1.5
Education		
0–11 years	21.9	46.1
12 years	39.4	32.1
13+ years	38.7	21.8
Employment status		
Unemployed	3.8	2.1
Not in labor force	31.5	74.1
Employed	64.7	23.8
Marital status		
Never married	19.1	7.8
Divorced/separated	9.3	7.7
Widowed	6.4	25.4
Currently married	65.3	59.1
Behavioral factors		
Cigarette smoking		
Current heavy	16.8	17.2
Current light	11.8	10.1
Former	21.3	31.7
Never	50.2	40.9
Deaths and person-years	189,685	2,056

Sources: Derived from NCHS 1989c, 1997b.

dance and general social participation are associated with adult mortality, net of demographic, social, health, and behavioral factors.

RELIGIOUS ATTENDANCE, GENERAL SOCIAL PARTICIPATION, AND ALL-CAUSE MORTALITY

The first two models of Table 6.2 display the baseline relationships between religious attendance, general social participation, and mortality, respectively, controlling only for age, sex, and race. Those who never attend services exhibit the highest mortality risks and those who attend more than once a week exhibit the lowest risks. Compared to those who attend services more than once a week, those who never attend exhibit 80% higher odds of death in the follow-up period, those who attend less than once a week exhibit 28% higher odds of death, and those who attend weekly exhibit 12% higher odds (also see Figure 6.1). Thus, like other research that has examined the association between religious variables and health (Levin 1994a), we find a graded relationship between religious attendance and U.S. adult mortality. That is, individuals who never attend church or services demonstrate significantly higher mortality in the follow-up period compared to people who attend services more often (also see Hummer et al. 1999a).

Like religious attendance, the lack of general social participation also exhibits a strong association with the odds of mortality (Model 2). Individuals who reported not participating in social activities at baseline have 49% higher odds of mortality than their more socially active counterparts. Thus, net of demographic factors, both types of social participation examined here—religious and general—are associated with lower odds of adult mortality in the follow-up period. Furthermore, Model 3 includes both the religious and general social participation variables and finds that, net of one another, the relationships with mortality remain strong. Nonetheless, because religious and general social participation are associated with one another, there is some attenuation of the effects of each.

Models 4 and 5 add health and social and economic variables, respectively, to control for selection effects underlying the relationships displayed in the first three models, and Model 6 includes cigarette smoking. Inclusion of the health variables (Model 4) alters the magnitude of the association between religious attendance and mortality to some degree, but does not change the overall pattern of the relationship. In fact, the mortality difference between those people who attend weekly and those who attend more than once a week becomes slightly wider and statistically significant. In addition, keep in mind that controlling for health factors may result in an underestimate of the association between religious attendance and mortality, because some of the impact of religious attendance may, in fact, be mediated by health factors (see House et al. 1988: 541). Thus, Model 4 demon-

TABLE 6.2 Odds Ratios of Religious Attendance, General Social Participation, and Mortality, U.S. Adults, 1987–1995

	Model 1	Model 2	Model 3	Model 4	Model 5	Model 6	Model 7
Religious attendance							
Never	1.80*		1.58*	1.54*	1.59*	1.45*	1.44*
<1 time per week	1.28*		1.21+	1.24*	1.27*	1.14	1.21+
Weekly	1.12		1.10	1.18+	1.13	1.08	1.16
>1 time per week	ref		ref	ref	ref	ref	ref
General social participation							
None		1.49*	1.32*	1.17*	1.20*	1.29*	1.11*
One or more activities		ref	ref	ref	ref	ref	ref
Demographic factors							
Age (continuous)	1.09*	1.08*	1.09*	1.08*	1.08*	1.09*	1.08*
Sex							
Male	1.51*	1.59*	1.52*	1.59*	1.73*	1.43*	1.64*
Female	ref	ref	ref	ref	ref	ref	ref
Race							
African American	1.63*	1.51*	1.59*	1.33*	1.44*	1.59*	1.30*
Other	ref	ref	ref	ref	ref	ref	ref
Health factors							
Activity limitations							
Limited				1.59*			1.52*
Not limited				ref			ref
Self-reported health (continuous)				1.29*			1.26*

Social and economic factors							
Income equivalence (continuous)					0.92*		0.98
Education							
<12 years					1.20*		1.10
12 years					1.11		1.09
13+ years					ref		ref
Employment status							
Unemployed					1.82*		1.71*
Not in labor force					1.65*		1.33*
Employed					ref		ref
Marital status							
Never					1.46*		1.60*
Divorced/separated					1.07		1.00
Widowed					1.16*		1.16*
Married					ref		ref
Behavioral factors							
Cigarette smoking							
Current heavy						1.74*	1.66*
Current light						1.44*	1.36*
Former						1.21*	1.17*
Never						ref	ref
−2*Log-likelihood	18,355.9	18,383.6	18,146.9	17,696.7	17,922.8	18,081.1	17,501.7

Sources: Derived from NCHS 1989c, 1997b.
+$p \leq .10$; *$p \leq .05$.

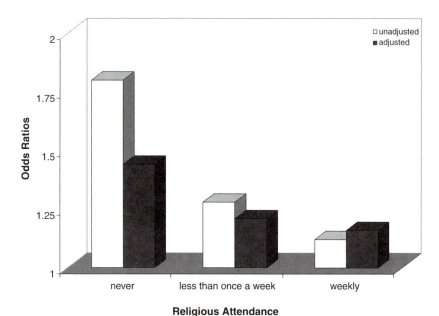

FIGURE 6.1   Odds ratios of dying by religious attendance, U.S. adults, 1987–1995. Note: Referent is those who attend more than once per week.

strates that the influence of religious attendance on mortality is not solely due to health selectivity.

Inclusion of the social and economic variables in Model 5 also has relatively little influence on the religious attendance association with mortality (compare Model 5 to Model 3). Thus, in contrast to Comstock and Tonascia (1977), we find little evidence that religious attendance is associated with mortality only because of confounding by social and economic factors. Note also that the religious attendance variable exhibits an association with mortality that is similar in magnitude to the social and economic variables—which receive far greater attention in the demographic and public health mortality literature. In contrast, the mortality difference between socially inactive and active individuals is reduced by about one-half once our model includes either social or health variables (compare Models 4 and 5 to Model 3). Thus, the relationship between general social participation and mortality is much more closely connected with the underlying health and social status of individuals than is the relationship between religious attendance and mortality.

Model 6 adds cigarette smoking. In this model, the association between religious attendance and mortality is somewhat weaker in comparison to that shown in Model 3. In other words, controlling for cigarette smoking produces a reduction in the mortality differential between the never and most frequently attending groups. A check of the smoking differences between religious attendance groups (data not shown) shows that more frequent attendees exhibit a very different pattern of smoking than those who attend less than once a week; in particular, they are far less likely to be heavy smokers. This finding provides some support to the idea that health behaviors, at least in part, are responsible for the association between religious attendance and mortality (Jarvis and Northcott 1987). Of course, data on a more inclusive range of health behaviors would help to further test this linkage. However, even net of cigarette smoking, those who never attend services exhibit 45% higher odds of mortality than those who attend more than once a week. Thus, it is clear that religious attendance exerts a strong net association with U.S. adult mortality.

When the complete set of variables is included (Model 7), the relationship between religious attendance and mortality remains moderately strong and graded. Particularly noteworthy is the 44% higher odds of death exhibited by those who never attend compared to those who attend more than once a week. In contrast, while the association between general social participation and mortality remains statistically significant, the magnitude of the difference (11% higher odds of mortality for socially inactive individuals) is small.

AGE- AND CAUSE-SPECIFIC MORTALITY

Table 6.3 considers the associations between religious attendance, general social participation, and all-cause mortality for younger adults and older adults, respectively. Model 1 for each age group includes only demographic controls, while Model 2 for each age group includes the complete set of independent variables. Most striking is the stronger association between religious attendance and the odds of mortality during the follow-up period for younger adults. In fact, younger adults who never attend services demonstrate over twice the odds of death than younger adults who attend more than once a week, even after controlling for health, social and economic, and behavioral factors. Substantial mortality differences also exist between those who attend less than once a week and weekly, in comparison to those who attend most frequently. Thus, frequent religious attendance seems to be especially protective for younger adults, but is also moderately protective for older adults. On the other hand, general social participation displays roughly the same relationship with mortality for both age groups. That is, social inactivity is moderately related to higher mortality, with the difference largely reduced with the inclusion of health and social variables.

Table 6.4 displays the results of models relating religious attendance and general social participation to cause-specific mortality. Similar to the modeling procedure used in the age-specific table, Model 1 for each cause in-

TABLE 6.3 Odds Ratios of Religious Attendance, General Social Participation, and Mortality for Two Age Groups, U.S. Adults, 1987–1995a

	Ages 18–64		Ages 65+	
	Model 1	Model 2	Model 1	Model 2
Religious attendance				
Never	2.58*	2.14*	1.34*	1.24+
<1 time per week	1.87*	1.83*	1.05	1.04
Weekly	1.66*	1.70*	0.97	1.02
>1 time per week	ref	ref	ref	ref
General social participation				
None	1.25*	0.93	1.34*	1.18+
One or more activities	ref	ref	ref	ref
−2*Log-likelihood	6,510.9	6,217.3	11,603.3	11,218.5

Sources: Derived from NCHS 1989c, 1997b.
^{a} Model 1 for each cause controls only for demographic factors. Model 2 additionally includes the health, social and economic, and behavioral factors.
$+p \le .10; *p \le .05.$

cludes only demographic controls, while Model 2 for each cause includes the complete set of independent variables. For all causes of death, individuals who attend services most frequently display the lowest odds of mortality. Interestingly, circulatory disease and cancer mortality differences across religious attendance groups are relatively small in magnitude, while the difference in respiratory disease mortality—which is strongly associated with cigarette smoking (e.g., Metropolitan Life 1990)—is wide. For example, compared to individuals who attend religious services more than once a week, individuals who never attend services are about twice as likely to die from respiratory disease, even net of cigarette smoking. Differences in mortality from social pathologies also pose an interesting pattern; compared to people who attend services more than once a week, those who attend less frequently or not at all exhibit two to three times higher odds of death (see Figure 6.2).

Finally, there is a substantial mortality difference between people who never attend religious services and those who attend frequently for the residual cause category. The heterogeneous nature of this cause-of-death category makes it difficult to even speculate on reasons for the linkage. Our check of the specific causes included in this category (not shown) demonstrated that diabetes mellitus (18%), infectious diseases (17%), and renal failure (6%) each account for a substantial share; however, about one-half of the deaths in this category are due to rather infrequent individual causes. Note also that there is a relatively strong association between social inactivity and mortality for this cause category.

TABLE 6.4   Odds Ratios of Religious Attendance, General Social Participation, and Cause-Specific Mortality, U.S. Adults, 1987–1995[a]

	Circulatory		Cancer		Respiratory		Social pathologies		Other causes	
	Model 1	Model 2	Model 1	Model 2	Model 1	Model 2	Model 1	Model 2	Model 1	Model 2
Religious attendance										
Never	1.35*	1.26	1.23	1.09	3.09*	2.31+	3.06*	2.48+	2.11*	2.14*
<1 time per week	1.09	1.11	1.11	1.04	2.01	1.72	3.55*	3.30*	0.99	1.15
Weekly	1.01	1.08	1.06	1.08	1.13	1.12	3.10*	2.86+	1.06	1.24
>1 time per week	ref	ref	ref	ref	ref	ref	ref	ref	ref	ref
General social participation										
None	1.39*	1.18*	1.07	0.93	1.63*	1.20	0.82	0.64*	1.84*	1.54*
One or more activities	ref	ref	ref	ref	ref	ref	ref	ref	ref	ref
−2*Log-likelihood	8,661.9	8,390.6	6,604.2	6,449.2	1,833.9	1,669.7	1,999.5	1,885.1	4,142.7	3,909.6

Sources: Derived from NCHS 1989c, 1997b.

[a] Model 1 for each cause controls only for demographic factors. Model 2 additionally includes the health, social and economic, and behavioral factors.

$+ p \leq .10$; $*p \leq .05$.

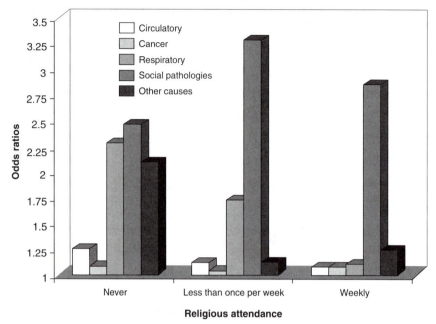

FIGURE 6.2   Odds ratios of cause-specific mortality by religious attendance, U.S. adults, 1987–1995. Note: Referent is those who attend more than once per week.

CONCLUSION

Our findings lend up-to-date nationally representative support to the idea that more frequent religious attendance is associated with better health and lower mortality (Levin 1994a, 1994b). We found this to be the case across the four categories of our religious attendance variable, although the mortality differences between those who attend once a week and those who attend even more frequently were only marginally significant. Thus, like socioeconomic status, religious attendance exhibits a graded association with U.S. adult mortality. In contrast to Comstock and Tonascia's (1977) often-cited study, we also found that religious attendance exhibited an effect on all-cause mortality net of social and health factors. Furthermore, at least part of this association is due to differences in behavior across religious attendance groups. This corresponds with the conceptual models of religion and health most recently put forth by Levin (1994a, 1994b) and Jarvis and Northcott (1987). Future work can help demonstrate how other mediating factors—such as instrumental support, volunteerism, and the alleviation of stress—may work to link religious attendance with lower mortality risks. In addition, recent work demonstrates that it will become increasingly important to understand the subjective aspects of social support that improve health and well-being, particularly for individuals who are tied into supportive religious networks (Ellison and George 1994). Such effects may also vary by religious denomination and region of the country.

We demonstrated a weaker association between general social participation and the risk of adult mortality during the follow-up period. To a much greater extent than religious attendance, general social participation is associated with both good health and high socioeconomic status, which help to account for the observed association between general social participation and mortality. An examination of more detailed measures of social participation is warranted to better specify the relationship between specific aspects of social participation and mortality. For example, Rogers (1996) recently revealed the importance of volunteerism; attending shows, movies, and concerts; socializing with friends and neighbors; and visiting with nonhousehold members in reducing the mortality prospects of U.S. individuals aged 55 and above.

Much stronger in our data, however, is the relationship between religious attendance and adult mortality. Given the long noted association between religion and suicide, the documented linkages between religion and various health and morbidity outcomes, and the multiple mechanisms by which religious involvement is thought to influence health and mortality, religion might best be conceptualized as a "fundamental cause" of mortality (Link and Phelan 1995, 1996). Fundamental causes of mortality—such as race and socioeconomic status—allow for access to important resources, affect various health and cause of death outcomes, and may even maintain an association with health and mortality when intervening mechanisms change over time (Link and Phelan 1995). Religious variables, however, have received far less attention in the mortality literature than race and socioeconomic status, and there is still a sense in the scientific community that religious effects are minor at best, or even irrelevant (see Levin 1994c, p. xvi). The findings demonstrated here (also see Hummer et al. 1999a) should help to dispel such a notion.

Clearly, additional research is warranted in this area—particularly when multi-factorial measures of religion can be included in national-level studies of health and mortality. We recognize, for example, that there are other very important dimensions of religious participation that we could not consider here. Our data set contained no information on religious affiliation, frequency of prayer or meditation, or belief in a god or the afterlife—all of which would allow for the improvement over our one-dimensional measure of religious participation. Thus, data needs are critical; simply, there have been few adequate data sources available at the national level to measure the impact of religiosity, religious affiliation, and religious beliefs on health and mortality.

The influence of religious attendance may also be stronger among some denominational groups or stronger among people who are both privately and publicly religious. More specific cause-of-death models may also prove fruitful. Our general cause-of-death models suggested that infrequent religious attendance was associated with higher mortality for all causes considered, including circulatory diseases and cancer, but especially so for respiratory diseases, social pathologies, and residual causes. These cause-of-death patterns were consistent with a seemingly stronger association between religious attendance and mortality among younger adults than among older adults.

In sum, religion is a major social institution and an important source of behavioral norms and social support for many people. Our analysis also revealed that religious attendance is a powerful force in understanding U.S. mortality patterns. Therefore, future studies on the health and mortality of the U.S. population must consider the effects which religion, preferably in its multiple dimensions, exhibits.

PART
III

SOCIOECONOMIC FACTORS

7

THE EFFECTS OF BASIC SOCIOECONOMIC FACTORS ON MORTALITY

Social stratification results in an uneven distribution of desirable resources among people, which in turn affects life chances: scant resources can shorten life. This chapter presents a more extensive model of the relations between socioeconomic status and mortality. We will examine the effects of education, income, and employment status—central measures in the construction of socioeconomic status—on mortality.

The research reported here is significant for three major reasons. First, the association between socioeconomic status and mortality, while generally well known, is not well understood because socioeconomic status is multidimensional and difficult to measure. Second, socioeconomic mortality differences are now recognized as a major U.S. public health problem, and important policy decisions depend on the scientific understanding of these differences. Finally, the apparent widening of U.S. socioeconomic mortality differences since 1960 lends urgency to the inquiries into how different socioeconomic factors influence mortality.

DATA AND MEASUREMENT PROBLEMS

The general pattern of socioeconomic mortality differentiation varies by the particular socioeconomic measure used, and most U.S. studies rely on measures so very limited and broad that the descriptive, scientific, and policy value of the studies is impaired (Moss and Krieger 1995). The United States continues to lag well behind other nations in collecting data on socioeconomic status and mortality. Moss and Krieger (1995: 302–303), in the summary report of a national conference on Measuring Social Inequalities in Health, state:

> Despite these well-known associations, we are hampered in our efforts to track, understand, and reduce socioeconomic inequalities in health for two reasons. First, U.S. vital statistics disease registries, and medical care utilization statistics, unlike those in many European countries, only report basic data about the health of the nation in terms of race, sex, and age, even when the socioeconomic data may be available. Yet the data reported often form the basis for policy. Second, the measures used are often inconsistent and inadequate for capturing the full range of socioeconomic disparity. For example, our focus on the poor and nonpoor obscures a whole range of socioeconomic differences that affect health.

The conference recommended collecting data on amount and sources of income, health insurance coverage, and completed educational level (Moss and Krieger 1995). Fortunately, all these items are available in our data and will be presented in this and subsequent chapters.

SCIENTIFIC AND POLICY RELEVANCE

In a review of socioeconomic and racial differences in U.S. health, Williams and Collins (1995: 380–381) write that "racial and socioeconomic inequality in health is arguably the single most important public health issue in the United States." In other reviews on the same topic, Link and Phelan (1996, 1995) contend that socioeconomic status is likely a fundamental cause of disease because it embodies access to important resources, has maintained an association with health and mortality over many years, and affects multiple disease outcomes. One of the three broad goals of the Healthy People 2000 campaign is to reduce health disparities among Americans (NCHS 1995c). Philip R. Lee (1995: 302), the Assistant Secretary for Health and head of the Public Health Service, argues that the deficiencies of socioeconomic health-related data "are no longer acceptable" and urges more in-depth collection and reporting of such data. Thus, the emphasis on socioeconomic differentials in mortality is well grounded in scientific and policy concerns.

THE WIDENING MORTALITY GAP

An inverse association between mortality and various measures of socioeconomic status dates back to early U.S. records and has been found in all countries researchers have examined (Krieger et al. 1993; Williams and Collins 1995). For many years, however, few U.S. studies reported on socioeconomic differentials in mortality, in part due to lack of data. But in the

1960s, demographers, sociologists, and epidemiologists began to focus on such differentials. One of the best known works is the study by Kitagawa and Hauser (1973), who used a sample of U.S. death certificates from 1960 matched to census data of that same year to estimate adult mortality differences across socioeconomic groups. They demonstrated that income and education each exhibited strong associations with mortality and that these associations were greater for persons between the ages of 25 and 64 than for those aged 65 and older. In short, the Kitagawa-Hauser study used an imaginative data linkage and created a descriptive foundation upon which future researchers can build. The use of multiple socioeconomic status indicators, even in methodologically simple fashion, alerted researchers to the need to measure both socioeconomic status and mortality inclusively. Using more sophisticated data sets and statistical analyses, a number of demographers and epidemiologists have since updated the work of Kitagawa and Hauser.

Alarmingly, most analyses have shown that socioeconomic differences in mortality have increased since 1960 (Feldman et al. 1989; Pappas et al. 1993; Preston and Elo 1995). For example, Pappas et al. (1993) found that the inverse relationship between mortality and socioeconomic status— as measured by education and broad income categories—were larger for women and men, whites and blacks, and people living with family members and those living with unrelated persons. More recently, Preston and Elo (1995), using the National Longitudinal Mortality Study, also found that education-related differences had widened for men in comparison to 1960, though they had narrowed for working-age women. These trends have raised the awareness of the scientific and government communities that such gaps need to be better understood and addressed.

CONCEPTUALIZING AND MEASURING SOCIOECONOMIC STATUS

Often, socioeconomic status is discussed and assessed as if it were a unidimensional concept, measurable by education, or current income, or occupational prestige. However, there is increasing awareness, some of which is recognized in the health and mortality literature, that socioeconomic status is a multidimensional construct; that is, several socioeconomic dimensions, in tandem, compose the bundle of characteristics that represent an individual's relative standing in society (Sorlie et al. 1995; Williams and Collins 1995). Important in such a conceptualization is the notion that each socioeconomic dimension, while overlapping with the others, carries a unique relationship with mortality.

EDUCATION

The inverse relationship between education and mortality is well documented. Not only do less educated groups have higher mortality, but a gradient persists, so that the most educated group is better off than groups directly below (see Adler et al. 1994). Kitagawa and Hauser (1973) found an inverse relationship between education and mortality for different age, race, and sex groups. Subsequent studies, with data from different times and different areas, have confirmed the education-mortality relationship, which persists, though it may be reduced by controlling for age, sex, race, marital status, cigarette smoking, adequacy of housing, and income (see Comstock and Tonascia 1977; Feldman et al. 1989). For example, Pappas et al. (1993) report that U.S. adults aged 25–64 with less than a high school education are more than twice as likely to die each year as similarly aged adults with a college education.

Some researchers argue that education is the best measure of socioeconomic status for mortality studies because it is usually determined early in life; can be assessed for all individuals; is important for employment, income generation, and information gathering; influences health behavior; affects health insurance coverage; and is critical for the use of health services (Christenson and Johnson 1995; Elo and Preston 1996; Preston and Taubman 1994; Rosenberg and Powell-Griner 1991). In short, education is a central socioeconomic measure, is easily determined, and must be considered in virtually all studies of socioeconomic status and mortality.

Educational attainment affects mortality directly through altered health behaviors and indirectly through its effect on income and occupation, which in turn can determine access to resources (Comstock and Tonascia 1977; Elo and Preston 1996; Feldman et al. 1989; Rosenberg and Powell-Griner 1991). Education provides the necessary knowledge, skills, information, and certification to qualify for more advanced jobs, for promotion, and for higher salaries. Although education, income, and employment status are interrelated, educational attainment usually precedes, and therefore most likely influences, income and employment status and their effects on mortality.

Education provides individuals a vast storehouse of knowledge about how to interact with others, how to intervene in crises, what to do in emergencies, how to gain access to medical care, and how to promote favorable health and prevent disease. Highly educated individuals are more likely to engage in positive health behaviors (abstain from smoking, drink moderately, eat nutritious meals, and wear seat belts), to regularly visit the doctor for health check-ups, to more quickly alert health personnel of health problems, to more clearly understand the communication with the doctor, and to better understand and to adhere to the treatment guidelines. Moreover, less educated people are more likely to exhibit negative psychosocial characteristics—risky health behavior, stress, social isolation, and lack of social control—that are important determinants of health and mortality (House, et al. 1988).

Education can be measured in a variety of ways. Generally, education is ascertained by degrees attained, years of schooling completed, or years of schooling attended. It would also be possible, for example, to include measures of on-the-job training, certifications, workshops, and vocational education. Such measures, however, are more difficult to compare and may vary by region of the country and type of work. Most studies employ years of schooling completed. Education is related to mortality and to age. Because of the increasing educational requirements over time, younger cohorts are more likely to have higher levels of education than older cohorts. Thus, it is advisable to control for age when examining the effects of education on mortality.

Although education is reported in years, there are general milestones that mark educational achievement. In the United States, schools are distinguished among elementary schools (kindergarten through fifth grade), middle school (sixth through eighth grade), high school (ninth through twelfth grade), and college. Educational philosophies have slightly modified the cut points between different schools. For example, there has been a general shift away from junior high to middle schools. There are also educational steps in college. College may be distinguished between a person who attends but does not graduate from college, and graduates with associate's (a two-year program past the high school degree), bachelor's (a 4-year program past the high school degree), master's (a 1- to 2-year post-baccalaureate program), and doctorate (a 4-year post-baccalaureate program) degrees. These distinctions suggest that specific cut points are more important than just cumulative years in school. Thus, there is generally a large educational gap between a person who completed 11 years of schooling and a high school graduate. The former completed many years of school, but stopped short of attaining a degree, while the latter completed high school and received a diploma that certifies minimal levels of accomplishments and skills.

FAMILY INCOME

Family income is one of the primary links between education and mortality, particularly for men (Elo and Preston 1996). The inverse relationship between income and mortality persists for women and men, the young and the old, majority and minority populations, and the married and the unmarried (Kaplan and Keil 1993; Kitagawa and Hauser 1973; Pappas et al. 1993; Rogers 1995a; Sorlie et al. 1992a, 1993). Most recently, Sorlie et al.

(1995) found that even after adjustment for education, occupation, and other demographic characteristics, increased family income was associated with lower mortality among adults in each age and sex group. For example, women aged 45–64 with a family income of more than $50,000 were 31% less likely to die during a recent follow-up period than similarly aged women with family incomes less than $5,000.

Critics suggest that poor health may be the cause, rather than the effect, of lower incomes—and that people in poor health are more likely to die (e.g., Illsley 1986; Morris 1996). But several papers have demonstrated that income has pronounced effects on mortality even after adjustments are made for health status (McDonough et al. 1994; Menchik 1993; D. G. Smith et al. 1996). Thus, while it is important to consider and adjust for the health status of individuals, family income remains a critical variable.

High income can increase survival chances by providing individuals access to health care, proper diet, adequate housing in safe neighborhoods, and reduced financial pressures and stresses. Moreover, high income is associated with healthy behaviors such as regular exercise and moderation in the use of alcohol and tobacco (Adler et al. 1994; Burstin et al. 1992; Cockerham 1988; Williams 1990).

As with education, income can be measured in a variety of ways. Frequently used measures of income include per capita income, poverty rates, income equivalence scales, family income, and respondent's income. Respondent's income overlooks other income sources within the family. Family income does not allow for differences in family size. Per capita income ignores the advantages of household economies of scale in the purchase and use of housing, health, and other goods and services.

Several measures have been developed to adjust income by taking into account family size. Many poverty measures assess poverty rather than general standards of living, are dichotomous (e.g., poor or not poor) rather than continuous, provide irregular adjustments by family size, and are based on the consumption of food rather than other household goods. Moreover, many poverty measures (see Orshansky 1963) make large adjustments of additional family members in large families but small adjustments in small families. Since economies of scale increase with increasing family sizes, these adjustments are unrealistic and counterintuitive (see Ruggles 1990).

Family income can be simply measured as a dichotomy of, say, less than $20,000 or $20,000 or more. Such a measure works well if the concern is with a threshold effect. For example, if the concern is with those who are considered poor, compared to those who are not poor, a dichotomy may work well. Moreover, respondents are more likely to respond to a broad income question rather than a question that asks for detailed information on income. In general, however, detailed measures are preferable to the conventional poor-nonpoor dichotomies (Moss and Krieger 1995; Ruggles 1990).

Income can also be assessed through a continuous measure, through logged income, or through income equivalence scales. Income equivalence scales address many of the concerns with other income measures by combining information on family size and family income to create a continuous measure of income that assesses family consumption patterns (see Rogers 1995a). Income equivalence scales represent the pooled resources of the family: larger families can share some goods and common food preparation, living, and dining areas, and can reduce expenses by purchasing products in bulk (Buhmann et al. 1988; Van der Gaag and Smolensky 1982). Further, these scales mathematically smooth the transition from one family size to the next, create a continuous measure of income, adjust for economies of scale, and measure different family consumption patterns (see Buhmann et al. 1988; Van der Gaag and Smolensky 1982).

EMPLOYMENT STATUS

Employment status is another crucial socioeconomic variable. Several studies have demonstrated the beneficial effects of working. Individuals who are employed benefit through the salaries they earn, the benefits that come with the job, the possibility of free or subsidized health insurance, and the social relations and camaraderie among co-workers.

Some individuals are still in the labor force, have worked in the past, but are no longer working. Individuals who are not currently employed, who were on lay-off, who were fired, or who had quit their jobs generally have higher mortality than those who are currently working. Furthermore, individuals who are not in the labor force represent a mixed group that generally experiences relatively high mortality. A small percentage of individuals not in the labor force may be independently wealthy and therefore not have to work. Some individuals, disproportionately females, work at home but do not have salaried work. Most studies have demonstrated that housewives have higher mortality than women who work. And some individuals who do not work are physically or mentally limited in their ability to work. For such individuals, it is the lack of the benefits that come from work, in addition to the higher mortality risk that comes from physical and mental limitations that places them at greater risk of death. This chapter is devoted to the basic socioeconomic status measures—income, education, and employment status. Chapters 8 and 9 examine the effects of occupational status and health insurance, respectively, on mortality.

METHODS

The National Health Interview Survey (NHIS) includes in the core questions information about employment, family income, and education. For this analysis, we use the 1991 NHIS, which provides enough cases (717,547 person years) and enough deaths (1,465) for the analysis. But any year of the NHIS would suffice. Although Chapter 2 summarizes the central covariates employed in this book, below we discuss in more detail the socioeconomic factors we examine in this chapter.

For education, NHIS obtains completed years of school attendance through a set of two questions. The first question asks, "What is the highest grade or year of regular school ___ has ever attended?" A specific year is filled in by the interviewer. The follow-up question asks "Did ___ finish the (grade/year)?" "Regular schooling is that which advances a person toward an elementary or high school diploma, or a college, university, or professional school degree" (NCHS 1992c). Thus, schools that are not part of the regular school system—vocational, business, and trade schools—are not included. Neither are on-the-job training, adult education classes, employment training, or military basic training. Individuals are considered to have graduated from high school if they completed 12 years of schooling, passed a high school equivalency test, or finished high school in the Armed Forces or at another time (NCHS 1992c).

In this chapter, we code education into six categories—less than 9 years, 9 to 11 years, 12 years, 13 to 15 years, 16 years, and 17 years or more. This distinguishes among individuals who have not attended high school, those who have attended high school but have not graduated, high school graduates, those who have attended college, college graduates, and those with college graduate school experience. We provide detailed education categories in this chapter because the focus is on socioeconomic status; later chapters include broader educational categories because the focus is on other factors and education is used as a control. Education is regularly used in mortality research because it changes little after the young adult years, is comparable across groups, like different races or sexes, helps predict mortality, and is usually reported: fully 98% of the respondents report their education. We drop the 2% of individuals who do not report their education.

Family income is more volatile than other measures of socioeconomic status and fluctuates over time with changes in household composition and with the employment and earnings of other household members (Hauser 1994). Nevertheless, income is a central socioeconomic measure and is strongly and consistently related to mortality. Family income is important for mortality analyses for the following reasons. First, all family members generally benefit by increased family income, even if they do not personally generate the income. Second, most previous mortality studies have examined family rather than individual income (e.g., Sorlie et al. 1995). Third, it is often difficult to separate individual from family income. Incomes from family businesses may be disbursed to family members to ensure the greatest disposable but lowest taxable income. Social security income distributed to married couples is based on the couple's previous earnings and marital status rather than individual earnings. Fourth, many family members adjust their work status (full time versus part time, flexibility in working hours, and number of vacation days) and their income to complement one another rather than to compete (Rogers 1996).

Family income includes two questions. The first question asks "Was the total combined FAMILY income during the past 12 months—that is, yours, (*read names, including Armed Forces members living at home*) more or less than $20,000? Include money from jobs, social security, retirement income, unemployment payments, public assistance, and so forth. Also, include income from interest, dividends, net income from business, farm, or rent, and any other money income received" (NCHS 1992c: D14–43). Not everyone is willing to report their incomes. But individuals are more likely to report broad rather than specific income groups. Thus, this question is important because it provides a general income group and avoids the larger number of refusals for more detailed questions. The follow-up question asks, "Of those income groups, which letter best represents the total combined FAMILY income during the past 12 months (that is, yours, (read names, including Armed Forces members living at home))? Include wages, salaries, and other items we just talked about" (NCHS 1992c: D14–43). This follow-up question asks for more income detail, which increases the refusal rate. To insure as high a compliance as possible, the interviewer hands the respondent a flashcard with letters corresponding to income ranges. Thus, the respondent answers with a letter instead of a specific income, which should increase the response accuracy and rate. The letters range from A (less than $1,000) to Z ($45,000–49,999), with the last category after Z listed as ZZ ($50,000 and over). The initial categories are grouped into $1,000 increments through $19,999, and then in $5,000 increments through $49,999.

Family income represents the income before deducting taxes, retirement, health insurance, and union dues. It does not include income "in kind," lump sum payments such as insurance payments or inheritances, occasional gifts from relatives not living in the household, money received from the sale of a house or personal property, savings withdrawals, or tax refunds.

Income can be measured in multiple ways. Income can be based on individuals or the family, can be dichotomous or continuous, can be logged, and can be converted into a scale. We computed income equivalences according to the formula of Buhmann et al. (1988), where economic well-being (W) relates to family income (I) and family size (S): $W = I/S^e$, where e, the equivalence elasticity, ranges from 0 to 1. Smaller equivalence elasticities signify larger economies of scale. Van der Gaag and Smolensky

(1982) suggest that an equivalence elasticity of .38 best adjusts for differences in consumption needs across families of different sizes. To illustrate, an income of $30,000 for a family of five would provide the same purchasing power as $16,275 for one individual (or $16,275 = $30,000 / $5^{.38}$). The income equivalences were computed from a detailed family income variable with a nonresponse rate of 13%. Assuming that persons with similar social, demographic, and educational characteristics will possess similar incomes, we imputed income values for the nonresponders on the basis of predicted values of age, sex, education, and marital status, stratified by the dichotomous family income measure (less than $20,000, or $20,000 or more). We excluded from the sample the 2% of the respondents who did not answer any income question. Analyses with and without imputed incomes yielded similar results. Because of the focus on socioeconomic status, this chapter examines income equivalence in $5,000 categories. Such detailed coding will more clearly reveal the effects of socioeconomic status on mortality, net of other controls. Other chapters control for income by using the midpoints of $10,000 income equivalence categories.

We ran analyses using a dichotomy of less than $20,000 or $20,000 or more, a continuous measure of income, and logged income to determine if a particular measure fit best. All income measures produced similar results on mortality. We retained the income equivalence scale because it provides a more substantive interpretation and directly adjusts for family size, another potentially important contributor to mortality differences.

Employment histories are ascertained through a series of core questions. First, the respondent is provided with a 2-week reference period from which to base the answers to a series of questions. The respondent is then asked, "DURING THOSE 2 WEEKS, did ___ work at any time at a job or business not counting work around this house? (Include unpaid work in the family (farm/business)." If the person did not work, a follow-up question asked, "Even though ___ did not work during those 2 weeks, did ___ have a job or business? (NCHS 1992c: D7-3). For those who replied that they had not worked, NCHS ascertained whether the person was looking for work or on layoff.

We code employment status as currently working, unemployed, or not in the labor force. Those who are currently working represent the referent; they have a job and either worked in the past 2 weeks or did not work but have not been formally laid off (they may be on vacation or may be looking for other employment opportunities). Those who are unemployed remain in the labor force; either they have been laid off temporarily, or they are looking for work. Those who are not in the labor force are not employed, are not on temporary lay-off, and are not looking for work.

Because socioeconomic status is affected by demographic, social, and health status, we also control for age, sex, race, marital status, and health status. We code health status as a continuous scale, which ranges from 1, excellent health, to 5, poor health. Perceived health status is widely used and considered a strong indicator of a person's general health (see Idler and Benyamini 1997; Kaplan and Camacho 1983; Peters and Rogers 1997; Singer et al. 1976). Because health status and socioeconomic status are interrelated, we run several models separately—first without controls for health status, and then with health status controlled. Further, because socioeconomic status varies by age, and because many researchers have focused on individuals below the age of 65, we present findings for the total adult population, as well as those aged 18 to 64.

RESULTS

Table 7.1 shows the percentages of all adults (Columns 1 and 2) and of adults aged 18 to 64 (Columns 3 and 4) who survived and who died during the period 1991 through 1995. Within both age groups, about the same proportions of alive individuals are high school graduates as have attended college (see Columns 1 and 3). Fewer than 10% of the population had an income equivalence of under $5,000, or of over $40,000. Moreover, about two-thirds of all adults and almost three-quarters of adults aged 18 to 64 are employed. Compared to the total adult population, individuals aged 18 to 64 have higher levels of educational attainment, higher rates of employment, and greater proportions of individuals in the income extremes— earning either less than $5,000 or more than $20,000 (compare Columns 1 and 3).

Mortality is more likely among those with low levels of education, those with lower incomes, and those who are not in the labor force (compare Columns 1 with 2, and 3 with 4). For example, only 22% of the total adult population who survived the period had less than a high school education, but almost one-half of those who died had less than a high school education. To examine the effects of socioeconomic status on mortality in a multivariate framework, we turn to Table 7.2.

THE EFFECTS OF EDUCATION ON MORTALITY

Table 7.2 focuses on educational differences in mortality for the general adult population. Model 1—which controls for age, sex, race, and marital status, but not income or employment status—displays a clear gradient: compared to individuals with 17 or more years of education, those with 16 years of schooling are 25% more likely to die, high school graduates are 60% more likely to die, and individuals with fewer than 9 years of schooling are almost twice as likely to die. Although education is related to mor-

TABLE 7.1 Descriptive Statistics of Socioeconomic Factors Related to Those Who Survived and Who Died, U.S. Adults, Various Age Groups, 1991–1995

	Ages 18 and over		Ages 18 to 64	
Socioeconomic factors	(1) Alive	(2) Dead	(3) Alive	(4) Dead
Education				
0–8 years	9.3	29.3	5.9	15.6
9–11 years	11.7	15.7	11.1	17.0
High school graduate	37.9	32.1	39.0	38.1
13–15 years	20.8	12.3	22.4	16.7
16 years	11.9	6.5	12.6	7.8
17 years or more	8.4	4.1	9.1	4.8
Income equivalence (U.S. dollars)				
Less than 5,000	5.8	6.7	6.1	8.8
5,000 to less than 10,000	14.8	30.2	12.4	20.6
10,000 to less than 15,000	15.2	22.2	13.5	17.7
15,000 to less than 20,000	10.9	10.8	10.8	10.4
20,000 to less than 25,000	14.4	11.5	14.8	14.0
25,000 to less than 30,000	10.9	6.0	11.9	8.8
30,000 to less than 35,000	12.6	4.8	14.1	7.8
35,000 to less than 40,000	7.5	3.1	8.4	6.2
40,000 or more	7.8	4.5	8.2	5.7
Employment status				
Employed	65.0	20.2	74.9	52.0
Unemployed	3.5	1.0	4.1	2.3
Not in labor force	31.5	78.8	21.0	45.7
Person years and deaths	717,547	1,465	323,210	945

Sources: Derived from NCHS 1993d and 1997b.

tality, it is also related to other socioeconomic variables. Education provides the knowledge, skills, and certification needed for entry into many jobs, and job income may be based not only on performance, but also on education. Thus, once other factors are considered, the apparent effect of education on mortality diminishes.

Subsequent models indicate that socioeconomic factors—education, income, and employment status—are indeed interrelated. Income, in Model 4, reduces the effect of education; and employment status, in Model 5, also reduces the effect of education, but to a lesser degree. Income and work status combine in Model 7 to dampen the effect of education on mortality. Nevertheless, the education-mortality gradient persists. Compared to those with 17 or more years of education, those with less than 9 years of education are over 40% more likely to die, controlling for age, sex, race, marital

TABLE 7.2 Odds Ratios Showing the Effect of Socioeconomic Status on Mortality, U.S. Adults Age 18 and Over, 1991–1995

Covariates	Model 1	Model 2	Model 3	Model 4	Model 5	Model 6	Model 7	Model 8
Socioeconomic status								
Education								
0–8 years	1.94*			1.53*	1.69*		1.44*	1.44*
9–11 years	1.85*			1.49*	1.61*		1.39*	1.39*
High school graduate	1.60*			1.37*	1.44*		1.30*	1.30*
13–15 years	1.41*			1.28*	1.30*		1.22*	1.22*
16 years	1.25*			1.21+	1.19		1.16	1.16
17 years or more	ref			ref	ref		ref	ref
Income equivalence (U.S. dollars)								
Less than 5,000		2.01*		1.69*		1.66*	1.44*	1.04
5,000 to less than 10,000		1.84*		1.57*		1.58*	1.37*	1.07
10,000 to less than 15,000		1.78*		1.57*		1.54*	1.39*	1.14
15,000 to less than 20,000		1.54*		1.37*		1.36*	1.24*	1.09
20,000 to less than 25,000		1.41*		1.27*		1.29*	1.19+	1.06
25,000 to less than 30,000		1.13		1.05		1.07	1.01	0.91
30,000 to less than 35,000		1.09		1.05		1.05	1.01	0.94

(*continues*)

TABLE 7.2 (continued)

Covariates	Model 1	Model 2	Model 3	Model 4	Model 5	Model 6	Model 7	Model 8
35,000 to less than 40,000		1.07		1.03		1.05	1.03	0.99
40,000 or more		ref		ref		ref	ref	ref
Employment status								
Employed			ref		ref	ref	ref	ref
Unemployed			1.07		1.02	0.96	0.96	0.88
Not in labor force			2.06*		1.94*	1.86*	1.84*	1.48*
Sociodemographic status								
Age (single years)	1.08*	1.08*	1.07*	1.08*	1.07*	1.07*	1.07*	1.07*
Sex (1 = male)	1.74*	1.78*	1.85*	1.77*	1.85*	1.87*	1.86*	1.80*
Race (1 = black)	1.19*	1.14*	1.23*	1.12*	1.17*	1.14*	1.13*	1.04
Marital status								
Currently married	ref	ref	ref	ref	ref	ref	ref	ref
Previously married	1.25*	1.20*	1.29*	1.20*	1.26*	1.23*	1.23*	1.27
Never married	1.66*	1.52*	1.59*	1.55*	1.58*	1.49*	1.51*	1.61*
Health status								
Health status								1.53*
-2*Log-likelihood	32,944	32,902	32,832	32,876	32,775	32,757	32,738	31,985

Sources: Derived from NCHS 1993d and 1997b.

$+ p \leq .10$; $* p \leq .05$.

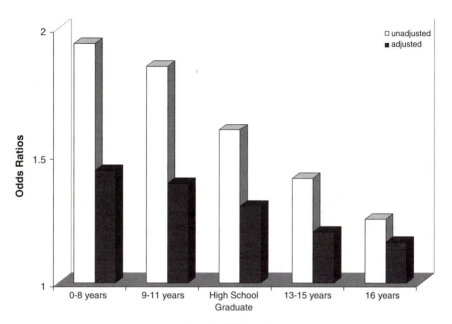

Level of Education

FIGURE 7.1   Odds ratios of dying by level of education, U.S. adults, 1991–1995. Note: Referent is 17 years or more of education.

status, income equivalence, and employment status. The introduction of perceived health status in the final model, Model 6, does not alter the education effect on mortality (see Figure 7.1). These results suggest that the effect of education on mortality is strong and persists even with the introduction of other controls. Furthermore, these results remain even with controls for health status (Model 8)

The effect of education on mortality for adults aged 18 to 64 is much stronger than for individuals aged 18 and over. Table 7.3 shows that compared to those with 17 or more years of education, those with less than a high school degree are about 80% more likely to die, even controlling for income, employment status, age, sex, race, and marital status. Controlling for health status dampens but does not eliminate the effect of education on mortality (Model 8).

THE EFFECTS OF INCOME ON MORTALITY

Table 7.2 also shows that income is strongly related to mortality for ages 18 and above. Indeed, Model 2 shows a strong mortality gradient. Income is predicated in part on education; the level of education forms the basis for job entry and also job advancement. Thus, controlling for education in

TABLE 7.3   Odds Ratios Showing the Effect of Socioeconomic Status on Mortality, U.S. Adults Ages 18 to 64, 1991–1995

Covariates	Model 1	Model 2	Model 3	Model 4	Model 5	Model 6	Model 7	Model 8
Socioeconomic status								
Education								
0–8 years	3.42*			2.03*	2.48*		1.78*	1.25
9–11 years	3.05*			2.00*	2.37*		1.80*	1.38+
High school graduate	2.13*			1.61*	1.86*		1.52*	1.30
13–15 years	1.97*			1.66*	1.80*		1.59*	1.42*
16 years	1.46*			1.38+	1.38+		1.33	1.29
17 years or more	ref			ref	ref		ref	ref
Income equivalence (U.S. dollars)								
Less than 5,000		3.72*		2.88*		2.41*	1.99*	1.28*
5,000 to less than 10,000		3.50*		2.74*		2.53*	2.11*	1.45*
10,000 to less than 15,000		2.74*		2.26*		2.23*	1.99*	1.47*
15,000 to less than 20,000		2.24*		1.89*		1.99*	1.74*	1.46*
20,000 to less than 25,000		2.06*		1.77*		1.91*	1.69*	1.43
25,000 to less than 30,000		1.54		1.36+		1.45*	1.31	1.16
30,000 to less than 35,000		1.26		1.18		1.22	1.16	1.06

35,000 to less than 40,000		1.34		1.28		1.32	1.27	1.21
40,000 or more		ref		ref		ref	ref	ref
Employment status								
Employed			ref		ref	ref	ref	ref
Unemployed			0.93		0.87	0.79	0.79	0.74
Not in labor force			2.68*		2.41*	2.22*	2.17*	1.62*
Sociodemographic status								
Age (single years)	1.09*	1.09*	1.08*	1.09*	1.08*	1.08*	1.08*	1.07*
Sex (1 = male)	1.72*	1.79*	2.04*	1.79*	2.03*	2.02*	2.02*	1.92*
Race (1 = black)	1.40*	1.25*	1.45*	1.23*	1.34*	1.26*	1.24*	1.18*
Marital status								
Currently married	ref	ref	ref	ref	ref	ref	ref	ref
Previously married	1.53*	1.32*	1.55*	1.33*	1.49*	1.36*	1.37*	1.32*
Never married	2.48*	2.14*	2.17*	2.18*	2.17*	2.01*	2.04*	2.08*
Health status								
Health status								1.64*
−2*Log-likelihood	11,841.4	11,793.4	11,740.0	11,771.7	11,696.36	11,675.8	11,661.3	11,404.2

Sources: Derived from NCHS 1993d and 1997b.

$+ p \leq .10$; $*p \leq .05$.

Model 4 reduces, though it does not eradicate, the effect of income. Income is also based on employment (see Model 6). Controlling for employment status and education in Model 7 further reduces the impact of income on mortality, but the effect remains strong and significant. For example, compared to those with an income equivalence of $40,000 or more, those with $20,000 to $25,000 are almost 20% more likely to die, and those with $15,000 or less income equivalence are about 40% more likely to die. Controlling for education, employment, and health status in Model 6 removes the statistical effect of income and mortality. Thus, income and health status are interrelated; once both are included in the model, the effect of income disappears for ages 18 and above.

But, again, the effect of income on mortality is stronger for individuals aged 18 to 64 (see Table 7.3). For instance, compared to those with an income equivalence of $40,000 or more, those earning less than $15,000 income equivalence are twice as likely to die, controlling for education, employment status, age, sex, race, and marital status (see Model 7). Controlling for health status in Model 8 dampens but does not remove the income gap in mortality for working age adults.

THE EFFECTS OF EMPLOYMENT STATUS ON MORTALITY

There are strong differences between those in and out of the labor force. Compared to adults aged 18 and over who are employed, those who are not in the labor force are more likely to die. Controlling for income and education (Model 7) reduces but does not eradicate the significant mortality difference between the employed and those not in the labor force: compared to adults aged 18 and over who are employed, those who are not in the labor force are 84% more likely to die.

The low mortality of the unemployed is puzzling. Common sense suggests that the unemployed suffer higher mortality than the employed because they lack the income to support themselves, but the results show little variation between those who are employed and unemployed. More detail about the unemployment status is needed to fully understand this relation, such as is offered in Chapter 8.

Model 8 reveals that health status dramatically attenuates the employment status gap, especially between those who are employed and those who are not in the labor force. This suggests that those who are not in the labor force may not have a choice about working; poor health may force them out of the labor force. From this model, we can see that health status strongly affects the relations between employment status and mortality. Similar but more pronounced relations are obtained for the working age population (ages 18–64).

THE EFFECTS OF SOCIOECONOMIC STATUS ON
CAUSE-SPECIFIC MORTALITY

Tables 7.4 (ages 18 and above) and 7.5 (ages 18 to 64) show the effects of education, income equivalence, and employment status on selected causes of death. Although respiratory diseases are included as a cause of death for individuals aged 18 and over, because of few cases, these deaths are combined with other causes for ages 18 to 64. Since previous tables showed a strong relation between socioeconomic status, health status, and mortality, each cause presents two models: one with and one without health status controlled. Different socioeconomic measures differentially affect causes of death. There is a strong mortality gradient between education and circulatory diseases and cancer, the top two causes of death. Indeed, compared to adults aged 18 and over with 17 years or more of schooling, those with less than 9 years of education are over 40% more likely to die from circulatory diseases (heart disease and stroke), and 70% more likely to die from cancer (Table 7.4, Model 1); compared to adults aged 18 to 64 with 17 years or more of schooling, those with less than 9 years of education are twice as likely to die from circulatory diseases, and over 70% more likely to die from cancer (Table 7.5, Model 1).

The effect of income is strongest for circulatory diseases and social pathologies, although there is not a clear income gradient with social pathologies. Compared to adults aged 18 and over earning $40,000 or more, those making less than $5,000 income are 55% more likely to die from circulatory diseases. Further, compared to adults aged 18 to 64 earning $40,000 or more income equivalence, those making less than $10,000 are three to four times more likely to die from social pathologies (Table 7.5).

Adults aged 18 and over who are not in the labor force experience high mortality due to all causes examined, but particularly high mortality from respiratory diseases. Compared to employed individuals, those aged 18 and over who are not in the labor force are two-and-one-half times more likely to die from respiratory diseases.

CONCLUSION

Education, income, and employment status all influence mortality in interrelated ways—controlling for any two measures dampens the effect of the other measure on mortality. In fact, controlling for education, employment status, and health status eradicates a separate effect of income on mortality. Such a finding suggests that income operates along with employment, education, and health status to influence mortality. But education and employment status retain separate independent effects on mortality, even with a variety of controls.

TABLE 7.4 Odds Ratios Showing the Effect of Socioeconomic Status on Mortality by Cause of Death, U.S. Adults, 1991–1995

	Circulatory		Cancer		Respiratory		Social Pathology		Residual	
Covariates	Mod 1	Mod 2	Mod 1	Mod 2	Mod 1	Mod 2	Mod 1	Mod 2	Mod 1	Mod 2
Socioeconomic status										
Education										
0–8 years	1.43*	1.19	1.70*	1.40+	1.14	0.90	0.83	0.79	1.29	1.01
9–11 years	1.37*	1.24	1.78*	1.57*	1.00	0.89	1.21	1.16	1.11	0.95
High school graduate	1.35*	1.30+	1.50*	1.41*	0.92	0.90	0.92	0.90	1.21	1.13
13–15 years	1.09	1.07	1.38+	1.34	0.94	0.94	0.92	0.91	1.45	1.42
16 years	1.23	1.27	1.13	1.15	0.69	0.73	0.63	0.63	1.651	1.70*
17 years or more	ref	ref	ref	ref	ref	ref	ref	ref	ref	
Income equivalance (U.S. dollars)										
Less than 5,000	1.55*	1.10	0.85	0.64*	1.27	0.77	2.69*	2.54+	2.03*	1.33
5,000 to less than 10,000	1.35*	1.04	0.96	0.78	1.53	1.03	3.14*	2.99*	1.76*	1.25
10,000 to less than 15,000	1.36*	1.10	1.06	0.90	1.51	1.11	2.76*	2.76*	1.75*	1.34
15,000 to less than 20,000	1.32+	1.13	0.98	0.88	0.92	0.72	3.27*	3.20*	1.33	1.10
20,000 to less than 25,000	1.23	1.08	0.92	0.84	1.48	1.23	2.66+	2.61*	1.12	0.97
25,000 to less than 30,000	1.07	0.95	0.82	0.75	1.02	0.85	2.72+	2.68+	0.88	0.77

30,000 to less than 35,000	0.92	0.85	1.06	1.00	1.00	0.88	1.69	1.68	0.99	0.91
35,000 to less than 40,000	0.96	0.92	1.15	1.12	1.00	0.96	2.03	2.02	0.68	0.65
40,000 or more	ref	ref	ref	ref	ref	ref	ref	ref	ref	ref
Employment status										
Employed	ref	ref	ref	ref	ref	ref	ref	ref	ref	ref
Unemployed	0.88	0.79	0.75	0.70	1.46	1.24	0.69	0.68	1.58	1.44
Not in labor force	1.55*	1.25*	1.54*	1.30	2.46*	1.79	1.54*	1.49*	2.81*	2.14*
Health status										
Health status		1.56*		1.44*		1.83*		1.10		1.71*
Sociodemographic status										
Age	1.10*	1.10*	1.07*	1.07*	1.10*	1.10*	1.02*	1.02*	1.05*	1.05*
Sex (1 = male)	1.83*	1.78*	1.68*	1.64*	2.44	2.33*	2.86*	2.85*	1.62*	1.54*
Race (1 = black)	1.16+	1.06	1.06	0.99	0.80	0.71+	0.96	0.95	1.46*	1.30*
Marital status										
Currently married	ref	ref	ref	ref	ref	ref	ref	ref	ref	ref
Previously married	1.20*	1.25*	1.02	1.05	1.02	1.09	1.69*	1.70*	1.42*	1.46*
Never married	1.27*	1.35*	1.03	1.08	1.36	1.48	2.74*	2.77*	1.90*	2.09*
−2*Log-likelihood	10,732	16,678	13,119	12,962	4,308	4,176	3,238	3,236	7,941	7,751

Sources: Derived from NCHS 1993d and 1997b.

+ $p \leq .10$; * $p \leq .05$.

135

TABLE 7.5 Odds Ratios Showing the Effects of Socioeconomic Status on Mortality by Cause of Death, U.S. Adults Ages 18 to 64, 1991–1995

	Circulatory		Cancer		Social Pathology		Residual	
Covariates	Mod 1	Mod 2	Mod 1	Mod 2	Mod 1	Mod 2	Mod 1	Mod 2
Socioeconomic status								
Education								
0–8 years	2.18*	1.49	1.73*	1.16	0.77	0.71	1.61	1.05
9–11 years	2.37*	1.79+	1.60	1.17*	1.37	1.28	1.11	0.82
High school graduate	1.97*	1.66	1.42	1.19*	1.00	0.96	1.15	0.96
13–15 years	1.52	1.33	1.61	1.41	0.97	0.94	1.55	1.38
16 years	1.60	1.55	0.90	0.88	0.59	0.58	2.16+	2.11+
17 years or more	ref	ref	ref	ref	ref	ref	ref	ref
Income equivalance (U.S. dollars)								
Less than 5,000	1.78	1.09	1.48	0.88	3.43+	3.17+	4.03*	2.35+
5,000 to less than 10,000	2.03*	1.38	1.34	0.88	4.91+	4.55*	4.17*	2.60*
10,000 to less than 15,000	1.89*	1.43	1.24	0.91	3.82*	3.63*	3.76*	2.64*
15,000 to less than 20,000	1.94*	1.63	1.12	0.92	3.14+	3.04+	2.68*	2.11
20,000 to less than 25,000	1.65+	1.38	1.34	1.12	3.71*	3.58*	2.51*	2.00
25,000 to less than 30,000	1.27	1.13	1.18	1.03	2.67	2.6	1.57	1.32

30,000 to less than 35,000	0.92	0.85	1.35	1.22	2.10	2.07	0.95	0.85
35,000 to less than 40,000	1.20	1.15	1.31	1.24	2.04	2.01	0.83	0.78
40,000 or more	ref	ref	ref	ref	ref	ref	ref	ref
Employment status								
Employed	ref	ref	ref	ref	ref	ref	ref	ref
Unemployed	0.63	0.59	0.69	0.66	0.64	0.62	1.13+	1.02
Not in labor force	1.91*	1.38*	1.99*	1.49	1.50+	1.42	2.62*	1.81*
Health status								
Health status	1.68*	1.68*		1.70*		1.13		1.86*
Sociodemographic status								
Age (single years)	1.11*	1.10*	1.11*	1.10*	1.21*	1.02*	1.07*	1.05*
Sex (1 = male)	2.59*	2.45*	1.45*	1.36*	2.86*	2.86*	1.79*	1.68*
Race (1 = black)	1.45	1.39*	0.89	0.84	1.17	1.16	1.69*	1.59*
Marital status								
Currently married	ref	ref	ref	ref	ref	ref	ref	ref
Previously married	1.40*	1.36*	1.05	1.02	1.67+	1.65+	1.84*	1.73*
Never married	1.67*	1.72*	1.37	1.4	2.82*	2.80*	2.55*	2.62*
−2*Log-likelihood	4,309.06	4,223.59	4,702.64	4,606.88	2,243.32	2,241.46	3,231.28	3,214.08

Sources: Derived from NCHS 1993d and 1997b.

+ $p \leq .10$; *$p \leq .05$.

137

Other results in this book and in other articles suggest that the effect of education is eradicated with controls for income and employment status. Thus, rather than asserting that one socioeconomic measure is superior to another in all analyses, we posit that socioeconomic measures are interrelated, are each important in mortality analyses, and that each can make separate, unique contributions. Education and income are important baseline variables and influence other health behaviors and social relations. For this reason, we include variants of both these measures in all subsequent analyses. Analyses that omit controls for education and income may be underspecified and thus overlook important relations.

Employment status is another important socioeconomic indicator of mortality. Employed individuals enjoy longer lives than those who are not employed. Although employment status is important, so too is occupational status. Occupational status is so central to mortality analysis that we devote the next chapter, Chapter 8, to its study. Another important socioeconomic factor is health insurance, which is featured in Chapter 9.

We found that different socioeconomic status measures contribute to different causes of death. This finding may be a statistical artifact—because the variables are interrelated, one variable raises the importance for one cause and another variable surfaces for a different cause—or the result may be accurate. If accurate, the results are rich with implications. First, this result helps explain that the measures operate differently to influence overall mortality: different socioeconomic status measures contribute to different reductions in specific causes of death, which then reduce overall mortality. Different mechanisms may be at work to reduce mortality. It seems reasonable that higher incomes would reduce circulatory diseases through reduced financial stress, which would reduce hypertension, but would have less impact on cancer: individuals cannot buy immunity from cancer. On the other hand, education can reduce the risk of cancer through increased knowledge about health practices that will reduce the risk of cancer, information about ways to screen for cancer, and insight into how to detect, diagnose, and treat cancer early. Individuals who are not in the labor force are more likely to die from respiratory diseases, possibly the very diseases that prevent them from working.

This analysis for socioeconomic status and mortality is based on all adults aged 18 and above and those aged 18 to 64. The effects of socioeconomic status on mortality are greater for younger (under 65) than older (65 and above) adults (see also Kitagawa and Hauser 1973). Indeed, compared to adults 18–64 with 17 years or more of schooling, comparable adults with less than a high school education are 80% more likely to die, even controlling for income, employment, age, sex, race, and marital status (see also Pappas et al. 1993). Similarly, compared to adults aged 18–64 with $40,000 or more family income equivalences, those earning less than $15,000 are twice as likely to die, net of education, employment, age, sex, race, and marital status. And, compared to employed adults aged 18–64, similar adults who are not in the labor force are also twice as likely to die, even net of education, income, age, sex, race, and marital status. Thus, socioeconomic status measures are central factors, and influence mortality both singly and jointly.

Basic socioeconomic factors—income, education, and employment status—are important predictors of mortality. But the importance of these results can be modified, as we will see throughout the book, through other important variables. For example, socioeconomic status affects functional limitations, perceived health status, mental health, and health behaviors (smoking, drinking, exercise), all of which have a bearing on survival prospects. In this chapter and throughout the book, we endeavor to paint a more complete picture of the full aspects of factors that impinge on the risk of death.

8

THE EFFECT OF
OCCUPATIONAL STATUS
ON MORTALITY

Apart from roles associated with the family, the worker role is arguably the most important social and economic role held by most adults (Hauser 1994). Jobs define how we spend much of our time. As we discussed in Chapter 7, people's educational level in part determines their occupation, which in turn affects their income. Because jobs require particular levels of technical and social skills and experience, they measure more than merely educational attainment (Blau and Duncan 1967). In addition to income, jobs provide social, psychological, and health benefits. In fact, in examining life expectancy differences between people with high and low levels of employment status, income, and education, Rogot, Sorlie, and Johnson (1992) found that the largest differences were those between employment categories. This chapter determines how occupation and employment status affects mortality for those currently working, those who have quit working, and those who have never worked.

Education and occupational status are interrelated: many managerial jobs require at least a bachelor's degree. Furthermore, most professional positions—accountants, doctors, dentists, lawyers, engineers—demand advanced degrees. Income and occupational status are also interrelated: high-status positions command high salaries. Thus, occupational positions can reduce mortality through providing the financial resources to buffer against the risk of death. Aside from income, occupations provide other forms of health-enhancing benefits. Many companies provide health insurance. Companies can further encourage good health through company-supported exercise programs, gyms, and exercise equipment.

Compared to high-status positions, low-status occupations tend to require less education, and to be plagued by lower income, lack of health in-surance, few company-supported health programs, less social interaction, more physically arduous labor, increased exposure to hazardous sub-stances, and emotionally draining working conditions (Demers et al. 1990; House et al. 1986; Loscocco and Spitze 1990; Marmot and Theorell 1988). Contact with poisons, dust, asbestos, smoke, acid, infectious agents, and explosives can cause illness, and, in more serious cases, death. High levels of routinized, monotonous work leads to boredom. Difficult working con-ditions with lack of personal control leads to stress and strain. Thus, it is important to fully illuminate the relations between occupational status and mortality.

Generally, the higher the occupational status, the lower the mortality. This relation persists even with controls for income and education, and applies to men and women, and both to the general working population and to working subpopulations, including the army (Liberatos, Link, and Kelsey 1988; Mare 1990; Marmot et al. 1984; Moore and Hayward 1990; Nam and Wu 1994; Preston and Taubman 1994). In fact, the army has a strong mortality gradient, from privates, to noncommissioned officers, to officers (Seltzer and Jablon 1977; Wilkinson 1986). Most mortality research shows that professionals and managers experience lower mortality than laborers, service workers, and private household workers (see Mare 1990; Moore and Hayward 1990).

Much of the literature asserts that compared to lower statuses, individu-als in higher occupational statuses engage in more healthful behaviors, and thus it is healthy practices rather than occupational status per se that is the driving force in mortality. Good health among the upper statuses may be fostered by effective coping strategies, personal control, and positive health behaviors (see Berkman and Breslow 1983). In fact, compared to clerical workers, professionals and executives are less likely to smoke and are more physically active in their leisure time (Marmot et al. 1984). If it is true that individuals who are in low-status jobs who have poor health experience higher mortality due to their poor health rather than their low occupational status, then controlling for health should eradicate mortality differences in occupational status.

There are difficulties in using occupation as the only index of socioeco-nomic status: occupations are not recorded for individuals who have never worked or who are not currently working. For example, in 1994, out of a total of 197 million individuals aged 16 and above, 123 million, or 63%, were employed. Those 74 million individuals who were not employed included students, homemakers, unemployed individuals seeking work, retirees, those with independent incomes, and those who were too disabled to work (U.S. Bureau of Labor Statistics 1995).

Sorlie and Rogot (1990) calculated standardized mortality ratios for em-ployed and unemployed individuals, controlling for family income and educational level. They found that the lowest mortality rates were for those who were employed, followed in order by those who were unemployed, retired, and unable to work. In fact, those who were unable to work exhibited over twice the average risk of death. Many of those who were unable to work may have been limited due to health problems (Wilkinson 1986). They also examined cause of death by employment characteristics. Generally, those who were employed exhibited low mortality from most causes, those who were unemployed had higher mortality from causes other than cancer or cardiovascular disease, and those who were retired or unable to work had higher mortality risks for most causes. This coincides with Marmot et al. (1987), who suggest that sick people are selected out of occupations and enter into nonworking statuses, and demonstrates that overlooking those not in the labor force not only excludes in excess of one-third of the population, but also excludes those with exceptionally high mortality rates.

HEALTHY WORKER EFFECT

The mortality gap between those who are working and those who are not is termed the healthy worker effect (Monson 1986; Sorlie and Rogot 1990): those who work are usually healthier than those not in the labor force. While workers may be hired because they are healthy, some individuals may be forced to leave the labor force because of health-related problems. There is continuing debate over whether jobs cause ill health and therefore job exits and higher mortality, or whether ill health creates greater risk of job exit and mortality (see Sorlie and Rogot 1990). Thus, it is important to assess whether those who cannot work for health reasons contracted ill health on or off the job.

OCCUPATIONAL STATUS AND
CAUSE OF DEATH

Occupational status is related to cause of death (see Preston and Taubman 1994). Although industries are subject to occupational regulations and therefore should maintain safe working environments for their employees, individuals who work in lower rather than higher status occupations are often exposed to greater risk of death from a number of causes. Rosenberg et al. (1993) examined cause of death for 46 selected occupations. Compared to all occupations, "architects, engineers, and scientists" (individuals working in high-status jobs), exhibited lower mortality risks due to infectious diseases, respiratory diseases, and social pathologies; average mortality due to heart disease; but higher rates due to cancer. On the other hand, construction laborers, or individuals working in lower status jobs, enjoyed lower mortality due to heart disease; average mortality due to most cancers, but higher mortality due to infectious diseases, respiratory diseases, and social pathologies. Although compared to all occupations, construction laborers are just 19% more likely to die from accidents overall, they are almost 50% more likely to die from industrial accidents (for similar results, see Lawson and Black 1993). These figures confirm the claim that lower status workers—because they are more likely to be exposed to hazardous materials and dangerous working environments—are more likely to die from respiratory diseases, infectious diseases, and external causes of death (Lawson and Black 1993; Marmot et al. 1987; Seltzer and Jablon 1977).

OCCUPATIONAL STATUS INDICES

Studies have used a number of methods to measure the impact of occupation. Researchers have examined selected occupations—comparing, say, architects to teachers to machine operators to laborers (see Rosenberg et al. 1993); types of work—professional, craft, skilled, and unskilled (see Pavalko et al. 1993; Smith and Waitzman 1994b); or classes of worker-employer relationships—private employment; federal, state, or local government employment; employment in incorporated businesses; or self-employment (Liberatos et al. 1988). Such classifications, however, do not take into account the crosscutting among categories. For instance, private workers range from unskilled cleaning and building service workers to executives, and skilled workers include advertising agents as well as butchers. To remedy these problems, social researchers have devised a number of unidimensional scales by converting the detailed three-digit occupational codes into status scores.

Two widely known and frequently used scales include Nam and Powers's (1983) Occupational SES Scores (OSS), and Duncan's (1961) Socioeconomic Index for All Occupations (SEI). Both of these scores have been updated over time to account for new occupations and/or new censuses. Duncan used the Census and NORC to combine measures of income, education, and prestige to rank occupations by socioeconomic-prestige scores. Thus, a person's SEI would show the percentage of respondents who would rank the occupation as having a favorable social standing.

The Nam-Powers' occupational status metric is a valuable measure of socioeconomic status that uses education requirements and income rewards to objectively determine status (Haug 1977). It averages information on median education and income distributions for individuals in each occupation to calculate socioeconomic status scores (for more information on the exact methods of calculation, see Nam 1996). It shows the percentage of persons in an occupation having combined average levels of income and education lower than the given occupation.

Because Duncan incorporated prestige rankings in his scores, and because prestige is more highly associated with education than with income, several occupations with relatively high education (and relatively high prestige) but low income, like teachers and sales workers, rank high on his scale. Such interplay between education and prestige leads to a more skewed distribution (Nam 1996). In contrast, the Nam-Powers measure of occupational status is based on objective referents from census data that are continuously updated, rather than on special surveys or public perception studies. Because the Nam-Powers index measures socioeconomic status rather than social desirability or prestige, provides a hierarchical ranking of occupations, is based on objective referents, is normally distributed, ascertains the ability for occupations to provide resources for individual incumbents, importantly differentiates by sex in a more consistent manner than the SEI, and has been refined over four decades, we use the Nam-Powers index for our analysis. Its power is partly demonstrated in the number of times it has been applied and in the findings it has generated (for examples, see Mutchler and Poston 1983; Stafford and Fossett 1991).

CENTRAL AIMS

This chapter is guided by two central aims. First, we test for an *occupational status score gradient*. We expect that increasing occupational scores reduces the risk of death. The occupational status score gradient will be most pronounced when examined in isolation, that is, without controls for other socioeconomic and health measures. Once income and education are introduced, the occupational status score gradient will persist, but will be attenuated, since all three socioeconomic measures are interrelated. Moreover, once health status is introduced, the mortality gap will close further. Cause-specific mortality results should show that, because lower status workers are more likely than higher status workers to be exposed to hazardous materials and conditions, those individuals who worked in low-status occupations and those who quit for job-related health reasons, will exhibit higher mortality due to some degenerative causes of death, notably respiratory diseases, infectious diseases, and social pathologies.

Second, we test for the *healthy worker effect:* those in the labor force should experience lower mortality than those out of the labor force. Most studies have focused either on those in the labor force or on those out of the labor force. Because poor health prevents some individuals from ever entering and encourages others to leave the labor force, we expect that those who are not in the labor force will generally experience higher mortality risks than those in the labor force. But by controlling for health status, we should be able to further close the mortality gap between workers and nonworkers.

DATA AND METHODS

To determine the relative importance of occupational status to mortality, we employ the 1988 National Health Interview Survey Occupational Health Supplement (NHIS-OHS), with detail on the work experience, work environment, and work-related injuries for 44,233 males and females aged 18 and above (NCHS 1993b), linked with information on 3,504 deaths (NCHS 1997b). We dropped 894 (2% of the sample) ineligible cases from subsequent analyses.

OCCUPATIONAL STATUS CODES

Almost all people know and are willing to report their occupations (Hauser 1994). Our first interest here is not in measuring the occupational risk per se but rather in measuring the socioeconomic status aspects of occupation. Accordingly, we recoded the detailed three-digit occupational codes for those males and females who reported their current job worked into the 1980 version of the Nam-Powers OSS (Nam and Powers 1983; Terrie and Nam 1994). These occupational status scores, which range from 0 to 100, are obtained by averaging the rankings of occupations arrayed by median education and income levels (for more information about the scoring algorithm, see Nam 1996). Each score reflects the status of the average person within that occupation (Terrie and Nam 1994).

We coded four occupational status groups: high (75–100), the referent, medium high (50–74), medium low (25–49), and low (0–24) for both current and longest job worked (for similar methods, see Nam and Wu 1994). Thus, each group is compared to the highest occupational status. Such categories are clear, are large enough for comparisons, are parsimonious, and can be compared with nonworking statuses.

We explored several occupational status score groupings. Occupational status scores can be measured as a continuous variable, ranging from 1 to 100, but such a variable produces small odds ratios, since it assesses the effect of a 1 out of 100-unit increase in occupational status scores on mortality. This variable can also be categorized on a 10-, 20-, 25-, or 33-point continuous scale. We tested each of these categories and found that the 25-point scale fit best: it provides a smooth gradient, relatively large differences between categories, large numbers of cases in each category, and robust estimates. But a continuous variable is more difficult to link and compare to nonworking statuses. The continuous occupational status score variable can be linked to dummy nonworking categories through interaction terms. Then, those not working would be compared to the average worker (the average occupational status score). But comparing workers with average (around 50) instead of high (75 and above) occupational status scores, artificially depresses the odds ratios and is more likely to lead to a conclusion of no statistically significant differences between workers and nonworkers, even when differences exist. Such a comparison is less direct than comparing all occupational categories. Thus, we rely on categories for those working and those not working to facilitate more direct, parsimonious comparisons, to enable comparisons between extremes instead of averages, and to uncover any statistically significant differences, should they exist.

Researchers have demonstrated that mortality can be high not only for those in the lowest occupational strata, but also for those who do not work (see Nam and Wu 1994; K. Smith and Waitzman 1994b). Although previous studies have separately examined "housewives," or "homemakers," these classifications are less prevalent today. Instead, we classify people as those who have never worked, or those who have stopped working. The latter group is subdivided by reasons for quitting: job-related health problems, nonjob-related health problems, retirement, lay-off, family reasons, or other reasons. Thus, we are able to compare mortality rates for all of those in and out of the labor force, whether never employed, currently employed, or previously employed. Moreover, we can separately assess whether the reason for not working is health-related, and whether health problems are work- or nonwork-related.

We recognize that quitting for job health and nonjob health reasons are self-reported and therefore subject to respondent recall and social desirability biases. Social desirability bias refers to the tendency to provide answers that others want to hear, even if they are incorrect (see Alreck and Settle 1985). Thus, individuals may respond that they quit for nonjob health reasons when in fact they were fired. Respondent recall may be inaccurate or the respondent's answers may be misleading if there were multiple steps toward final nonwork status. For instance, some individuals with work-related disability may first move to a less demanding job within the company, then to part-time work, then temporary work, until finally they quit work through retirement or through disability (see for example, Hayward et al. 1989).

We control for four sociodemographic variables: age, sex, race, and marital status. Age is a continuous variable, measured in individual years. Race compares blacks to all other respondents. Small cell sizes preclude further race and ethnic disaggregation. Marital status is coded into never, previously, and currently married, with the latter category selected as the referent.

We also control for health status, which may be especially important in occupational status research. Individuals may base their occupational status in part on their health status. For example, individuals may not currently work because of poor health. And health status may mediate the effects of occupational status on mortality: individuals in low status jobs who have poor health may experience higher mortality due to the poor health rather than the low occupational status.

Because occupational status is linked to education and income, it is important to examine occupational status net of these other socioeconomic factors (Rosenberg et al. 1993). We coded education into four categories— 0 to 8 years, 9 to 11 years, 12 years, and 13 or more years. As in Chapter 7, we examine income equivalence, based on family income and family size. This income equivalence could prove especially useful for examining occupational differences in mortality because of the potential variations in occupational status, income, and family size. In our cause-specific analyses, 1,564 individuals died of circulatory diseases, 892 from cancer, 330 from respiratory diseases, 150 from social pathologies, 107 from infectious diseases, 87 from diabetes, and 374 from other causes.

RESULTS

Table 8.1 presents the distribution of occupational statuses for those who survived the period from 1988 through 1995 and those who died during the period. Occupational statuses for those currently working are generally well distributed, but with few people working in the lowest strata. Over 20% of the population was engaged in occupations defined as in the second lowest occupational status. Fewer than 2% of the sample quit work because of job health problems, a relatively high percentage of individuals quit work for family reasons, at 7%, and fewer than 4% of the sample has never worked. Among those not currently employed, a large proportion is retired. Comparing the two columns shows that mortality is higher for those who quit for job health reasons, quit for nonjob health reasons, retired, quit for family reasons, and never worked. Although this table demonstrates that several variables are related to mortality, it does not simultaneously adjust for age (hence, the disproportionately high mortality for retired individuals) or for other covariates of mortality. For such analyses, we turn to Table 8.2.

TABLE 8.1 Percentage Distributions of Occupational Status for Survivors and Decedents Aged 18 and above in the United States, 1988–1995[a]

Occupational status	Alive (%)	Dead (%)
Currently working		
0–24 Nam-Powers score	9.5	3.9
25–49 Nam-Powers score	22.0	7.4
50–74 Nam-Powers score	14.9	4.4
75+ Nam-Powers score	17.9	4.4
Not currently employed because of		
Job health problems	1.6	4.0
Nonjob health problems	3.9	14.0
Retired	10.7	38.8
Lay-off	1.6	1.1
Family reasons	7.1	8.6
Other reasons	7.2	7.3
Never worked	3.7	6.2
Total	100.1	100.1

Source: Data derived from NCHS 1993b, 1997b.
[a] Columns may not sum to 100% due to rounding.

COMPARISONS AMONG THOSE CURRENTLY WORKING

Table 8.2 focuses on occupational status and reports the covariates' effects on mortality. Because education typically occurs prior to occupation, we include its effect on mortality in Model 1. The models then build by examining occupational status, adding measures of education, income, and health status, and ending with the full model of all covariates. Models 1 and 2 display significant mortality differences first between educational levels and then between occupational statuses.

For example, Model 2 reveals an occupational status gradient: compared to those in the highest occupational status, the reference category, those in the lowest occupational status, statuses 0–24, are 59% more likely to die (an odds ratio of 1.59), those in the second lowest category are 44% more likely to die, and those in the second highest category are 42% more likely to die (for similar results, see Nam and Wu 1994).

Mutchler and Poston (1983) demonstrated that females are overrepresented among those in the lower occupational statuses and among those who have never worked. Many females who have never worked are homemakers. And Ross and Mirowsky (1995) have demonstrated that compared to the average full-time worker, homemakers possess a greater health risk.

TABLE 8.2 Odds Ratios of Socioeconomic Status and Mortality, with a Focus on Occupational Status, Controlling for Other Covariates: U.S. Adults Aged 18 and above, 1988–1995

	Model 1	Model 2	Model 3	Model 4	Model 5	Model 6
Socioeconomic						
Occupation						
Currently working						
0–24 Nam-Powers score		1.59*	1.44*	1.33*	1.31*	1.25+
25–49 Nam-Powers score		1.44*	1.34*	1.27*	1.25*	1.21+
50–74 Nam-Powers score		1.42*	1.36*	1.32*	1.31*	1.26+
75–100 Nam-Powers score		ref	ref	ref	ref	ref
Not currently working because of						
Job health problems		3.25*	2.94*	2.65*	2.59*	1.69*
Nonjob health problems		4.65*	4.25*	3.79*	3.72*	2.40*
Retirement		2.23*	2.09*	1.90*	1.88*	1.68*
Lay-off		2.15*	1.94*	1.74*	1.70*	1.43
Family reasons		2.62*	2.43*	2.21*	2.17*	1.90*
Other reasons		2.47*	2.29*	2.06*	2.03*	1.78*
Never worked		3.00*	2.70*	2.48*	2.42*	1.98*

Education						
≤8 years	1.45*		1.20*		1.06	.94
9–11 years	1.51*		1.27*		1.15*	1.06
12 years	1.18*		1.07		1.01	.97
13 or more years	ref		ref		ref	ref
Income equivalence				.87*	.88*	.93*
Health						
Health status						1.39*
Demographic						
Age (continuous)	1.10*	1.09*	1.09*	1.09*	1.09*	1.08*
Sex (male = 1)	1.92*	2.14*	2.12*	2.15*	2.14*	2.15*
Race (black = 1)	1.14*	1.11+	1.07	1.04	1.03	.95
Marital status						
Currently married	ref	ref	ref	ref	ref	ref
Previously married	1.36*	1.38*	1.37*	1.32*	1.32*	1.36*
Never married	1.44*	1.37*	1.37*	1.30*	1.31*	1.36*
−2*Log-likelihood	29,012.0	28,711.4	28,691.2	28,667.4	28,660.8	28,290.0

Source: Data derived from NCHS 1993b, 1997b.

$+p \leq .10$; $*p \leq .05$.

151

Thus, the odds ratio for sex increases from 1.9 in Model 1 to 2.1 in Model 2 once the "at-risk" females are controlled by including job status.

Education is linked to mortality and to occupational status. As Chapter 7 and previous studies have demonstrated, more educated individuals enjoy lower mortality than less educated ones (see Comstock and Tonascia 1977; Elo and Preston 1996; and Feldman et al. 1989). Because education is related to occupational status, once it is included in the model, the relations between occupational status and mortality diminish. Indeed, the 60% gap between the two occupational status extremes closes to 44% once we discount education (Model 3). Similarly, the 45% gap between the two education extremes closes to 20% once we discount occupation. This suggests that part of the effect of occupation on mortality is due to education effects, but further, that net of education effects, occupational differences in mortality persist.

The relations between income and occupational status parallel the relations between education and occupational status, but with income demonstrating more profound effects on the relation between occupational status and mortality. For example, the 60% gap between the two occupational extremes closes to just a 33% difference once we adjust for income (Model 4). And the combined influences of education and income further attenuate that relationship. This again demonstrates the ties between the three socioeconomic status measures. (Note that controls for socioeconomic status remove the significance of the race gap in mortality, consistent with some previous research [see Rogers 1992]).

Controlling for health status, in Model 6, further reduces the gap in occupational statuses. Compared to those in the highest status, those in the lowest status experience a 25% greater risk of death, even with controls for education and income (Model 6).[1] Among those currently working in various occupations, education and especially income exhibit strong effects on their relation to mortality; the introduction of health status only modestly changes this relation. Thus, health status modestly mediates but does not eradicate the relation between occupational status and mortality.

Figure 8.1 graphically depicts the relations between occupational status and mortality when few other socioeconomic variables are included (the unadjusted odds ratios) and when other socioeconomic factors are included (the adjusted odds ratios). Once income, education, and health status are controlled, we see a difference between the highest occupational status and the lower three statuses, but lose the mortality gradient for the occupational statuses illustrated by the unadjusted rates (see also Model 2).

---

[1] To determine how occupational status and mortality were related by age group, we re-analyzed Model 6 for Table 8.2 and Table 8.3 for ages 18–44, 45–64, and 65 and above. The results generally parallel the relations found in the tables.

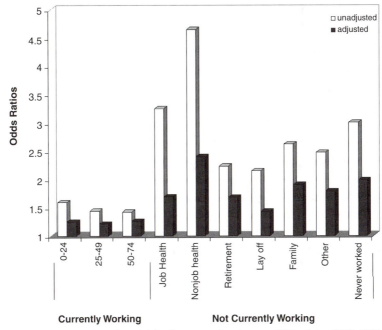

FIGURE 8.1   Odds ratios of dying by occupational status, U.S. adults, 1988–1995. Note: Referent is individuals with occupational status scores 75–100.

COMPARISONS AMONG THOSE
NOT CURRENTLY WORKING

Most studies have stopped at examining the effects of occupation on mortality for those in the labor force. But equally important is demonstrating mortality risks for those not in the labor force. Returning to Model 5, which examines socioeconomic effects, those who were never in the labor force and those who left the labor force experience at least 70% higher mortality risk than those who are currently in the labor force in the highest occupational status, and higher mortality than those who are in the lowest status jobs (for similar results, see Sorlie and Rogot 1990; Wilkinson 1986). These findings support the healthy worker effect.

Previous literature asserts that compared to individuals in higher status positions, those in lower status jobs often retire earlier and are more likely to leave a job because of health problems (Hayward et al. 1989). This suggests that such individuals will experience high mortality both because of their previous low status position and their current health problems. Our findings support this claim. Comparing Models 5 and 6 shows that the gaps between occupational statuses and mortality close substantially with the introduction of health status. Many individuals either leave their jobs because of health problems or are in statuses that are more likely to have health problems. For example, some individuals leave explicitly for job or nonjob-related health problems. Thus, controlling for health status reduces the effects of these categories. Compared to those in the highest occupational status, individuals who are not currently working because of job health problems are 2.6 times more likely to die in Model 5, but just 70% more likely to die in Model 6, where health status is controlled. Compared to those currently in the highest status jobs, those who left the labor force because of job-related health problems experience a 70% greater risk of death, and those who left the labor force because of nonjob-related health problems experience a 2.4-fold greater risk of death (for similar results, see Moser et al. 1987). Those who retired experience mortality intermediate to those still in the labor force, and others no longer in the labor force (see also Moore and Hayward 1990; Sorlie and Rogot 1990).

There persists a gap between the highest occupational status and those who have never worked. Thus, compared to those in the highest occupational strata, those who have never worked are 2.4 times more likely to die, even controlling for education and income. This gap, however, closes with the introduction of health status. This indicates that many individuals who have never worked possess poor health that prevents them from working, and that their poor health largely accounts for their higher mortality.

CAUSE-SPECIFIC MORTALITY

Table 8.3 shows which specific causes of death contribute to differences in mortality by occupational status. Those in the lower rather than higher socioeconomic status exhibit an almost fourfold mortality excess for social pathologies (for similar results, see Rosenberg et al. 1993). Lower occupational statuses also exhibit higher mortality for respiratory diseases. Those who have never worked have higher mortality from most all causes, but especially due to circulatory and respiratory diseases and social pathologies. Indeed, compared to those who are in high-status positions, those who have never worked are three-and-one-half times more likely to die from social pathologies. Compared to those who work in high-status occupations, those who are not currently working are more likely to die of degenerative diseases. For example, compared to those in high-status occupations, those who were not currently working because of nonjob-related health problems experience over two times the risk of death due to circulatory diseases, cancer, respiratory diseases, social pathologies, and residual causes of death.

CONCLUSION

This chapter sheds light on how occupational status contributes to mortality. High occupational status—which bestows respect, prestige, a choice place in the labor force, and access to social and political circles—can encourage healthy behavior and long life. Even after controlling for income and education, those currently in the lowest status jobs experience a 25% excess risk of death compared to those in the highest status jobs. But large mortality gaps also exist between those in the highest status jobs and those who have left the labor force for nonjob-related health reasons (an almost fourfold difference), and between those in the highest status jobs and those who quit for family, retirement, lay off, or other reasons, and those who never worked at all (about a twofold difference) (Table 8.2, Model 5).

Part of the mortality gap between individuals who are currently working and who quit work may be attributed to the healthy worker effect (see Monson 1986; Nam and Wu 1994; Sorlie and Rogot 1990). The healthy worker effect may emerge for four reasons. First, employers most likely prefer to hire and retain healthy individuals. Second, either sick workers may quit, or their employers may fire them or provide medical retirement for them. Thus, those not in the labor force include some individuals who did not fit into the working world because they were physically ill and/or emotionally troubled. Third, businesses may provide extrinsic health benefits: health insurance, company gyms, health screening, and alcohol and drug detoxification and rehabilitation programs. Fourth, work may provide intrinsic life-promoting benefits: a sense of worth, accomplishment, and camaraderie and community.

Individuals who are injured on the job may have access to resources that blunt the seriousness of injuries, including health insurance, and may qualify for medical disability benefits, worker's compensation, or medical retirement. Compared to individuals with job-related health problems, individuals who possess a nonjob-related health problem exhibit higher mortality risk and most likely have access to fewer health resources and benefits. Indeed, compared to current workers in the highest status jobs, those who are not currently working for nonjob-related health reasons are over two times as likely to die from degenerative diseases—diseases that are chronic and that often require expensive follow-up treatment and management.

Occupations provide more than a position within a company. They are also related to general styles of life. They help determine the neighborhoods where people live, the types of housing they live in, and the natural and built environment of their location. All of these factors are tied to health and survival.

Several studies have employed longitudinal data to examine the effects of career changes on mortality (see Mare 1990; Moore and Hayward 1990; Pavalko et al. 1993). While important, many of these studies are limited by sample size, region of the country, age, or sex. Moreover, many cannot examine detailed occupational statuses or nonworking statuses. This chapter examines a large nationally representative sample of men and women with a variety of working and nonworking occupational statuses using prospec-

TABLE 8.3 Odds Ratios of Socioeconomic Status and Cause-Specific Mortality, Controlling for Other Covariates: U.S. Adults Aged 18 and Above, 1988–1995

	Circulatory	Cancer	Respiratory	Social Pathology	Infectious	Diabetes	Residual
Socioeconomic							
Occupation							
Currently working							
0–24 Nam-Powers score	1.06	1.16	2.77	3.70*	.37+	1.29	.78
25–49 Nam-Powers score	1.01	1.31	1.56	2.27+	.51+	1.59	1.50
50–74 Nam-Powers score	1.05	1.21	4.25+	1.71	.62	2.02	2.20+
75–100 Nam-Powers score	ref	ref	ref	ref	ref	ref	ref
Not currently working because of							
Job health problems	1.81*	1.23	9.38*	.96	.47	1.53	1.50
Nonjob health problems	2.31*	2.04*	8.52*	3.83*	1.01	1.96	2.79*
Retirement	1.36+	1.36+	7.00*	3.87*	.58	1.43	3.67*
Lay-off	1.42*	1.03	7.87+	1.19	@	@	3.86*
Family reasons	1.67*	1.27	7.14+	3.20+	1.64	4.44*	2.15*
Other reasons	1.46*	1.52+	4.78*	2.45	1.13	1.05	2.95*

Never worked	2.48*	3.02	@	3.53+	8.60*	1.25	1.75*
Education							
≤8 years	.93	.41*	.71	1.35	.92	.95	.96
9–11 years	.83	.85	1.21	1.92*	1.36	1.01	1.02
12 years	.83	.68	.90	1.17	1.09	.98	1.02
13 or more years	ref	ref	ref	ref	ref	ref	ref
Income equivalence	.90	1.13	1.00	.79*	.97	.97	.93*
Health							
Health status	1.52*	2.16*	1.46	1.12	1.64*	1.32*	1.35*
Demographic							
Age (continuous)	1.08*	1.08*	1.03*	.99	1.11*	1.08*	1.11*
Sex (male = 1)	1.80*	1.34	4.37*	6.11*	2.47*	1.57+	2.13*
Race (black = 1)	1.06	2.48*	1.95*	.86	.48*	.95	.92
Marital status							
Currently married	ref	ref	ref	ref	ref	ref	ref
Previously married	1.81*	.85	3.41*	1.86*	1.22	1.11	1.23*
Never married	1.61+	.66	5.54*	1.08	.98	.77+	1.18

Source: Data derived from NCHS 1993b, 1997b.
[a] @ indicates fewer than two deaths.
+$p \le .10$; *$p \le .05$.

157

tive data. Thus, combining the findings from both sets of analyses—longitudinal and prospective—can further contribute to the literature on occupational status and mortality.

From a public policy point of view, it is important to examine the size of the groups affected as well as the relative mortality gaps. Small mortality differences for proportionately large groups may numerically affect the population as a whole as much as large mortality differences for proportionately small groups. For example, we revealed that, compared to individuals working in the highest status jobs, individuals working in the lowest status jobs experience a 70% greater risk of death, and individuals who have never worked experience a twofold greater risk of death (Table 8.2). But intervention programs that intend to reduce mortality should also be aware that there are three times as many people working in low status jobs, at 19 million, as there are people who have never worked, at 6 million (calculations not shown). Thus, policy decisions must be based on numerical representation as well as mortality risk.

The effect of occupation on mortality is mediated by health status. People who are employed in lower-status occupations often work more physically demanding jobs, with greater exposure to industrial hazards (Williams and Collins 1995). Moreover, individuals who work in the lower-status occupations may face increased stress in work and at home that may manifest itself through drinking, smoking, and risky behaviors, which in turn can increase their risk of circulatory diseases, cancers, and social pathologies (see, for instance, Lawson and Black 1993). Thus, future studies should examine the effects of other factors, including specific health behaviors, on occupational status and mortality. This chapter illuminates how occupational status affects people's chances of staying alive.

9

HEALTH INSURANCE
COVERAGE
AND MORTALITY

Although socioeconomic status differences in mortality have long persisted in the United States, in the past, the array of possible socioeconomic status variables used by researchers has been constrained, often to education and income. We expand this set to include health insurance, Medicare, and Medicaid. We also consider the extent to which the relations among health insurance variables and mortality vary across broad age groups.

This research on health insurance is significant for several reasons. First, the association between socioeconomic status and mortality is not fully understood because socioeconomic status is multidimensional; the inclusion of health insurance in models of mortality contributes to a fuller understanding of the total effects of socioeconomic status and mortality. Second, our research directly addresses one of the central recommendations raised in the 1995 National Institutes of Health conference, Measuring Social Inequalities in Health, namely, including health insurance as an additional dimension in the examination of socioeconomic status and mortality (Moss and Krieger 1995).

There is enormous national concern about the relatively high mortality among the uninsured, who may number from 30 to 40 million (Franks et al. 1993). Many individuals cannot afford health insurance because it is too expensive or because they lose their coverage through layoffs or poor health. Their high mortality may be due to their inability to get appropriate care because of lapses in insurance or gaps in coverage, or to other socioeconomic factors, including underemployment, unemployment, and lack of education. Individuals who lack health insurance may delay seeking medical care for current health conditions, thus reducing the likelihood of timely diagnosis, treatment, and remedy, and increasing the chances that these health conditions will persist, worsen, and become life-threatening. The continuing national debate over health insurance underscores the need to understand who is adequately insured, what factors affect peoples' ability to get insurance, and how insurance affects subsequent mortality.

In one of the few nationwide studies that have examined insurance status and subsequent mortality, Franks and colleagues (1993) found that uninsured people were about 25% more likely to die in a 12-year follow-up period than were those who were insured at baseline. This increased risk was net of education, income, and occupational differences between the insured and uninsured groups. Compared to insured hospital patients, uninsured patients are twice as likely to sustain negligent injury through substandard medical care (Burstin et al. 1992). The uninsured are also more likely than the insured to have limited access to preventive and curative health care, to receive treatment by emergency center personnel who may act more quickly than private health center and clinic personnel but less thoroughly, and to receive improper diagnosis and treatment (Burstin et al. 1992). Thus, it is especially important to include the effects of insurance status in studies of socioeconomic factors and mortality; our inclusion of Medicare and Medicaid receipt will make the analysis even more comprehensive.

As debate continues about national health insurance, millions of Americans remain uninsured. In 1992, 98.8% of individuals aged 65 and above were covered by private or government health insurance. But many governmental insurance programs are limited to the elderly, or the poor, or the disabled. The youngest adults are the least likely to be insured. For example, private health insurance covers 77% of individuals aged 55 to 64, 79% of individuals aged 45 to 54, and 77% of individuals aged 35 to 44, but only 69% of individuals aged 25 to 34, and just 60% of individuals aged 18 to 24 (U.S. Bureau of the Census 1994).

Like income sources, insurance sources may vary in their effects on mortality. Medicare is a federal program of health insurance that covers almost all people aged 65 and over, as well as younger disabled individuals. In 1986, Medicare spent $2,100 per covered person (Atchley 1991). It consists of hospital insurance, for which practically all elderly people are eligible, and supplementary medical insurance, which is optional. Supplementary medical insurance covers, for a premium, health care, diagnostic tests, and laboratory services, but it does not cover long-term health care, eyeglasses, hearing aids, dental care, physical examinations, or immunizations; also, it requires deductibles or copayments with some services. Many elderly purchase private health insurance to cover such "medigaps" (Atchley 1991).

Medicaid can cover poor individuals who are otherwise uninsured. But coverage usually does not begin until someone has demonstrated a dire need for financial assistance with medical care. Medicaid provides health care—including physicians' services, diagnostic tests, outpatient hospital services, and, importantly, long term care—to the poor of any age. To be eligible, individuals must have low incomes as well as few assets that could be converted into income. Thus, poor uninsured individuals may have to forgo preventive and even palliative care until a health problem becomes an emergency—at which point it is less easily treated and more life-threatening. Moreover, because of Medicaid price caps, some physicians will not treat patients with Medicaid insurance, and others provide hurried examinations to compensate for the lower payments (see Preston and Taubman 1994). Generally, poor young adults use Medicaid to cover physicians' services and short-term hospitalizations, while poor people aged 65 and over are more likely to use Medicaid for the more expensive long-term care. This explains why, in 1987, that only 14% of the Medicaid recipients were 65 or older, while 36% of the funds were used by the elderly (Atchley 1991).

DATA AND METHODS OF ANALYSIS

In the past, mortality research has been hampered by lack of detail on socioeconomic factors (Moss and Krieger 1995). At best, most studies were designed around one or two facets of socioeconomic status and included summary measures such as dichotomous indicators of family income and/or two or three educational categories. The release of the Health Insurance (HI) Supplement of the National Health Interview Survey (NHIS), linked to mortality information from the National Death Index, has expanded mortality research frontiers. We use the 1986 HI Supplement of the NHIS, matched to death information from the National Death Index (NDI) (NCHS 1989b, 1997b). The socioeconomic variables from the core NHIS include education and family income, along with standard demographic and health status information. In addition, the HI contains information on health insurance coverage as well as details on Medicare and Medicaid.

Socioeconomic characteristics are important determinants of mortality because they indicate access to resources that foster good health and long life (Kitagawa and Hauser 1973; Rogot et al. 1992). Although different measures of socioeconomic status are correlated with one another, they tap different features that are each related to mortality (Preston and Taubman 1994). In this chapter, we examine the effects of health insurance on mortality, controlling for education and income, two central measures of socioeconomic status.

Private health insurance coverage is linked to mortality and to other socioeconomic factors. Compared to those who are well insured, those who are uninsured or underinsured are often less educated, poorer, and either in lower status occupations or unemployed. Limited studies have also demonstrated that, net of other social and demographic factors, the uninsured have higher mortality risks because they get less timely, less consistent, and poorer health care (Franks et al. 1993). We measure health insurance coverage first by whether an individual has private health insurance. Granted, health insurance companies, such as Blue Cross, Blue Shield, and HMOs, vary in what they cover—hospitalization, well check-ups, doctor visits, dental services, and emergency room costs—how much they cover, and whether there are deductibles or copayments. But we argue that the source of insurance should be less important than whether someone is insured. A substantial proportion of individuals have no health insurance because they cannot afford it, they are not covered through their employers, or they do not think that they need it. Thus, health insurance coverage should be a crucial variable.

We code individuals as covered or not covered by Medicare and by Medicaid. Since Medicaid is known by different names in different states, like Medi-cal in California, NHIS interviewers showed respondents flashcards to ensure correct responses to their questions on Medicaid receipt (NCHS 1989b). We expect that receipt of Medicaid, because it indicates both poverty and health-care needs, will be associated with an increased risk of death. Medicare receipt, on the other hand, is most often based on age, rather than poverty or ill health. Since practically all individuals aged 65 and over qualify for Medicare, we expect that Medicare receipt among the elderly will not radically affect the risk of death. However, Medicare receipt among younger adults indicates a special, documented health need; we expect such individuals to exhibit higher mortality risks than younger adults who do not receive Medicare.

Health insurance coverage, Medicare and Medicaid, education, and income, are all influenced by age. Income and education exhibit stronger associations with mortality for persons between the ages of 25 and 64 than for those 65 and older (Elo and Preston 1996; Kitagawa and Hauser 1973; Pappas et al. 1993). Most individuals do not qualify for Medicare unless they meet certain age eligibility requirements (at ages below 65, individuals can qualify for support through some of these programs through survivorship or disability benefits). Because mortality, income, health, and health insurance coverage are all interrelated by age, we examine these relations separately for those less than 65 years of age and for those aged 65 and over. Thus, we examine 324,250 person-years and 1,554 deaths for young adults, and 77,142 person years and 2,446 deaths for older adults.

Education affects mortality directly through altered health behaviors and indirectly through its effect on income and occupation, which, in turn, can determine access to resources, including health insurance (Rosenberg and Powell-Griner 1991). We measure education in years completed, using a four-category scheme: less than 9 years, 9 through 11 years, 12 years, and 13 or more years. We expect that highly educated individuals will experience lower risks of mortality than less educated individuals, but that this effect will be reduced with the inclusion of other socioeconomic factors, such as income and health insurance. High *income* can increase survival chances through its association with quality housing, improved nutrition, safer transportation, and access to health care. We measure income through an income equivalence scale (for more discussion and justification of income equivalence scales and the coding of education, see Chapter 7).

To determine the net effects of health insurance coverage on mortality, each model we test controls for demographic and health status variables that have been shown to be critical for the analysis of U.S. adult mortality patterns. Sex is included as a conventional dummy variable, and we generally expect to find higher mortality among males. Age is measured in single-year age groups. Because race is not the focal point of this chapter, it is specified as black and nonblack, rather than into more detailed categories. We expect blacks to exhibit higher mortality than nonblacks, although more comprehensive socioeconomic measurement should narrow the racial mortality differences (Hummer 1996).

Marital status is also strongly linked to mortality and to socioeconomic status (Rogers 1995a; Smith and Zick 1994) and is therefore included as a control variable. In general, we expect that married individuals will exhibit lower mortality risks than the unmarried because they engage in more positive health behavior and are linked to tighter-knit social support networks (Lillard and Waite 1995). We measure marital status using a three-category scheme: currently, previously (widowed or divorced), or never married.

Mortality, and to some extent socioeconomic position, is also influenced by a person's state of health. Health status is self-reported in the NHIS and is measured on a five-point scale ranging from excellent to poor. Recent research has highlighted the importance and accuracy of self-reported health (Montgomery et al. 1996; Rogers 1995b), and the same measure has been used as a health status control in similar research (e.g., Franks et al. 1993). We examine the effects of health insurance with and without controls for health status, since lack of health insurance may contribute to poor health status, which in turn could affect mortality.

Consistent with previous chapters, we examine overall, then cause-specific mortality. The causes include circulatory diseases, cancer, respiratory diseases, social pathologies, and residual causes of death. For more detail on coding decisions or International Classification of Disease (ICD) codes, see Chapter 2.

RESULTS

The descriptive statistics in Table 9.1 provide a number of comparisons. First, we can compare younger (column 1) and older (column 3) adults who survived from 1986 through 1995. Compared to younger adults, older adults possess the same percentage of private health insurance coverage, substantially more Medicare, and slightly more Medicaid. Further, they are less likely to have attained the same educational level, and they earn lower incomes. Although about the same percentage of older and younger adults have private health insurance, there are large differences between these two groups in Medicare coverage: less than 2% of those under 65 rely on Medicare, compared to 95% of the older adults.

Both older and younger adults are more likely to die if they have low family income or are less educated—the usual associations seen in most studies of this type (compare columns 1 to 2 and 3 to 4). In addition, people who rely on Medicaid—a government program for the poor—and who lack private health insurance are more likely to die than their more socioeconomically advantaged counterparts. Although Medicare receipt is associated with mortality among younger adults—indicating specialized need for governmental health insurance and higher health risks—Medicare receipt among the elderly—which is more commonplace—displays less association with mortality. Not only does this simple table show the associations between classic dimensions of socioeconomic status and mortality, it also demonstrates the associations between health insurance and mortal-

TABLE 9.1   Percentage Distributions of Health Insurance and Other Socioeconomic Factors for Younger and Older U.S. Adults, 1986–1995[a]

	Less than 65 years		Ages 65 and above	
	Alive	Dead	Alive	Dead
Socioeconomic status measures	(1)	(2)	(3)	(4)
Health insurance measures				
Private health insurance (uninsured = 1)	22.3%	32.8	22.0	28.1
Medicare (yes = 1)	1.3	8.8	94.7	98.5
Medicaid (yes = 1)	4.1	9.2	5.5	7.7
Socioeconomic status controls				
Education				
Less than 12 years	19.1	38.7	44.7	53.6
12 years	40.7	38.1	32.9	27.7
Over 12 years	40.3	23.2	22.4	18.7
Income equivalence	1.9	1.6	1.5	1.4

Source: NCHS 1989b, 1997b.

[a] Income equivalence is mean income equivalence measured in $10,000s.

ity, albeit without controls for other factors. To examine these relations in a multivariate framework, we turn to Tables 9.2 (for younger adults) and 9.3 (for older adults), which simultaneously model these factors with mortality.

YOUNG AND MIDDLE-AGED ADULTS

Table 9.2, which displays the results for adults under the age of 65, shows that the effect of socioeconomic status on mortality includes more than income and education. Model 2 shows that compared to those with health insurance, those without private health insurance are 35% more likely to die. Individuals without private health insurance can still seek medical treatment through other programs, including Medicare and Medicaid, but those below age 65 must qualify for these programs through survivorship, disability, or poverty. Thus, it is not surprising to find that young adults who are enrolled in Medicare and Medicaid are twice as likely to die as those who are not (see Models 3 and 4).

Many socioeconomic status measures are interrelated, so that their combined net effects are smaller than the sum of their individual effects on mortality (see Model 10). For example, individuals who lack private health insurance may try to get health coverage through Medicare or Medicaid. Thus, the 35% gap between insured and uninsured in Model 2 drops to a 9% gap once other insurance and income sources are included in the model (compare Model 2 to Models 7 through 10). Even in Model 10, young and middle-aged adults who receive Medicare and Medicaid support are almost 40% more likely to die than those who do not.

It is interesting to note that marital status is affected by health insurance. Never married individuals experience high mortality, in part, because they lack the ability to obtain health care. For instance, compared to married individuals, individuals who have never married are 75% more likely to die when health insurance is not controlled, but just 55% more likely to die with controls for private health insurance and Medicare and Medicaid receipt (Model 9).

OLDER ADULTS

Almost all elderly qualify for Medicare. Thus, there is no difference in mortality between elderly who are and are not on Medicare (see Table 9.3, Model 3). Because of the gaps in Medicare coverage, some elderly also choose private health insurance. Compared to those elderly with private health insurance, those without private coverage experience an 11% higher risk of death. Those who get Medicaid experience a 39% higher risk of death than others (Model 4). Thus, elderly who are ill and who rely on

TABLE 9.2 Odds Ratios of Private Health Insurance and Medicare and Medicaid Receipt on Mortality, U.S. Adults under Age 65, 1986–1995

Socioeconomic status measures	Model 1	Model 2	Model 3	Model 4	Model 5	Model 6	Model 7	Model 8	Model 9	Model 10
Health insurance measures										
Private health insurance (1 = uninsured)		1.35*			1.28*	1.16	1.23+	1.11	1.18	1.09
Medicare receipt (1 = yes)			2.35*		2.23*	1.41*			2.15*	1.39*
Medicaid receipt (1 = yes)				1.94*			1.76*	1.41+	1.66*	1.39+
Socioeconomic status controls										
Education										
Less than 12 years	1.74*	1.69*	1.68*	1.71*	1.65*	1.29*	1.68*	1.30*	1.64*	1.29*
12 years	1.34*	1.35*	1.34*	1.35*	1.35*	1.20*	1.35*	1.20*	1.36*	1.21*
Over 12 years	ref	ref	ref	ref	ref	ref	ref	ref	ref	ref
Income equivalence	.75*	.79*	.77*	.78*	.80*	.89*	.80*	.89*	.81*	.89*
Sociodemographic controls										
Sex (1 = male)	1.80*	1.80*	1.74*	1.87*	1.74*	1.78*	1.86*	1.85*	1.80*	1.82*
Age (single years)	1.09*	1.09*	1.09*	1.09*	1.09*	1.08*	1.09*	1.08*	1.09*	1.08*
Race (1 = black)	1.28*	1.26*	1.29*	1.24*	1.27*	1.16	1.23*	1.14	1.25*	1.15
Marital status										
Currently married	ref	ref	ref	ref	ref	ref	ref	ref	ref	ref
Previously married	1.14	1.10	1.11	1.10	1.08	1.09	1.08	1.09	1.06	1.08
Never married	1.75*	1.67*	1.65*	1.66*	1.60*	1.60*	1.62*	1.59*	1.55*	1.57*
Health status						1.56*		1.58*		1.55*
−2*Log-likelihood	13,793.99	13,777.80	13,745.41	13,763.63	13,735.13	13,485.99	13,756.72	13,486.22	13,718.19	13,478.46

Source: NCHS 1989b, 1997b.
+$p \leq .10$; *$p \leq .05$.

TABLE 9.3 Odds Ratios of Private Health Insurance and Medicare and Medicaid Receipt on Mortality, Among U.S. Adults Ages 65 and Above, 1986–1995

Socioeconomic status measures	Model 1	Model 2	Model 3	Model 4	Model 5	Model 6	Model 7	Model 8	Model 9	Model 10
Health insurance measures										
Private health insurance										
(1 = uninsured)		1.11+			1.11+	1.02	1.06	1.00	1.06	1.00
Medicare receipt (1 = yes)			1.02		1.02	.96			1.02	.97
Medicaid receipt (1 = yes)				1.39*			1.35*	1.13	1.35*	1.13
Socioeconomic status controls										
Education										
Less than 12 years	1.18*	1.17*	1.18*	1.18*	1.17*	1.06	1.17*	1.07	1.17*	1.07
12 years	1.08	1.08	1.08	1.08	1.08	1.06	1.08	1.06	1.08	1.06
Over 12 years	ref	ref	ref	ref	ref	ref	ref	ref	ref	ref
Income equivalence	.95	.96	.95	.96	.96	1.03	.97	1.03	.97	1.03
Sociodemographic controls										
Sex (1 = male)	1.83*	1.82*	1.83*	1.85*	1.82*	1.89*	1.84*	1.89*	1.84*	1.89*
Age (single years)	1.08*	1.08*	1.08*	1.08*	1.08*	1.08*	1.08*	1.08*	1.08*	1.08*
Race (1 = black)	1.25*	1.22*	1.25*	1.23*	1.22*	1.18*	1.21*	1.18*	1.21*	1.18*
Marital status										
Currently married	ref	ref	ref	ref	ref	ref	ref	ref	ref	ref
Previously married	1.19*	1.18*	1.20*	1.18*	1.18*	1.23*	1.18*	1.23*	1.18*	1.23*
Never married	1.19+	1.17+	1.19+	1.18+	1.17+	1.24*	1.17+	1.24*	1.17+	1.24*
Health status						1.34*		1.34*		1.34*
−2*Log-likelihood	24,512.35	24,507.39	24,512.27	24,496.53	24,507.27	24,204.19	24,495.00	24,202.57	24,494.83	24,202.17

Source: NCHS 1989b, 1997b.

$+p \leq .10$; $*p \leq .05$.

Medicaid are at greater risk of death, not because of Medicaid receipt, but because of what it represents—illness, lack of private health insurance, and poverty.

The next two tables focus on private health insurance among young (Table 9.4) and older adults (Table 9.5) and cause-specific mortality. Compared to young adults with health insurance, those without insurance are more likely to die from every cause examined, save cancer. For example, compared to young insured adults, uninsured adults are 26% more likely to die from circulatory disease (the major cause of death), are 30% more likely to die from respiratory diseases, and are 58% more likely to die from social pathologies, including accidents.

Older adults again show less variation in health insurance and cause-specific mortality than younger adults (Table 9.5), but there is a significant difference between older insured and uninsured individuals and circulatory diseases. Compared to older insured adults, comparable uninsured adults are 11% more likely to die from circulatory diseases. The difference, although small in magnitude, is important because it deals with the major cause of death.

TABLE 9.4   Odds Ratios of Private Health Insurance on Cause-Specific Mortality among U.S. Adults under Age 65, 1986–1995[a]

	Circulatory	Cancer	Respiratory	Social pathology	Residual
Private health insurance (1 = uninsured)	1.26*	1.04	1.30*	1.58*	1.84*
Socioeconomic status controls					
Education					
Less than 12 years	1.63*	1.96*	2.09*	1.91*	1.79*
12 years	1.44*	1.54*	1.47*	1.39*	1.24*
Over 12 years	ref	ref	ref	ref	ref
Income equivalence	.75*	.89*	.70*	.91*	.81*
Sociodemographic controls					
Sex (1 = male)	2.53*	1.51*	1.11	3.09*	1.71*
Age (single years)	1.12*	1.11*	1.13*	1.02*	1.07*
Race (1 = black)	1.65*	1.06	.90	1.11	1.70*
Marital status					
Currently married	ref	ref	ref	ref	ref
Previously married	1.27*	1.18*	1.26+	1.47*	1.50*
Never married	1.34*	1.15+	1.95*	1.38*	1.94*

Source: NCHS 1989b, 1997b.
[a] −2*Log-likelihood is 94,156.60; person years is 324,250.
+$p \leq .10$; *$p \leq .05$.

TABLE 9.5   Odds Ratios of Private Health Insurance on Cause-Specific Mortality among U.S. Adults Ages 65 and above, 1986–1995[a]

	Circulatory	Cancer	Respiratory	Social pathology	Residual
Private health insurance (1 = uninsured)	1.11*	.96	1.01	1.04	1.00
Socioeconomic status controls Education					
Less than 12 years	1.36*	1.19*	1.33*	.83*	.80*
12 years	1.07+	1.15*	1.21*	.73*	.72*
Over 12 years	ref	ref	ref	ref	ref
Income equivalence	.86*	.96*	.81*	1.01	.84*
Sociodemographic controls					
Sex (1 = male)	1.88*	2.50*	2.68	3.07*	1.36*
Age (single years)	1.09*	1.04*	1.09*	1.06*	1.09*
Race (1 = black)	1.09*	1.33	.45	1.63	1.21*
Marital status					
Currently married	ref	ref	ref	ref	ref
Previously married	1.48*	1.17*	1.82*	1.34*	1.47*
Never married	1.08	1.34*	1.58*	1.28	.92

Source: NCHS 1989b, 1997b.
[a] −2*Log-likelihood is 129,433.34; person years is 77,142.
+$p \leq .10$; *$p \leq .05$.

CONCLUSION

Previous studies have highlighted the effects of income and education, two socioeconomic factors—on mortality. But income by itself does not reduce the risk of mortality. Mortality risks are reduced when income is used to purchase health insurance and to buy goods and services that will promote health and prevent disease. Similarly, education reduces the risk of death by providing the knowledge necessary to find insurance coverage, either private or governmental, and to know what is covered and what insurance gaps exist.

Private health insurance affects mortality. This relation persists even net of income and education effects. Compared to young adults with health insurance, those without health insurance are 35% more likely to die. This figure is more disturbing when the number of uninsured individuals is considered: in 1986, almost 31 million individuals aged 18 to 64 lacked private health insurance (calculations not shown). These 31 million young adults are 35% more likely to die than their insured peers during the follow-up period.

Young and middle-aged adults who use Medicare or Medicaid are also more likely to die. Such results are rich with implications. First, individuals who qualify for government insurance programs indicate through their high mortality that they do indeed require social health support to combat their high risk of death. Many of these individuals have been laid off work and are already sick and/or disabled. To further exacerbate their problems, individuals who are laid off work may lose access to group medical insurance; individuals who become disabled may lose their health insurance. And individuals who lose their jobs, who are self-employed but with low incomes, or who are just poor may not be able to afford health insurance. Second, many of these programs do in part compensate for lack of private health insurance. Still, Medicare and Medicaid cannot fully ameliorate the mortality risks associated with lacking private health insurance, and they cover only a few individuals, often only during medical emergencies. Among those young adults who remained alive between 1986 and 1995, 22.3% lacked private health insurance, but only 1.3% had Medicare and only 4.1% had Medicaid support.

The mortality gap between insured and not insured people is greater for younger than for older adults. Part of this difference between younger and older ages may be due to differences in government programs. Virtually all older adults are covered by Medicare, whereas many younger adults are without health insurance of any kind. Thus, older adults may use private health insurance mainly to cover gaps in Medicare, so that the gap between those who have and do not have private health insurance is much smaller for older than younger adults. Similarly, the majority of elderly are guaranteed a minimum level of income: most qualify for and receive social security. If social security or other sources of income do not place elderly above the poverty level, they can request other support, including SSI. These mortality differentials by age suggest that we, as a nation, should give the young the same support we provide for the old. The United States should reconsider a national health insurance that would cover all ages.

Both young and older adults who lack private health insurance experience greater risk of death from circulatory diseases, the major cause of death in the United States. Uninsured individuals may not possess the resources to receive proper diagnoses and treatments of existing conditions. For example, hypertension may be unrecognized and untreated, or even recognized but still untreated, which can increase the chances of death due to circulatory diseases. Moreover, the shear stress associated with lacking health insurance and realizing that chronic conditions may lead to disabling and possibly fatal outcomes may in itself further increase the risk of circulatory disease mortality. Social programs could work to reduce circulatory disease mortality through national health insurance, or through specific screening programs for the uninsured.

Young uninsured individuals are more likely to die from social pathologies. Individuals involved in accidents can look forward to hasty recoveries if they are treated thoroughly and promptly. But many uninsured individuals wait longer before being examined by health-care personnel, may be treated less thoroughly, are more likely to receive improper diagnosis, and are at increased risk of sustaining negligent injury because of the substandard medical care (Burstin et al. 1992).

Overall, this chapter expands the socioeconomic status factors responsible for high and low mortality risks. We have demonstrated that socioeconomic status includes income and education, the conventional measures, in addition to employment and occupational status, important but often overlooked factors, and now health insurance as well as Medicare and Medicaid receipt. Clearly, access to health insurance is a central socioeconomic variable that affects whether we live or die.

HEALTH CONDITIONS AND HEALTH STATUS

10

PERCEIVED HEALTH STATUS AND MORTALITY

Death is the end point of a lifetime in which an individual has experienced various threats to continuing existence. Some such threats are of short-term and/or mild in their consequences. Others may be longer-term and/or severe in nature. Life threats can be the result of cataclysmic events or accidents or illnesses from genetic or environmental sources. We describe states of living that are free of severe threats as generally healthy ones, and talk about life periods subject to severe threats as unhealthy ones. Clearly, however, health is a relative concept that can be variously defined and measured. In this chapter, we focus on a prime indicator of health and examine its linkage to death for a representative sample of U.S. adults, taking into account other associated factors.

The mortality transition of societies has been related to an epidemiologic transition, during which patterns of disease and illness (or morbidity) are observed to change structurally and thereby alter the risks of death among the people. Among developed nations, the epidemiologic transition has been traced historically from a stage when infectious and parasitic diseases were predominant causes of death to one when chronic, degenerative, and other noncommunicable conditions became more prevalent determinants of mortality (Omran 1971). Yet, patterns of illness are not necessarily matched to patterns of death. According to Riley and Alter (1989), while the risk of death declined sharply during the 19th century, the age-specific *incidence* of disease and injury has not declined as markedly, and the age-specific *duration* of disease and injury has increased. Thus, the tie between relative health status and mortality in a population can be quite complex and multifaceted.

For a long time, demographers and epidemiologists inferred the health status of a population from reported causes of death in that population. Today, we attempt to measure health status more directly at different points in a person's lifetime, using surveys and health and medical records. Still, the concept of "health" is an evasive one and has more than one dimension.

First of all, we can observe that poor health can interfere with the normal routines of everyday life and, as a result, place limitations on daily activity. These may range from inability to drive a car to pursuing a full-time job to not being able to dress oneself. People with such limitations suffer from some types of ailments that result from disease or normal aging processes, and their risks of mortality are greater than for those who do not have those limitations. We concentrate on that relationship in Chapter 11 on functional limitations, but we incorporate some aspects of it in this chapter.

Second, there is the distinction between physical and mental health. While the latter is increasingly regarded as part and parcel of one's total health status, most analysts separate the two, ostensibly because they derive from differing principal sources. We have chosen, in this book, to maintain the distinction. Chapter 12 deals exclusively with mental and addictive disorders and their association with mortality. The present chapter does not deal with mental health explicitly, but aspects of mental health may be part of more general conceptions of health measured in this chapter.

Third, assessment of one's health can be made in various ways. In modern societies, to determine our health status, we rely most often on the judgments of physicians who have examined our bodies and thereby determine what are our ailments and how severe they are. But we may not see a physician until we have decided ourselves (or a family member decides) that we are ill and need to be examined. In the case of many poor persons, appointments with physicians may be too costly or otherwise inaccessible. Hence, assessment of population health by physicians is generally incomplete.

At the same time, individuals are not always good judges of their state of poor health. Biraben (1982) described a study by two British biologists, Scott-Williamson and Pearce, of a socially heterogeneous area of southeast London during the late 1930s. They examined 3,911 individuals from 1,206 families and found that 90% of them had one or more of the pathological deficiencies generally recognized by doctors at that time. But only 21% of the persons were aware of any deficiency, and 69% thought they were in perfect health. Many of the deficiencies may have been quite minor ones and not severely life-threatening, yet the patients were not expert judges of their health conditions.

General assessments of one's own health status may be at variance with one's own recognition of medical conditions. In the 1989 U.S. National Health Interview Survey (NHIS), 40% of civilian noninstitutionalized adults assessed their health as "excellent," 28% as "very good," and 22% as "good"—a combined 90% in these three categories (Adams and Benson 1990). Roughly 7% regarded their health as "fair" and less than 3% as "poor." Yet 62% reported acute conditions (illnesses or injuries of less than 3 months duration that required physician attention or interrupted daily activity). Because we decided to use the variable of one's own "perceived health status" as a prime measure of general health status, in our analysis we turned to the existing research literature to establish how useful that variable would be. (This will be reported below.)

In the context of our broader concerns with factors affecting adult mortality, a measure of health status is important to our overall analysis of adult mortality in two respects. First, we want to determine the nature of the linkage between health status throughout life to the risks of mortality by cause of death. Moreover, we would like to know how that linkage is affected by a range of demographic, social, and behavioral variables. Second, we recognize that the relationship between several demographic, sociocultural, and behavioral factors and mortality, examined in this book, depend on how health conditions of the individual might introduce a selectivity dimension to our analysis. To the extent that such selectivity exists, we may be erroneously attributing determinations of mortality to factors that happen to be correlated with health status and that the relationship of those factors to mortality is spurious. (This will be discussed further in the section below.)

PAST STUDIES OF HEALTH STATUS

The epidemiologic transition in the United States, as in other parts of the world, transformed the society from one with high risk of infectious and parasitic diseases from the country's establishment through the turn of the 20th century to one of predominant chronic and degenerative diseases by midcentury. Early settlers in America often suffered from malnutrition and a variety of communicable diseases. At times, these assumed epidemic proportions. As living conditions improved during the 18th and 19th centuries, so did the health of Americans (Leavitt and Numbers 1997). The crowded conditions of emerging cities set back health improvements for a while, but better living arrangements and organized health programs served to counter disease and illnesses and led the nation, through healthier environments and medical progress, to higher life expectancies. Public health programs more than matched medical contributions in the early 20th century, and better diets, more favorable housing, and personal hygiene contributed to further reductions in mortality (McKeown 1976a, 1976b).

As the 20th century evolved, heart diseases and stroke became leading causes of adult deaths in the United States, followed by various forms of cancer. Most infectious and parasitic diseases had been receding in importance. In recent years, better medical practice and public and private health programs were complemented by more favorable health behaviors on the part of individuals, although continued smoking, inadequate eating habits, and lack of good exercise sustained morbidity and mortality levels.

Throughout the history of the United States, health levels remained uneven. Variations existed by social class, race and ethnicity, and other demographic and social categories. While the records show that every population category exhibited gains in health and survival, one cannot describe a national picture of health and mortality without considering the disparities that existed in each.

In recent decades, we have become much more aware than before that health conditions of people have been determined not only by the influences of governments, health organizations, and the medical profession, but also by the actions of individuals. These actions have been the result of changing personal concepts of health, health as a value, and the consequences of risk taking (Illsley 1980; Calnan 1987). At the same time, individuals have become more conscious of their own health conditions and more sensitive to what they learn from doctors and media information.

Every person knows that determinations of sickness are officially made by physicians after medical examinations and tests, but that these usually take place after the individual has felt suspicious symptoms and has arranged to see a doctor. Moreover, there are times when a person feels ill but does not see a physician, and times when what a person feels does not jibe with what the doctor's diagnosis indicates. It is customary to assume that medical evaluation is the standard for a person's health condition. Yet, individuals' own judgments about their health have some validity as well.

Individuals may be able to collate previous diagnoses by physicians with a personal assessment of their own nervous, endocrine, immunologic, and psychological conditions to more fully determine their own general health status (see Kaplan and Camacho 1983). The significance of perceived health status argues for a greater focus not only on the clinical but also on the social assessment and treatment of disease, health conditions, and social environment of individuals.

Increasingly, surveys related to health have included some form of self-assessments of health by respondents. Such a self-rating is part of the NHIS in the United States and is a measure we find convenient to use as a health indicator in this study. What, then, is the utility of such a measure?

Idler and Benyamini (1997) examined 27 studies of global self-ratings of health, along with other health status indicators, in their ability to predict mortality. If these self-ratings were to have an independent effect, they would "provide a simple, direct and global way of capturing perceptions of health using criteria that are as broad and inclusive as the responding individual chooses to make them" (Idler and Benyamini 1997: 22). The studies examined ranged in the form of the question asked, the locations, elapsed survival time, and the kind of other health indicators and covariates included in the analysis. Still, there was a great deal of commonality in the components of the studies.

The researchers discovered that self-ratings of health (generally a judgment of health on a five-point scale) reliably predicted survival in populations even when known health risk factors were accounted for. The effect was more apparent for men than women, seemingly because men typically had more serious illnesses and were thus more aware of them and were more likely to die prematurely from those illnesses.

Idler and Benyamini (1997) put forth several possible interpretations of these findings. First, self-rated health is a more inclusive and accurate measure of health status and health risk factors than the covariates used, covering the full array of illnesses a person has and possibly even symptoms of disease as yet undiagnosed but present in preclinical and prodromal stages. Furthermore, they represented complex human judgments about the severity of current illness as well as family history. Second, self-rated health is a dynamic evaluation, judging trajectory and not only current level of health. Third, self-rated health influences behaviors that subsequently affect health status. For example, poor perceptions of health may lead to less engagement in preventive practices or health care. Also, poor perceptions of health may produce nonadherence to screening recommendations, medication, and treatment. Fourth, self-rated health reflects the presence or absence of resources that can attenuate decline in health. In summary, health self-assessment combines myriad factors from many different domains of life to indicate the relative prospect of survival at any adult age.

Mossey and Shapiro (1982) found that, over a 2-year period, when age, sex, life satisfaction, income, place of residence, and objective health status were controlled, elderly individuals with poor self-rated health were still almost three times more lkely to die than those with excellent self-rated health. Kaplan and Camacho (1983), who examined the relationship between perceived health and mortality in a 9-year follow-up of the Alameda County Human Population Laboratory cohort, found that the association between perceived health and mortality persisted net of controls for age, sex, income, education, physical health, health practices, social network participation, and emotional well-being. In fact, net of other factors, people who perceive their health as poor rather than excellent are about twice as likely to die during follow-up periods of various studies (see also Idler and Kasl 1991; McGee et al. 1999; Peters and Rogers 1997; Rakowski et al. 1991; Schoenfeld et al. 1994; Singer et al. 1976).

Although we will use self-rated health as a prime measure of the respondent's health status, as subsequently indicated in our analysis, we will also include a number of other health-related variables, encompassing measures of activity limitation, bed sick days, and medical causes of death, and four specific health measures, including hypertension, diabetes, current heart condition, and stroke.

MEASUREMENT AND METHODS

Our approach in this chapter is to examine the relationship between self-reported health status and mortality, taking into account various demographic, social, and behavioral factors and looking at causes of death. We use the 1990 NHIS—Health Promotion and Disease Prevention supplement, involving 41,104 respondents (or 237,929 person-years), matched to the Multiple Cause of Death (MCD) file through 1995, which incorporates 2,388 deaths (NCHS 1993c, 1997b).

The self-reported health variable is based on the question: "Would you say your health in general is excellent, very good, good, fair, or poor?" (Respondents answer for themselves and, in many interviews, for other family members.) In this chapter, we maintain the five different categories of the health status variable to best judge how each category relates to the odds of mortality. In other chapters, however, we measure the health status variable on an interval level because of parsimony, because it is not the focal variable in other analyses, and because our preliminary runs suggested that little statistical power is lost with this continuous measurement. The subjectiveness of the health context of the question allows the respondent to define *health*, and it may be oriented to just physical health or that combined with psychological or mental health.

Two other general health variables are measured. "Activity limitations" stems from a series of questions relating to what the person's major activity was (i.e., work, school, housework, etc.) and how they might be limited in performing that activity or other kinds of activities. This information is then collapsed into four categories—unable to perform major activity, limited in amount/kind of major activity, limited in other activities, not limited (or unknown limitation). "Bed sick days" is based on a question, "During the past 12 months, that is, since DATE a year ago) ABOUT how many days did illness or injury keep you in bed more than half of the day? (include days while an overnight patient in a hospital)." We dichotomized this continuous variable into less than 30 days and 31 or more days, a split that serves to differentiate mortality risks well.

Several other health-related variables were obtained from the survey and included in the analysis. One item asks about high blood pressure or "Current Hypertension." About 11% of the respondents answered affirmatively. Another item inquired about "Current Diabetes." Only 4% responded "Yes," although some who responded "No" may have had it in the past and still have some effects of it. Still another item had to do with a "Current Heart Condition." About 9% answered positively on that item. Finally, an item was included on "Ever Have Stroke." Just 2% responded "yes" to that item. These items were used as additional health covariates in the analysis.

In addition to these general and specific health variables, all analyses were controlled for age, sex, and race, and several social, economic, and behavioral variables were incorporated into the analytical models. These are measured as in earlier chapters of this book and include employment status (unemployed, not in labor force, employed); income equivalence (measured as a continuous variable in $10,000 increments); education (less than 12 years, 12 years, 13 or more years); marital status (never married, divorced or separated, widowed, married); cigarette smoking (current heavy, current light, former, never); exercise (not regular, regular); and body mass (top 10%, bottom 10%, remainder of distribution). In the case of each of these variables, the last category mentioned is the reference category in logistic regression analysis to obtain odds ratios of death across categories of various measures.

Because it is generally believed that mortality effects vary between younger and older adults, we conduct the analysis for all adults as well as for those 18 to 64 and those 65 and over separately. Also, because different causes of death reflect varying illness episodes during life, we examine the odds ratios of dying by health factors and other covariates separately for five cause-of-death categories: circulatory diseases (heart diseases and stroke), cancer (all types combined), respiratory diseases, social pathologies, and other causes.

RESULTS

The distribution of general health factors (measured in 1990) in the study population is portrayed in Table 10.1, separately for those remaining alive and those who had died by the end of 1995. Understandably, survivors were much more likely than decedents to have reported a favorable health condition at the time of the 1990 survey. Roughly 90% of those who were still alive at the end of 1995 had earlier stated that their health was excellent, very good, or good, compared with a little over 60% of subsequent decedents. Survivors were three times as likely to report an excellent health condition as were eventual decedents. Those who remained alive over the 5-year period were also much less likely than those who died in that period to have activity limitations (16 vs. 48%). Considering how many sick days were spent in bed, only 3% of survivors indicated 31 or more days as compared to 10% of decedents.

TABLE 10.1   Descriptive Statistics for General Health Factors Related
to Overall Mortality, U.S. Adults, 1990–1995

General health factors	Alive (%)	Dead (%)
Health status		
Poor	2.7	16.1
Fair	7.9	22.3
Good	24.7	31.1
Very good	29.4	16.9
Excellent	35.2	13.4
Activity limitation		
Unable to perform major activity	4.4	17.9
Limited in major activity	5.9	14.7
Limited in other activities	5.6	15.5
Not limited	84.1	51.9
Bed sick days		
0–30	97.1	90.3
31 or more	2.9	9.7
Person-years and deaths	237,929	2,388

Sources: Derived from NCHS 1993c, 1997b.

We proceed, in Table 10.2, to calculate odds ratios of dying for the whole adult population in the study, focusing on self-reported health status and taking account of the other variables in seven successive analytical models. Model 1 provides odds ratios for the health status categories, controlling only for age, sex, and race. The disparities among categories is sharp, with those indicating poor health status five times more likely to die in the time span covered than those who reported excellent health status (see also Figure 10.1). Even those with an assessment of their health as fair had odds ratios of dying that were two to three times greater than for reporters of excellent health. The odds ratio for those reporting good health status was 1.70 and also statistically significant. The disparity in mortality chances for responses of very good versus excellent health was not significant. Hence, respondents' self-reports of health were indeed related to mortality consequences in a predictable and graded fashion.

A parallel examination of the activity limitation variable is given in Model 2. Controlling for age, sex, and race, those who could not perform a major activity in 1990 were between three and four times more likely than those who were not limited in any way to die in the ensuing 5-year period. Those who had some limitation in performing a major activity were also more likely to die in the next 5 years, although the risks were not as great as for those who could not perform a major activity at all.

TABLE 10.2 Odds Ratios for General Health Differences in Mortality, Controlling for Demographic, Social, Economic, Behavioral, and Specific Health Covariates, U.S. Adults, 1990–1995[a]

	Model 1	Model 2	Model 3	Model 4	Model 5	Model 6	Model 7
Health status							
Poor	5.01*			3.06*	2.82*	2.65*	2.32*
Fair	2.61*			2.01*	1.87*	1.78*	1.63*
Good	1.70*			1.54*	1.47*	1.41*	1.32*
Very good	1.10			1.07	1.04	1.03	0.98
Excellent	ref			ref	ref	ref	ref
Activity limitations							
Cannot perform major activity		3.44*		1.99*	1.81*	1.72*	1.66*
Limited in major activity		2.11*		1.49*	1.45*	1.43*	1.35*
Limited in other activities		1.60*		1.27*	1.24*	1.23*	1.19*
Unlimited		ref		ref	ref	ref	ref
Bed sick days							
31+/year			2.60*	1.19*	1.19*	1.12	1.11
<31/year			ref	ref	ref	ref	ref
Social and economic factors							
Employment status							
Unemployed					1.75*	1.74*	1.70*
Not in labor force					1.35*	1.36*	1.34*
Employed					ref	ref	ref
Income equivalence (continuous in $10,000s)					0.97	0.98	0.98
Education							
Less than 12 years					1.21*	1.12+	1.13+
12 years					1.20*	1.12+	1.14+
13+ years					ref	ref	ref

(continues)

TABLE 10.2 (continued)

	Model 1	Model 2	Model 3	Model 4	Model 5	Model 6	Model 7
Marital status							
Never married					1.34*	1.39*	1.47*
Divorced/separated					1.25*	1.15+	1.15+
Widowed					1.16*	1.14*	1.16*
Married					ref	ref	ref
Behavioral factors							
Cigarette smoking							
Current heavy (20+/day)						2.03*	2.08*
Current light (<20/day)						1.94*	1.95*
Former						1.34*	1.32*
Never						ref	ref
Exercise							
No regular exercise						1.25*	1.25*
Regular exercise						ref	ref
Body mass							
Top 10%						1.09	1.00

	(1)	(2)	(3)	(4)	(5)	(6)	(7)
Bottom 10%						1.21*	1.25*
Remainder of distribution						ref	ref
Specific health factors							
Current hypertension							
Yes							1.11+
No							ref
Current diabetes							
Yes							1.60*
No							ref
Current heart condition							
Yes							1.17*
No							ref
Ever have stroke							
Yes							0.91
No							ref
−2*Log-likelihood	21,764.7	21,867.2	21,980.3	21,471.4	21,298.7	20,643.7	19,810.7

Sources: Derived from NCHS 1993c, 1997b.
[a] All models control for age, sex, and race.
+$p \leq .10$; *$p \leq .05$.

185

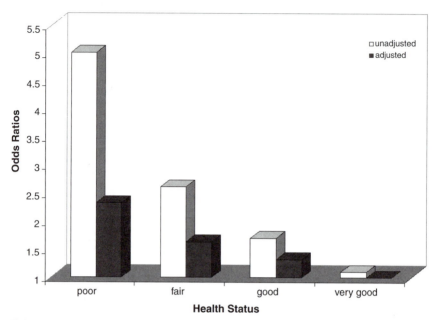

FIGURE 10.1   Odds ratios of dying by general health differences, U.S. adults, 1990–
1995. Adjusted odds ratios control for demographic, social, economic, behavioral, and specific
health covariates. Note: Referent is excellent health.

The mortality risks associated with bed sick days are shown in Model 3.
Again controlling for age, sex, and race, respondents who were sick in bed
for at least 31 days during the year were two to three times more apt to be
decedents by 1995 than were those who did not have so many bed sick days.

Each of these general health variables is associated with the chances of
dying, but clearly the extreme categories of self-reported health status
(poor) and activity limitations (cannot perform major activity) generate
very high odds ratios of dying, and even less extreme categories are associated with significant risks of dying (at least twice that of the reference category).

What happens when all three general health variables are examined
simultaneously in their relationship with mortality, and controlling for age,
sex, and race (shown in Model 4)? The magnitude of odds ratios for each
category of each variable is reduced somewhat, but the statistical significance is maintained. This seems to reflect the fact that self-reports of health
are partly based on activity limitations and days sick in bed, but that there
is a considerable dimension of each of the variables that persists beyond the
effects of the other variables. The bed days variable loses much of its predictive power when health status and activity limitations are also included
in the model. Thus, while health status and activity limitations remain

strong, bed days is only weakly associated with mortality when the other two general health factors are considered.

Introducing other variables into the analysis serves to dampen the effects of the general health variables; yet, the statistical significance of most of the categories of the health variables remains. Thus, in Model 5, the further introduction of social and economic variables provides a small reduction in the odds ratios of the health categories. The still further inclusion of behavioral factors in Model 6 provides another modest reduction in the odds ratios, although it eliminates the statistical significance of bed sick days. Last, adding the four specific health factors (current medical conditions) drops the odds ratios a bit more.

What is most relevant from this table is the robustness of both self-reported health status and self-reported activity limitation with regard to mortality chances. The effect of all of the other variables is to blunt somewhat the effects of the health variables. In other words, some part of the initial effect of the health variables is due to the mortality risks that are associated with being characterized demographically, socioeconomically, and behaviorally, but the greater part of the health status and activity limitations variables is due to the impact of their performance as influential forces regarding survival prospects (see also Figure 10.1).

Are these findings similar for persons 18 to 64 years of age and those 65 and over? Tables 10.3 and 10.4 examine the relationships of health status and the other variables in their mortality consequences separately for those two age categories. (The age controls used in the analysis operate within those broader age ranges.) The results are significant for both age groups: self-reported health and activity limitations are potent variables for survival among pre-senior adults as well as among seniors. The effects of the health variables are greater for pre-senior adults, the odds ratios of dying being larger for that age group. As additional factors are entered into the analysis, especially employment status, the age difference persists for the self-reported health status variable but diminishes for the activity limitations variable. It is possible that activity limitations prevent individuals from working, which combines to increase the risk of death, particularly for younger adults. These results suggest that, once other factors are accounted for, activity limitations are just as likely to be a mortality predictor for older as younger adults, whereas self-reported health status is a good predictor of mortality for both age groups but is somewhat stronger for younger adults.

Are the effects of general health factors on mortality the same, independent of the eventual cause of death, or are the effects more pronounced for some causes than others? In Table 10.5, we look at the full models (all variables included) for each of the cause-of-death groups specified earlier. In the case of self-reported health status, magnitudes of odds ratios are found for each cause category, but they are not statistically significant for

TABLE 10.3 Odds Ratios for General Health Differences in Mortality among U.S. Adults Aged 18–64, Controlling for Demographic, Social, Economic, Behavioral, and Specific Health Covariates, 1990–1995[a]

	Model 1	Model 2	Model 3	Model 4	Model 5	Model 6	Model 7
Health status							
Poor	7.84*			3.89*	3.26*	3.12*	2.78*
Fair	3.58*			2.47*	2.15*	2.07*	1.90*
Good	2.17*			1.95*	1.84*	1.78*	1.67*
Very good	1.06			1.03	1.02	1.00	0.95
Excellent	ref			ref	ref	ref	ref
Activity limitations							
Cannot perform major activity		4.74*		2.29*	1.80*	1.72*	1.60*
Limited in major activity		2.44*		1.64*	1.56*	1.50*	1.40*
Limited in other activities		1.70*		1.30	1.21	1.25	1.30
Unlimited		ref		ref	ref	ref	ref
Bed sick days							
31+/year			3.49*	1.23	1.24	1.22	1.29+
<31/year			ref	ref	ref	ref	ref
Social and economic factors							
Employment status							
Unemployed					2.03*	1.99*	1.93*
Not in labor force					1.34*	1.36*	1.36*
Employed					ref	ref	ref
Income equivalence (continuous in $10,000s)					0.93+	0.96	0.94
Education							
Less than 12 years					1.14	1.01	1.01
12 years					1.07	0.99	1.02
13+ years					ref	ref	ref
Marital status							
Never married					1.74*	1.82*	1.90*
Divorced/separated					1.24+	1.14	1.16

188

Widowed				1.43*	1.36+	1.38+
Married				ref	ref	ref
Behavioral factors						
Cigarette smoking						
Current heavy (20+/day)					2.19*	2.14*
Current light (<20/day)					2.06*	2.00*
Former					1.45*	1.36*
Never					ref	ref
Exercise						
No regular exercise					1.20*	1.21*
Regular exercise					ref	ref
Body mass						
Top 10%					0.95	0.90
Bottom 10%					1.27+	1.29+
Remainder of distribution					ref	ref
Specific health factors						
Current hypertension						
Yes						1.21+
No						ref
Current diabetes						
Yes						1.41*
No						ref
Current heart condition						
Yes						1.16
No						ref
Ever have stroke						
Yes						0.89
No						ref
−2*Log-likelihood	8,125.1	8,175.1	8,278.8	8,039.4	7,965.1	7,735.8	7,414.9

Sources: Derived from NCHS 1993c, 1997b.
[a] All models control for age, sex, and race.
+$p \leq .10$; *$p \leq .05$.

TABLE 10.4 Odds Ratios for General Health Differences in Mortality among U.S. Adults Aged 65 and Above, Controlling for Demographic, Social, Economic, Behavioral, and Specific Health Covariates, 1990–1995[a]

	Model 1	Model 2	Model 3	Model 4	Model 5	Model 6	Model 7
Health status							
Poor	4.06*			2.70*	2.56*	2.43*	2.08*
Fair	2.23*			1.80*	1.70*	1.62*	1.48*
Good	1.46*			1.33*	1.28*	1.24*	1.16
Very good	1.07			1.04	1.02	1.01	0.96
Excellent	ref			ref	ref	ref	ref
Activity limitations							
Cannot perform major activity		2.99*		1.86*	1.79*	1.73*	1.69*
Limited in major activity		1.99*		1.44*	1.42*	1.40*	1.32*
Limited in other activities		1.55*		1.26*	1.25*	1.22*	1.17*
Unlimited		ref		ref	ref	ref	ref
Bed sick days							
31+/year			2.29*	1.15	1.16	1.08	1.04
<31/year			ref	ref	ref	ref	ref
Social and economic factors							
Employment status							
Unemployed					0.54	0.56	0.59
Not in labor force					1.31*	1.30*	1.28*
Employed					ref	ref	ref
Income equivalence (continuous in $10,000s)					1.00	1.01	1.02
Education							
Less than 12 years					1.25*	1.17*	1.20*
12 years					1.27*	1.20*	1.22*
13+ years					ref	ref	ref
Marital status							
Never married					0.99	0.98	1.03
Divorced/separated					1.25*	1.14	1.13

	Model 1	Model 2	Model 3	Model 4	Model 5	Model 6	Model 7
Widowed					1.09	1.06	1.06
Married					ref	ref	ref
Behavioral factors							
Cigarette smoking							
Current heavy (20+/day)						1.97*	2.10*
Current light (<20/day)						1.92*	1.96*
Former						1.33*	1.33*
Never						ref	ref
Exercise							
No regular exercise						1.28*	1.28*
Regular exercise						ref	ref
Body mass							
Top 10%						1.19*	1.08
Bottom 10%						1.18*	1.24*
Remainder of distribution						ref	ref
Specific health factors							
Current hypertension							
Yes							1.08
No							ref
Current diabetes							
Yes							1.68*
No							ref
Current heart condition							
Yes							1.20*
No							ref
Ever have stroke							
Yes							0.91
No							ref
−2*Log-likelihood	13,607.4	13,671.0	13,689.0	13,401.7	13,288.6	12,858.6	12,341.3

Sources: Derived from NCHS 1993c, 1997b.

[a] All models control for age, sex, and race.

$+p \leq .10$; $*p \leq .05$.

TABLE 10.5 Odds Ratios for General Health Differences in Cause-Specific Mortality, Controlling for Demographic, Social, Economic, Behavioral, and Specific Health Covariates, U.S. Adults, 1990–1995[a]

	Circulatory	Cancer	Respiratory	Social pathologies	Other
Health status					
Poor	2.08*	2.43*	2.97*	1.79	2.93*
Fair	1.47*	1.75*	1.81+	1.45	2.20*
Good	1.32*	1.31*	1.19	1.39	1.63*
Very good	1.09	0.73*	1.09	0.94	1.54+
Excellent	ref	ref	ref	ref	ref
Activity limitations					
Cannot perform major activity	1.61*	1.81*	3.69*	1.18	1.52*
Limited in major activity	1.30*	1.22	2.24*	1.07	1.47*
Limited in other activities	1.22*	0.98	2.05*	1.11	1.18
Unlimited	ref	ref	ref	ref	ref
Bed sick days					
31+/year	0.87	1.07	1.17	3.26*	1.35
<31/year	ref	ref	ref	ref	ref
Social and economic factors					
Employment status					
Unemployed	1.78+	1.05	1.92	1.63	3.29
Not in labor force	1.45*	1.06	1.04	0.98	2.52*
Employed	ref	ref	ref	ref	ref
Income equivalence (continuous)	0.94	1.06	0.94	0.94	1.00
Education					
<12 years	1.19+	1.02	0.87	1.68*	1.08
12 years	1.19+	1.20+	1.11	0.93	1.03
13+ years	ref	ref	ref	ref	ref
Marital status					
Never married	1.35*	0.90	0.91	1.50+	2.45*
Divorced/separated	0.88	1.16	1.83*	1.32	1.47+

Widowed	1.22*	0.76*	1.14	1.77+	1.46*
Married	ref	ref	ref	ref	ref
Behavioral factors					
Cigarette smoking					
Current heavy (20+/day)	2.02*	2.82*	4.70*	1.16	1.51*
Current light (<20/day)	1.95*	2.34*	2.82*	1.21	1.82*
Former	1.15+	1.83*	3.37*	0.41*	1.16
Never	ref	ref	ref	ref	ref
Exercise					
No regular exercise	1.27*	1.15	1.52*	1.04	1.52*
Regular exercise	ref	ref	ref	ref	ref
Body mass					
Top 10%	1.16	0.94	0.29*	1.04	1.18
Bottom 10%	0.98	1.24+	1.76*	0.98	1.78*
Remainder of distribution	ref	ref	ref	ref	ref
Specific health factors					
Current hypertension					
Yes	1.28*	0.88	1.07	1.12	1.14
No	ref	ref	ref	ref	ref
Current diabetes					
Yes	1.56*	1.50*	1.18	0.96	2.49*
No	ref	ref	ref	ref	ref
Current heart condition					
Yes	1.86*	0.59*	0.98	0.68	1.02
No	ref	ref	ref	ref	ref
Ever have stroke					
Yes	1.18	0.59*	0.58	0.94	1.69
No	ref	ref	ref	ref	ref
$-2*$Log-likelihood	9,238.5	7,542.8	2,050.2	2,361.0	3,934.8

Sources: Derived from NCHS 1993c, 1997b.
[a] All models control for age, sex, and race.
$+p \leq .10; *p \leq .05.$

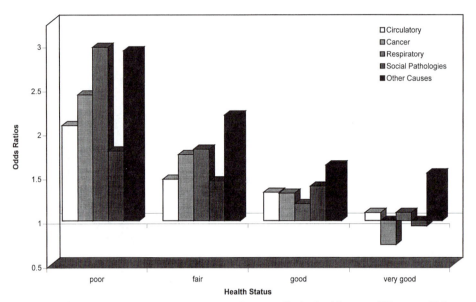

FIGURE 10.2   Odds ratios of cause-specific mortality by health status differences, U.S. adults, 1990–1995. Controls for demographic, social, economic, behavioral, and specific health covariates. Note: Referent is excellent health.

social pathologies (for a graphic representation of these relations, see Figure 10.2). The same phenomenon is found for activity limitations; however, in this case, the effect on mortality is especially large for those dying from respiratory diseases. With regard to bed sick days, the only significant effect on death is for social pathologies. The different pattern of effects for social pathologies may be due to the differing characteristics of persons in this grouping, including a higher mortality risk for the poorly educated among them and a lesser mortal effect of cigarette smoking. It also suggests that those who are victims of social pathologies are more apt to perceive their health status as poor even when their illness does not have as great a mortal risk. Apart from social pathologies, however, it seems that self-reported health status and activity limitations are good mortality predictors regardless of the morbidity track leading to death.

CONCLUSION

It is clear that health status is a multidimensional concept that can incorporate elements of physical as well as mental or psychological health and states of disability. In the analysis carried out in this chapter, we have focused on physical health status while recognizing that other health elements may creep into accepted definitions.

In choosing a critical measure of health status, we adopt an indicator of self-perceived health, as opposed to medical determinations of a person's health. This selection was mandated by the availability of that indicator in the major data set we used and the unavailability of medical evaluations in the same source. Self-rated health status, however, has been validated as a measure of general health in terms of its relationship to the prospects of death. A review of existing studies (Idler and Benyamini 1997; also see McGee et al. 1999) confirms the power of that measure and its effectiveness as a personal health marker.

The self-rated health measure is based on responses to a question as to whether one's health is poor, fair, good, very good, or excellent. The analysis we undertook further confirmed the linkage between self-rated health and mortality, even when taking into account a range of demographic, social, and behavioral variables, as well as different causes of death. By introducing covariates successively in the analysis, we were able to determine if the effect of self-perceived health is robust in its association with mortality.

Our results indicate that, indeed, self-perceived health relates strongly to the risk of dying and that other variables introduced into the analysis reduce the effect somewhat but that the effect persists with statistical significance. The observed relationship obtains for all cause-of-death categories, except that it is not statistically significant for persons dying from social pathologies.

These findings lead to three general implications for the use of a self-rated health status measure in mortality research. First, our analysis supports the findings of previous studies about the effectiveness of such a health indicator as a predictor of mortality status. Second, it leads us to stress the importance of including a health measure as part of any analysis of the process linking demographic, sociocultural, and behavioral factors to mortality. This is so both because health conditions mediate the effects of other variables with regard to the risks of dying and because examinations of other variables in their effects on mortality must take account of possible selectivity of health conditions in producing those effects. Third, we are cognizant of the limited way in which we define and measure health status in this analysis, and understand the need for greater specificity and distinctions among health components in definition and measurement. This is especially the case where we examine both younger and older adults, whose age levels may suggest different patterns of influence of factors affecting mortality (Casselli and Lopez 1996; Crimmins 1997). Perceived health status taps crucial survival prospect dimensions.

11

FUNCTIONAL LIMITATIONS
AND MORTALITY

While most adults are active, independent, and healthy, those who fall ill and who develop functional limitations endure increased risk of death. It is important to provide preventive health-care support not only to promote health, but also to lengthen life. It is imperative that health planners and policy makers anticipate the future adult population's functional status and mortality risks. Individuals with limitations may require extra mechanical and social support. With the passage of the Americans with Disabilities Act (ADA), more institutions have become sensitized to the needs of disabled individuals at home, school, work, and worship. To understand the mechanisms that contribute to long life, we examine in this chapter the effects of health and activity limitations on mortality.

AGE AND FUNCTIONAL LIMITATIONS

Although individuals at any age can be and/or become disabled, the chances of experiencing limitations in activities increases with age (Verbrugge 1989). As the U.S. population ages, health care demands will escalate. Between 1980 and 2040, it has been projected that the total population will increase by 40%, while the number of noninstitutionalized elderly needing assistance in activities of daily living (ADLs) will double (Rice and Feldman 1983).

Much of the extensive literature on functional status has focused on the elderly. This is understandable in light of the fact that compared to younger individuals, the elderly are more likely to be disabled. But functional limitations at younger ages may impart additional difficulties. Young disabled adults may be limited in the types of jobs they can find and the amount of work that they can do; they may not have had the opportunity to accrue the resources necessary to support themselves. Young disabled adults will contribute more years of disability than older adults. Moreover, young disabled adults may experience higher risks of death at earlier ages than other individuals. Such factors underscore the importance of understanding the relationship between functional status and mortality among young and older adults.

FUNCTIONAL STATUS MEASURES

Over the years, researchers have developed, modified, and refined several measures of health and functional status. Most of these measures assess the ability of an individual to maintain independence in activities that are required on a weekly if not day-to-day basis. Katz et al. (1963) developed a scale of ADLs that assesses the functional ability of individuals. Some activities are essential to daily life, such as bathing, dressing, transferring from bed to chair, using the toilet, eating, and getting around inside the home.

More complicated activites, which may not be relied on as frequently as ADLs include Instrumental ADLs (IADLs). IADLs include the ability by oneself to shop, prepare meals, do light housework, manage money, use the telephone, and get around outside.

Individuals who are limited in activities experience lower life expectancies than those not limited. Rogers (1995b), calculating life expectancies at age 55 for those with and without limitations, found that those who expressed no limitations in using the toilet, an ADL measure, had life expectancies at age 55 of 26.1 years, while those who were limited could only expect to live another 11.4 years. Similarly, at age 55, those who could prepare their own meals, an IADL measure, could expect to live another 26.5 years, compared to 11.4 years for those who were limited in preparing meals.

Because there is heterogeneity in rates of aging and within functional statuses (Manton 1988), and because many researchers and policy makers are more concerned with multiple rather than single dimensions of health, it is important to examine combinations of health statuses. Rogers (1995b) found high life expectancies among those with no chronic conditions and no limitations. At age 55, individuals can expect to live 32 additional years, or 7 years longer than average, if they report their health as excellent to very good, report no limitations in daily activities or in physical performance, and report no major chronic conditions. On the other hand, individuals who report multiple limitations and conditions experience higher mortality.

Many studies have combined ADL measures into a single index of disability or functional limitation and have thereby obscured important information. For example, Katz et al. (1983) condensed four ADL measures (bathing, dressing, transferring from bed to chair, and eating) into a summary index of dependent or independent ADLs. Such a summary measure loses important detail about each individual measure and overlooks the effects of combined limitations. In the Katz et al. scheme, a person with one limitation is treated the same as a person with limitations on all four ADLs. We examine both individual and joint contributions of functional statuses.

Functional limitations are important in mortality research in part because those individuals who experience limitations may be more likely to be socially disconnected, to be depressed, and to engage in less healthy behaviors. Individuals form expectations about their future health and longevity prospects on the basis of their current health status, and these expectations can alter their health behaviors and ultimately either hasten or retard their death (Nam and Harrington 1986).

This chapter examines how limitations in ADLs are associated with higher mortality, both individually and together. We expect that including all ADLs into one model will dampen individual ADL effects, because some of the limitations are interrelated. For the same reason, we expect to see a functional health gradient in mortality: those individuals with more limitations will have higher risk of earlier death. Finally, we will examine these differences for adults ages 65 and above, and younger adults, those aged 18–64.

DATA AND METHODS

For this analysis, we use the 1991 National Health Interview Survey-Health Promotion and Disease Prevention Supplement (NHIS-HPDP; NCHS 1993e) matched to the death information from the National Death Index (NCHS 1997b). This supplement is well suited for our purposes, since it includes individuals of all ages, rather than only older adults. Thus, we will be able to produce national estimates of the relations of functional limitations to mortality for the noninstitutionalized population in 1991. Because NCHS does not include the institutionalized population in the sample, the data will most likely underestimate functional limitations and mortality rates among the total institutionalized and noninstitutionalized population. Thus, we generalize our results to those who are initially noninstitutionalized in the U.S. population.

We classify respondents as being limited or not limited on the basis of their responses to several sets of ADL and IADL measures. The ADL measures include the abilities to bathe, dress, eat, get in and out of bed, get around inside the home, and use the toilet, all without difficulty. The interviewer asked "Because of any physical or mental condition, do you have difficulty bathing or showering, dressing, eating, getting in or out of bed or chairs, getting around INSIDE the home, or using the toilet, including getting to and from the toilet?" (NCHS 1993e). ADLs measure a person's ability to conduct basic physical functions on a daily basis.

IADLs are less basic, may not be required as frequently, and call on both physical and cognitive abilities. IADLs include the abilities to prepare meals, shop for personal items, do light housework, manage money, use the telephone, and get around outside the home—again, without difficulty. The interviewer asked "Because of any physical or mental condition, do you have difficulty preparing your meals, using a telephone, shopping for personal items, such as food or medication, doing light work around the house, such as washing dishes or doing light yard work, managing your money, such as keeping track of expenses or paying bills, or going OUTSIDE the home ALONE, such as to shop or visit a doctor's office?" (NCHS 1993e). Clearly, several of these activities could be performed monthly, weekly, or biweekly instead of daily. Although such operations are not required daily, they do affect the ability to live independently.

The original IADLs also included the ability to do heavy housework (see Wolinsky and Johnson 1991). We did not include this measure because previous analysis has empirically shown that the other IADL measures loaded together in a factor analysis but did not load with heavy housework (see Rogers 1995b). Moreover, others contend that the ability to do heavy housework is sensitive to sex differences (older females may report that they cannot do heavy housework because they consider heavy housework to include, say, moving furniture, whereas older males may report that they have never done heavy housework, even if they were physically able to conduct the work).

There are a variety of ways to assess limitations in ADLs. The National Center for Health Statistics ascertains whether a person has difficulty performing a particular task, how much difficulty the respondent experiences, and whether the respondent receives help from another person or from special equipment (Verbrugge 1990). Difficulty indicates how hard a task is to accomplish; dependency indicates whether a person requires the assistance of another person to complete the task. We examine difficulty instead of dependency because we focus on the broader notion of respondent health (Verbrugge 1989). We code each measure as (1) yes, had difficulty with the task, or (0) did not express difficulty with the task.

We deleted individuals who did not respond to any question regarding limitations. There are fewer individuals who did not respond to a particular question regarding limitations, or who do not perform the tasks for reasons other than difficulty. For example, some individuals noted that they do not manage money, but did not indicate whether doing so would be difficult for them. We coded such individuals as not limited in managing money. This coding decision may slightly reduce the mortality gap between those with and without limitations, because some of those who state that they do not perform the tasks for reasons other than difficulty might in fact have difficulty if required to perform the task.

For our analyses, we first examine the individual effects of each ADL and IADL measure on mortality. Some individuals, however, are limited in more than one activity. Thus, within clusters of activities (within ADLs and IADLs), we examine the effect of multiple limitations on overall mortality. And last, because some individuals may be limited in more than one cluster of activities, we combine our two clusters into one category to assess the effect of kinds of multiple limitations on mortality.

Because the prevalence of functional limitations increases with age (Verbrugge 1989), it is important to control for age in our analyses of limitation and mortality. We code age in single-year age groups. Because most studies have focused on functional limitations for the elderly only, we also examine functional limitations and mortality for ages 65 and over, but also introduce similar results for young adults, those 18-64. We also control for sex and for marital status. Marriage, one of the key sources of social support, provides a sense of meaning and importance to life and thus promotes health and reduces the risk of death (see House 1987).

Education can reduce functional limitations through better knowledge of health promotion and disease prevention practices. Education also provides a means to acquire higher income; and education and income both reduce disability and the risk of death. In fact, the middle and upper classes are more likely than the lower classes to adopt new health practices, to have access to health aids like gyms, and to have better knowledge of, access to, and use of medical information (Susser et al. 1985). Compared to nonpoor elderly, poor elderly are about twice as likely to have ADL limitations. For example, only 6% of those who are not poor experience difficulty bathing, compared to 12% of poor elderly (Longino et al. 1989). We also adjust for functional limitations by income equivalence.

We code health status as a continuous measure, from 1 (excellent health status) to 5 (poor health status). Despite being self-reported, health status seems to reflect a person's general health condition well (see Kaplan and Camacho 1983; Mossey and Shapiro 1982; Robine and Michel 1992).

We determine whether individuals interviewed in 1991 died between 1991 and 1995. Some individuals may change their functional health or institutionalized status over this 4-year period. This may lead to competing outcomes. The effects of activity limitation on mortality may be initially dampened because the population is select (noninstitutionalized) and because individuals are aging over this time period (with 20 year olds in 1991 becoming 24 year olds in 1995), while we have no update on their functional status. On the other hand, the effects may be greater over time as more individuals risk institutionalization and mortality because of their limitation. Although the sample is well suited for overall mortality analyses, it is too small for cause-specific analyses.

RESULTS

FUNCTIONAL LIMITATIONS FOR ADULTS
AGES 65 AND OVER

We first discuss the effects of functional limitations for individuals over age 65 because this is the common age group that studies report. In the later section, we present information on functional limitations for adults under age 65. Table 11.1 provides general descriptive statistics for functional limitations for older adults. Individuals who are physically limited are disproportionately more likely to die than others.

In general, few elderly report functional limitations. Among those who survived the period, fewer than 3% had difficulty with many ADL measures: dressing, getting around inside the home, toileting, or eating (Column 1). Similarly, fewer than 3% experienced difficulty with managing money or using the telephone, IADL measures. Thus, an overwhelming majority of elderly lead active lives. A relatively large proportion, however (over 8%), do have difficulty shopping for personal items and getting around outside the home. Individuals who are functionally limited are disproportionately more likely to die than others. For example, only 4.5% of individuals in the sample had difficulty bathing, but 13.9% of those who died had such difficulties. Individuals who have difficulty shopping for personal items and getting around outside are disproportionately represented as decedents. About 8% of the elderly who survived the period

TABLE 11.1   Percentage Distributions of Activity Limitations among U.S. Adults Ages 65 and over Who Survived and Who Died between 1991–1995

	Alive (%)	Dead (%)
Activities of daily living		
Bathing	4.49	13.86
Dressing	2.66	8.23
Getting around inside home	2.23	9.02
Transferring	6.12	13.26
Toileting	2.17	7.26
Eating	0.79	3.24
Instrumental activities of daily living		
Shopping	8.30	22.64
Preparing meals	3.50	12.22
Light housework	4.85	16.01
Managing money	2.97	8.92
Using telephone	1.58	4.77
Getting around outside	8.63	24.47

Source: Derived from NCHS 1993e, 1997b.

but over 22% of the decedents had earlier reported difficulty shopping or getting around outside.

Table 11.2 compares able elderly to those who exhibit one or more limitations. In every category of ADLs, more older adults are able than disabled. For example, about 90% of all individuals who survived the period reported no limitations in ADLs, and close to 90% expressed no limitations in IADLs. The bottom section of the table provides a summary of individuals who report 0 to 11 or more limitations of either ADLs or IADLs. Among those who survived the period, about 85% reported no difficulty. Among those who have difficulty, most have difficulty in only one or two activities. For example, out of the entire sample of difficulty in ADL or IADL measures, 8.7% report one or two limitations, 3.2% report three or four limitations, and fewer than 1.7% report five or six limitations.

Not surprisingly, those who report limitations comprise a larger proportion of the decedent than the survivor population, and increase with the

TABLE 11.2   Percentage Distributions of Activity Limitations among U.S. Adults Ages 65 and over Who Survived and Who Died between 1991–1995

	Alive (%)	Dead (%)
Activities of daily living (ADL)		
No limitations	91.55	80.38
1 limitation	4.33	7.12
2 limitations	1.52	3.75
3 limitations	0.80	2.31
4 limitations	0.73	2.25
5 limitations	0.66	2.43
6 limitations	0.41	1.76
Instrumental activities of daily living (IADL)		
No limitations	87.35	68.01
1 limitations	4.84	9.63
2 limitations	2.84	6.29
3 limitations	2.25	5.38
4 limitations	1.46	5.08
5 limitations	0.83	3.29
6 limitations	0.43	2.32
All limitations (ADL and IADL)		
No limitations	84.57	64.37
1–2 limitations	8.66	15.50
3–4 limitations	3.20	7.62
5–6 limitations	1.67	5.35
7–8 limitations	0.94	2.28
9–10 limitations	0.55	2.74
11–12 limitations	0.40	2.14

Sources: Derived from NCHS 1993e, 1997b.

numbers of limitations. Although over 80% of individuals who survived the period reported no limitations in ADLs or IADLs, among those who died, only 64% reported no limitations. Compared to those who survive, persons with one or two ADL or IADL limitations are about 1.8 times as likely to die (8.7 compared to 15.5%), persons with three to four limitations are twice as likely to die (3.2 compared to 7.6%), persons with five or six limitations are over three times as likely to die (1.7 compared to 5.4%), and persons with nine or more limitations are about five times as likely to die. To fully compare functional status and mortality, we must control for other covariates, as is done in Table 11.3.

Models 1 through 6 in Table 11.3 show the effects of individual ADL limitations on mortality, net of demographic, social, economic, and health status factors. Compared to individuals who do not report difficulty in ADLs, individuals who cannot perform individual ADLs are at least 30% more likely to die. Indeed, compared to those who can feed themselves, those who cannot feed themselves are over twice as likely to die during the follow-up period (see also Figure 11.1).

Those with IADL limitations also experience high mortality, as demonstrated in Models 7 through 12. As each model shows, any limitation in activity increases the risk of death. Compared to those without such limitations, those who have difficulty preparing meals, doing light housework, or getting around outside are each over 80% more likely to die (Models 8, 9, and 12).

Socioeconomic status, when considered in conjunction with functional health status, has little effect on mortality. Generally, in each model shown, neither education nor income is significantly related to mortality. The socioeconomic status variables may be working through functional health status to influence mortality (see Blane et al. 1993; House et al. 1988).

Some individuals are limited in more than one activity. Table 11.4 first presents combinations of limitations within specific categories of daily activities, and then combines activities. Model 1 compares individuals who report no limitations in ADLs to those who are limited. Those with more limitations generally experience higher mortality. The mortality gradient by functional status is not completely consistent because of small sample sizes: fewer individuals are limited with multiple limitations, which contributes to increased variability in the odds of death. Nevertheless, compared to individuals with no ADL limitations, individuals with one limitation are 17% more likely to die, those with two limitations are 43% more likely to die, and those with five or six limitations are 2.8 times more likely to die (Model 1). Thus, mortality is tied to the activity limitation as well as the numbers of limitations. Similar results are obtained for numbers of limitations in IADLs (Model 2).

Many of the different daily activities are interrelated. Thus, combining ADLs and IADLs wipes out all of the effects of ADLs, except for those

TABLE 11.3 Odds Ratios of Detailed Functional Statuses and Mortality among U.S. Adults Ages 65 and over, 1991–1995

	Model 1	Model 2	Model 3	Model 4	Model 5	Model 6	Model 7	Model 8	Model 9	Model 10	Model 11	Model 12
Activities of daily living												
Bathing	1.67*											
Dressing		1.68*										
Getting around inside home			2.22*									
Transferring				1.33*								
Toileting					1.85*							
Eating						2.13*						
Instrumental activities of daily living												
Shopping							1.74*					
Preparing meals								1.89*				
Light housework									2.04*			
Managing money										1.52*		
Using telephone											1.68*	
Getting around outside												1.81*

(*continues*)

TABLE 11.3 (Continued)

	Model 1	Model 2	Model 3	Model 4	Model 5	Model 6	Model 7	Model 8	Model 9	Model 10	Model 11	Model 12
Sociodemographic factors												
Age	1.07*	1.08*	1.08*	1.08*	1.08*	1.08*	1.07*	1.07*	1.08*	1.08*	1.08*	1.07*
Sex (1 = male)	1.72*	1.68*	1.70*	1.69*	1.69*	1.66*	1.76*	1.70*	1.70*	1.68*	1.66*	1.78*
Race (1 = black)	0.95	0.94	0.94	0.95	0.94	0.96	0.93	0.93	0.93	0.94	0.96	0.94
Marital status												
Currently married	ref	ref	ref	ref	ref	ref	ref	ref	ref	ref	ref	ref
Previously married	1.16*	1.17*	1.18*	1.17*	1.17*	1.17*	1.14+	1.15*	1.15*	1.17*	1.17*	1.15*
Never married	1.26+	1.31*	1.29+	1.31*	1.30+	1.31	1.27+	1.30*	1.32*	1.30*	1.31*	1.29+
Education												
Less than 12 years	1.07	1.07	1.09	1.07	1.08	1.07	1.07	1.08	1.08	1.06	1.06	1.07
12 years	1.13	1.13	1.15+	1.13	1.14	1.13	1.14	1.15+	1.15+	1.13	1.13	1.14
13 or more years	ref	ref	ref	ref	ref	ref	ref	ref	ref	ref	ref	ref
Income equivalence	0.99	0.99	0.99	0.98	0.99	0.99	0.98	0.99	0.99	0.99	0.99	0.98
Health status	1.46*	1.47*	1.45*	1.48*	1.48*	1.49*	1.42*	1.45*	1.42*	1.49*	1.50*	1.42*
−2*Log-likelihood	12,893	12,905	12,872	12,917	12,899	12,909	12,870	12,880	12,854	12,912	12,914	12,859

Sources: Derived from NCHS 1993e, 1997b.

+$p \leq .10$; *$p \leq .05$.

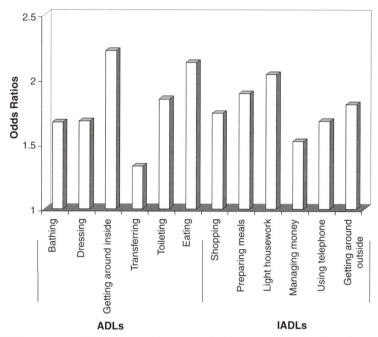

FIGURE 11.1   Odds ratios of dying by detailed functional statuses, U.S. adults, ages 65 and over, 1991–1995. Note: Referent for each activity is the ability to perform that activity without difficulty.

individuals with five or more limitations, but has little effect on IADLs (Model 3). There is a hierarchical nature to the ADLs and IADLs such that individuals generally lose IADLs before ADLs, or more specifically, individuals lose the ability to manage money before they lose the ability to feed themselves. Thus, once IADLs are controlled, only additional losses in ADLs become important. To examine the combined effects of losses in either ADLs or IADLs, we turn to Table 11.5.

Table 11.5 shows a clear functional limitation gradient in mortality. Compared to those with no limitations, those with one or two limitations in any activity studied are over 40% more likely to die, those with three or four limitations are about 70% more likely to die, and those with five or more limitations are over twice as likely to die. Undoubtedly, it is important to include both the type and the number of functional limitations in mortality analyses.

FUNCTIONAL LIMITATIONS FOR ADULTS
UNDER AGE 65

Most studies have overlooked the effects of disability on mortality for younger adults. But younger adults have limitations and risk higher mor-

TABLE 11.4   Odds Ratios of Functional Status Categories and Mortality among U.S. Adults Ages 65 and over, 1991–1995

	Model 1	Model 2	Model 3
Activities of daily living			
No limitations	ref		ref
1 limitation	1.17		0.99
2 limitations	1.43*		1.02
3 limitations	1.22		0.81
4 limitations	1.33		0.89
5–6 limitations	2.77*		1.59*
Instrumental activities of daily living			
No limitations		ref	ref
1 limitation		1.54*	1.53*
2 limitations		1.51*	1.50*
3 limitations		1.77*	1.76*
4 limitations		2.09*	1.93*
5–6 limitations		2.73*	2.30*
Sociodemographic factors			
Age	1.08*	1.07*	1.07*
Sex (1 = male)	1.70*	1.75*	1.74*
Race (1 = black)	0.93	0.92	0.92
Marital status			
Currently married	ref	ref	ref
Previously married	1.17*	1.14*	1.15*
Never married	1.31*	1.31*	1.33*
Education			
Less than 12 years	1.09	1.07	1.07
12 years	1.15	1.15+	1.15*
13 or more years	ref	ref	ref
Income equivalence	0.99	0.99	0.99
Health status	1.45*	1.39*	1.39*
−2*Log-likelihood	12,872	12,834	12,822

Sources: Derived from NCHS 1993e, 1997b.
$+p \le .10$; $*p \le .05$.

tality because of their limitations. For example, while less than 1% of adults aged 18-64 have limitations in bathing (Table 11.6), compared to 4.5% of older adults (Table 11.1), over 7% of these young adults died. Thus, compared to older adults, younger adults exhibit lower prevalences of functional limitations, but higher risk of death for those who are limited.

Over 97% of young adults report no limitations in ADLs or IADLs (see Table 11.7). Furthermore, only a small fraction of young adults mention multiple limitations. For example, only 1.2% of the sample has one limitation in IADLs, .5% of young adults have two IADL limitations, and about

TABLE 11.5   Odds Ratios of Functional Limitations
and Mortality among U.S. Adults Ages 65 and over,
1991–1995

	Odds ratios
All limitations (ADL and IADL)	
No limitations	ref
1–2 limitations	1.44*
3–4 limitations	1.71*
5–6 limitations	2.09*
7 or more limitations	2.35*
Sociodemographic factors	
Age	1.07*
Sex (1 = male)	1.77*
Race (1 = black)	0.92
Marital status	
Currently married	ref
Previously married	1.15*
Never married	1.29+
Education	
Less than 12 years	1.07
12 years	1.14+
13 or more years	ref
Income equivalence	0.98
Health status	1.38*
-2*Log-likelihood	12,844

Sources: Derived from NCHS 1993e, 1997b.
$+p \leq .10$; $*p \leq .05$.

.3% of young adults have three or four IADL limitations, respectively. Still, young adults with limitations display disproportionate risk of death.

Table 11.8 displays the risk of death from limitations, controlling for other demographic, social, and health factors. Note that functional limitations among young adults increase their mortality. Compared to individuals who are not limited, individuals who are limited in their ability to dress or get around inside the home, ADL measures are about twice as likely to die (see also Figure 11.2). Compared to those who are not similarly limited, individuals are over twice as likely to die if they cannot prepare their own meals or go outside the home alone. Thus, functional limitations drastically curtail young adults' activities and dramatically increase their risk of death.

In fact, compared to older adults who are similarly limited, younger adults generally experience a higher relative risk of death. For instance, compared to those who can, young adults who cannot dress themselves are twice as likely to die; older adults who cannot dress themselves are 68%

TABLE 11.6   Percentage Distributions of Activity Limitations among U.S. Adults under 65 Years of Age Who Survived and Who Died between 1991–1995

	Alive (%)	Dead (%)
Activities of daily living		
Bathing	0.63	7.17
Dressing	0.63	7.28
Getting around inside home	0.38	4.25
Transferring	1.51	10.02
Toileting	0.34	1.54
Eating	0.24	2.59
Instrumental activities of daily living		
Shopping	1.45	12.04
Preparing meals	0.71	7.96
Light housework	1.13	8.49
Managing money	0.61	3.17
Using telephone	0.23	1.22
Getting around outside	1.15	12.16

Sources: Derived from NCHS 1993e, 1997b.

more likely to die. Thus, although compared to older adults, younger adults are less likely to be physically limited, those who are limited suffer relatively high mortality.

Young adults who have multiple functional limitations experience higher mortality (Table 11.9). For example, compared to those who have no ADL functional limitations, those who have one limitation are 59% more likely to die, those who have two limitations are 90% more likely to die, and those who have three or four limitations are over twice as likely to die. Thus, as in older adults, increasing numbers of limitations increases the risk of death. Furthermore, including limitations in IADLs eradicates the effects of ADLs.

Generally, the more functional limitations, the greater the risk of death (see Table 11.10). Among young adults, compared to those with no limitations, those who have one or two ADL-IADL limitations are over 40% more likely to die, and those with three or more limitations are over twice as likely to die. Thus, functional limitations, even among young adults, can be life threatening.

CONCLUSION

Functional limitations represent the central forces that prevent individuals from remaining independent, staying in their residences, living alone if desired, and continuing social interaction in the community. Individuals

TABLE 11.7 Percentage Distributions of Activity Limitations among U.S. Adults under 65 Years of Age Who Survived and Who Died between 1991–1995

	Alive (%)	Dead (%)
Activities of daily living (ADL)		
No limitations	98.23	86.25
1 limitation	0.90	4.49
2 limitations	0.32	3.85
3 limitations	0.23	2.19
4 limitations	0.14	2.11
5 limitations	0.12	1.00
6 limitations	0.06	0.11
Instrumental activities of daily living (IADL)		
No limitations	97.50	82.22
1 limitations	1.21	6.33
2 limitations	0.46	2.88
3 limitations	0.35	3.16
4 limitations	0.32	3.71
5 limitations	0.10	1.58
6 limitations	0.06	0.12
All limitations (ADL and IADL)		
No limitations	96.78	79.14
1–2 limitations	1.98	7.85
3–4 limitations	0.59	6.23
5–6 limitations	0.34	3.62
7–8 limitations	0.18	2.48
9–10 limitations	0.08	0.58
11–12 limitations	0.05	0.11

Sources: Derived from NCHS 1993e, 1997b.

who cannot by themselves bathe, dress, and, especially, use the toilet, often become institutionalized. And institutionalization, although necessary and appropriate for many individuals, can remove them from their friends and neighbors and steal away their social identity. Some people's misgivings about institutions result from these potential social losses—the physical distancing of friends, neighbors, social landmarks, neighborhood businesses, and the entire social milieu.

People with one or two limitations can often compensate for their restricted ability through the use of mechanical devices or through short-term personal assistance. For example, individuals who cannot manage money can request periodic help from family, friends, or organizations. But individuals who are limited in multiple activities require more long-term, constant care.

An overwhelming majority of studies that have examined functional limitations have focused exclusively on the elderly. Thus, these results contribute to the literature by expanding the study of functional limitations to the adult population. Although compared to older adults, younger adults

TABLE 11.8 Odds Ratios of Detailed Functional Statuses and Mortality among U.S. Adults under 65 Years of Age, 1991–1995

	Model 1	Model 2	Model 3	Model 4	Model 5	Model 6	Model 7	Model 8	Model 9	Model 10	Model 11	Model 12
Activities of daily living												
Bathing	1.82*											
Dressing		1.98*										
Getting around inside home			2.45*									
Transferring				1.55*								
Toileting					1.06							
Eating						1.64						
Instrumental activities of daily living												
Shopping							1.81*					
Preparing meals								2.29*				
Light housework									1.59*			
Managing money										1.40		
Using telephone											1.57*	
Getting around outside												2.36*

Sociodemographic factors												
Age	1.08*	1.08*	1.08*	1.08*	1.08*	1.08*	1.08*	1.08*	1.08*	1.08*	1.08*	1.08*
Sex (1 = male)	1.81*	1.79*	1.82*	1.80*	1.80*	1.79*	1.83*	1.81*	1.81*	1.79*	1.80*	1.83*
Race (1 = black)	1.25+	1.26*	1.26*	1.26*	1.25+	1.25+	1.25+	1.25+	1.25+	1.25+	1.26*	1.27*
Marital status												
Currently married	ref	ref	ref	ref	ref	ref	ref	ref	ref	ref	ref	ref
Previously married	1.34*	1.33*	1.34*	1.34*	1.33*	1.33*	1.31*	1.32*	1.33*	1.33*	1.33*	1.31*
Never married	2.29*	2.28*	2.29*	2.27*	2.27*	2.27*	2.27*	2.28*	2.27*	2.25*	2.27*	2.28*
Education												
Less than 12 years	1.07	1.07	1.06	1.07	1.06	1.06	1.06	1.06	1.07	1.06	1.06	1.05
12 years	1.10	1.09	1.09	1.09	1.08	1.09	1.10	1.09	1.09	1.08	1.08	1.10
13 or more years	ref	ref	ref	ref	ref	ref	ref	ref	ref	ref	ref	ref
Income equivalence	0.92+	0.92+	0.92+	0.92+	0.92+	0.92+	0.93+	0.92+	0.92+	0.92+	0.92+	0.92+
Health status	1.66*	1.65*	1.66*	1.65*	1.70*	1.68*	1.62*	1.63*	1.65*	1.68*	1.69*	1.59*
−2*Log-likelihood	5,730	5,728	5,726	5,731	5,737	5,735	5,724	5,721	5,731	5,735	5,736	5,712

Sources: Derived from NCHS 1993e, 1997b.

+$p \leq .10$; $p \leq .05$.

213

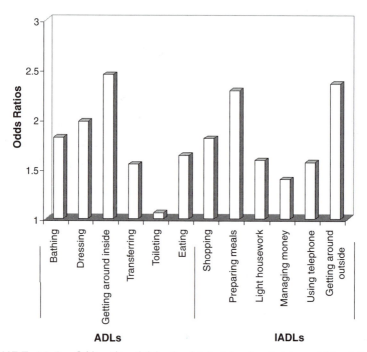

FIGURE 11.2   Odds ratios of dying by detailed functional statuses, U.S. adults under age 65, 1991–1995. Note: Referent for each activity is the ability to perform that activity without difficulty.

have fewer limitations, the limitations they do have are more life threatening. The greater mortality among young adults with limitations could be caused by a variety of factors. Many young adults lack health insurance, and thus may wait for or forgo diagnosis, treatment, and rehabilitation; older adults are more likely to have access to Medicare and other health insurance programs. Younger adults may have obtained their limitations through accidents and other forms of trauma that are more devastating, more disruptive, and less amenable to treatment and rehabilitation. Automobile accidents cause many short- and long-term limitations and may be difficult to recover from. And older adults may experience a slower, more gradual onset of limitations, which could afford them more time to accommodate and adjust to their limitations. Whatever the causes, these results call for additional research into the causes and consequences of functional limitations in older, but especially younger adults.

Recall that individuals from the NHIS come from the noninstitutionalized population. This means that some individuals are remaining in the community despite extreme limitations on their own activities, through heroic efforts of family and friends, and/or the concerted efforts of public and private organizations. The family is a strong, resilient social institution

TABLE 11.9 Odds Ratios of Functional Status Categories and Mortality among U.S. Adults under 65 Years of Age, 1991–1995

	Model 1	Model 2	Model 3
Activities of daily living			
No limitations	ref		ref
1 limitations	1.59*		1.31
2 limitations	1.90*		1.32
3 limitations	2.02*		1.28
4 limitations	2.23*		1.26
5–6 limitations	1.76		0.82
Instrumental activities of daily living			
No limitations		ref	ref
1 limitation		1.59*	1.48+
2 limitations		1.39	1.27
3 limitations		1.85*	1.67+
4 limitations		2.73*	2.43*
5–6 limitations		2.90*	2.82*
Sociodemographic Factors			
Age	1.08*	1.08*	1.08*
Sex (1 = male)	1.79*	1.81*	1.80*
Race (1 = black)	1.26+	1.27*	1.27*
Marital status			
Currently married	ref	ref	ref
Previously married	1.33*	1.31*	1.31*
Never married	2.28*	2.27*	2.27*
Education			
Less than 12 years	1.07	1.06	1.06
12 years	1.10	1.10	1.10
13 or more years	ref	ref	ref
Income equivalence	0.93	0.93	0.93
Health status	1.62*	1.58*	1.57*
−2*Log-likelihood	5,723	5,714	5,712

Source: Derived from NCHS 1993e, 1997b.
$+p \leq .10$; $*p \leq .05$.

that may rearrange itself to accommodate functionally limited family members (Rogers 1996). Parents may allow functionally limited grown children back into their home; husbands and wives may encourage an older disabled parent to move in with them, and brothers and sisters may move in with ill siblings.

Note that we considered only the existence/nonexistence of difficulty, not its severity, which is also important (Verbrugge 1990). Some individuals may "have difficulty" dressing themselves, while others may experience so much pain and distress that it is virtually impossible for them to dress

TABLE 11.10   Odds Ratios of Functional Limitations
and Mortality among U.S. Adults under 65 Years of Age,
1991–1995

	Odds ratios
All limitations (ADL and IADL)	
No limitations	ref
1–2 limitations	1.43*
3–4 limitations	2.37*
5–6 limitations	2.10*
7 or more limitations	2.50*
Sociodemographic factors	
Age	1.08*
Sex (1 = male)	1.82*
Race (1 = black)	1.26*
Marital status	
Currently married	ref
Previously married	1.31*
Never married	2.27*
Education	
Less than 12 years	1.06
12 years	1.10
13 or more years	ref
Income equivalence	0.93
Health status	1.56*
−2*Log-likelihood	5,713

Source: Derived from NCHS 1993e, 1997b.
$+p \leq .10$; $*p \leq .05$.

themselves. Thus, future research could explore mortality differences related to severity.

The importance of maintaining independence in both ADLs and IADLs
suggests that we should support programs that increase independence at
home. Meals on Wheels can help individuals who can no longer prepare
their own meals. Special Transport and grocery delivery can assist individuals who can no longer shop for personal items. The Retired Senior Vol-
unteer Program (RSVP) can help individuals manage their money. These
programs can preserve people's independence, increase their chances of
remaining in the community, and may also prolong their lives.

Functional limitations reported at one point in time affect the mortality
of individuals for several years. Torres-Gil (1992) cautions that as people
live longer, the United States and other countries will have to contend with
increased frailty, disability, and dependency. It is true that not all individuals
see continued health declines. A large minority regain their ability, become

healthier, and are more active (see Rogers et al. 1989). But some limitations persist, and even when the associated health conditions are treated and ameliorated or the limitations are compensated for with mechanical devices, some vestigial effects may remain. For example, the divorce from or death of her husband may contribute to a woman's difficulty in getting in or out of bed, or in dressing. Although mechanical devices—say, button pulls—or visiting or live-in aides may reduce the woman's problems, the central problem—the loss of her husband—persists. Policy makers must realize that programs that treat the conditions with mechanical devices may not solve the larger social problems.

Much of the previous literature has treated functional limitations as a result of chronic conditions. But as the previous example demonstrates, some limitations originate through social or psychological events. In surveys, individuals are now asked whether the limitation is caused by a "physical or mental condition" (NCHS 1993e). Such mental disorders as Alzheimer's disease and depression can limit the ability to maintain ADL and IADL functioning. For more information on the effects of mental disorders, physical functioning, and mortality, see Chapter 12.

This data set ascertains health status of adults in 1991 and follows those individuals for 4 years to determine whether they die. Thus, there are several offsetting factors that are operating in our analyses. First, ADL and IADL limitations are fixed with the 1991 responses, even though over time a minority of the sample will recover and experience fewer limitations and better health, while a larger proportion will experience health declines and more limitations. Therefore, we will slightly underestimate the actual degree of limitation in the population. Meanwhile, these individuals are aging. Some individuals will decline in health and may become institutionalized, and will thus experience higher death rates, contributing to an overestimate of our reported risk of mortality. We hope that these countervalences will cancel any biases they otherwise introduce. Future research could better model the effects we present with a long-term longitudinal data set that includes both the institutionalized and the noninstitutionalized population, and a hazards model with time-dependent covariates that adjusts for age and directly examines duration, net of age.

Information on long-term residents in nursing homes would be useful and could be calculated with such data as the National Nursing Home Survey Followup (NNHSF). But many residents will have been in the nursing home for long periods, and the time spent in nursing homes must be considered. Lewis et al. (1990) found that first admissions to nursing homes are different from readmissions. Compared to first-time patients, readmitted patients are more debilitated and less likely to return home. To fully consider functional status and mortality requires combining institutionalized and noninstitutionalized populations.

Socioeconomic status when considered in conjunction with functional health status has very little effect on mortality, especially for the elderly. This suggests a number of different dynamics. First, the effect of income in older ages may be muted by national social programs—Social Security, Medicare, Medicaid, and Supplemental Security Income. Second, the effect of education on mortality may be diminished since there is little variation among the elderly, and since the effects of education for young adults may act through income. And last, lower socioeconomic status at younger ages may predispose some individuals to functional limitations and thus work through health status to affect mortality (see Blane et al. 1993).

Rowe and Kahn (1987) discuss the factors that contribute to long lives. They note that individuals live longer when they engage in few risky behaviors and maintain strong physical health. We have found that compared to individuals with no reported limitations, those who are limited in ADLs or IADLs all can expect shorter lives. Thus, maintaining physical health clearly contributes to longer life. But what causes these limitations? Some limitations are certainly due to biological aging and degeneration, and to accidents. But some are due to previous detrimental health behaviors, including cigarette smoking, which can also alter the risk of death (Rogers et al. 1994). Armed with information on the causal factors, we should pursue research and policy directions that will improve health, reduce functional limitations, and extend life.

12

MENTAL AND ADDICTIVE DISORDERS AND MORTALITY

Mental and addictive disorders affect the personal, social, and economic relations of a sizable portion of the population. Mental disorders can prevent people's full time employment, limit their effectiveness at work, affect family relationships, cloud their judgment, increase their susceptibility to illness, increase their risk of disability, and ultimately increase their risk of death. But surprisingly few studies, particularly at the national level, have examined the effect of mental and addictive disorders on mortality. This chapter attempts to highlight some of the central relations between mental health and mortality at the national level.

Mental and addictive disorders are often costly to individuals and the larger social system. Personal costs include limitations on working, remaining employed, managing money, maintaining strong social ties to friends and family, and enjoying life to the fullest extent possible. Mental disorders can precipitate divorce, separation from siblings, social distancing from children, and soured friendships. Societal costs include increased healthcare costs, lost productivity, increased law enforcement costs, losses from crimes, and expensive prevention and treatment efforts.

There is a rich history of documenting mental disorders, with demographers playing an instrumental role in the formative years. In fact, the 1840 Census is considered the first official attempt to enumerate individuals with mental illness in the United States with a single category of idiocy/insanity (American Psychiatric Association [APA] 1994). By 1880, the U.S. Census Bureau expanded the number of categories on mental illness to seven. In the 1950s and early 1960s, many mental health studies were based on clinical interviews on small numbers of patients in the army or in mental hospitals. Now, many estimates of the prevalence of mental disorders are based on local or national surveys.

Despite vast improvements in survey methods of mental disorders, it is difficult to assess the prevalence of mental disorders for several reasons. First, not everyone who has a disorder is diagnosed. Individuals with mental disorders who have not been clinically diagnosed are a large and heterogeneous lot, including individuals with mild problems, but also individuals with more severe problems who may not have access to health-care resources, have not come to the attention of health care personnel, or have been examined by health care personnel but not classified with a mental disorder. Psychiatrists do not have a gold standard for diagnosing mental disorders (Mirowsky and Ross 1989a), which may lead to variations in diagnosis and in incorrectly defining a mentally ill person as mentally healthy. Some homeless individuals have mental problems and have been overlooked by the health-care system or are not presented to health-care workers. Second, some people are selected out of the population before being counted. For example, some individuals may commit suicide before mental health personnel realize that those individuals had mental disorders (Brown and Birthwhistle 1996). Furthermore, some individuals with severe mental disorders are institutionalized and so are not enumerated in surveys of the noninstitutionalized population. Thus, community-based surveys will not include 255,000 individuals in mental hospitals and residential treatment centers (U.S. Bureau of the Census 1987), as well as other individuals with mental disorders who reside in correctional institutions. Third and interrelated, many studies are clinically based and therefore examine only those individuals who sought or were referred for clinical help. Although such individuals have been identified as having a mental disorder, many may actually be healthier than other people in the general population since they have undergone evaluation and/or treatment (see Eastwood et al. 1982). Fourth, many disorders are interrelated and therefore may be double-counted. Last, while many mental disorders are chronic, others are cyclical, and still others are of limited duration; once they run their course, or once they are treated, they are no longer a problem. Short-term disorders may develop through a specific event, say divorce or bereavement. Once the person comes to terms with the loss or disruption, the mental disorder should dissipate if not disappear completely. On the other hand, prolonged stress, as might be associated with long-term unemployment and/or dealing with a dysfunctional family, can also lead to mental and addictive disorders. Thus, it is important when estimating the prevalence of mental conditions to examine the type reported and to follow individuals for a period that is long enough to capture any increased risk of death.

Although many mental disorders are similar and interrelated, others differ by etiology, manifestation, age at onset, treatment, and potential outcome. Most of the disorders, if untreated, result in dysfunctional relations at work, in school, and within interpersonal relations. Below, we review some of the major disorders and discuss how they are treated. More detailed definitions are available in the *Diagnostic and Statistical Manual of Mental Disorders* (DSM-IV) (APA 1994). Mental and addictive disorders can be broadly grouped into four major categories: cognitive disorders, affective disorders, alcohol abuse, and substance abuse.

DEFINITION OF TERMS

Cognitive disorders include schizophrenia and paranoia. Paranoia/delusional disorder is an extreme and unwarranted tendency to suspect that the remarks or actions of others are deceiving, threatening, or demeaning. Paranoid individuals are quick to anger but slow to confide in others. Paranoid individuals are often difficult to interact with and have problems forming and maintaining close personal and social relationships (APA 1994). The average age of onset for paranoid disorders is between 40 and 55 (Kahn and Fawcett 1993).

Delusional individuals may firmly hold a false belief—such as being followed, persecuted, or cheated—that is contradicted by social reality and is not shared by others (Campbell 1981). They are unable to differentiate fact from fiction and cannot be convinced through any amount of information that their fantasies are false. Extremely delusional individuals will have difficulty interacting in society, but some delusional individuals exhibit normal behavior when their delusions are not discussed. Such individuals can engage in more impersonal social relations, such as working and attending school, but may have difficulty with closer personal relationships, including marriage (APA 1994).

Schizophrenia, which is described as a deterioration in basic mental processes, often has a paranoid component (Mirowsky and Ross 1989b). Schizophrenia may be triggered through stress and can start slowly but then escalate. Schizophrenics may be confused, hallucinate, hear voices, withdraw from reality, regress in their behaviors, speak in bizarre ways, demonstrate irrational thinking, and repeat tasks compulsively. Disorganized thinking may be the single most important symptom of schizophrenia and can result in disorganized speech that is severe enough to prevent effective communication (APA 1994). Schizophrenics are often isolated, asocial, and estranged (Campbell 1981). The prevalence of schizophrenia is approximately 150 per 100,000 individuals (Kahn and Fawcett 1993). As many as 80 percent of schizophrenics respond to antipsychotic drugs and psychosocial interventions (Institute of Medicine [IOM] 1985).

Affective disorders include manic episodes, depression, and the combination of the two, bipolar disorder, or manic depression. Depression is the most common adult mental illness. It is characterized by feelings of sadness, discouragement, pessimism, discontent, hopelessness, and helplessness. It may be caused by stress or by social or financial loss. Depression may manifest itself mentally in anxiety, fear, and an inability to concentrate and/or physically in headaches, backaches, stomachaches, malaise, weight loss or gain, and insomnia (Ingram and Scher 1998). Severely depressed individuals may be unable to function socially or occupationally, may have difficulty performing minimal self care, and may attempt suicide. During their lifetimes, approximately 15% of the population will experience at least one episode of depression (IOM 1985). Specific mental symptoms, duration (e.g., lasting at least 2 weeks), and functional impairment usually define major depression (Kahn and Fawcett 1993). Depression may produce marital, job, and academic problems, as well as abuse of alcohol and drugs (APA 1994). Individuals who experience physiological effects due to drug and alcohol abuse, chronic health conditions, or medications are not clinically defined as depressed (APA 1994).

Manic (unipolar) individuals may exhibit transitory periods of euphoria, elation, overconfidence, optimism, and hyperactivity, but these moods are often unstable and can quickly switch to irritability (IOM 1985). Invariably, manic individuals experience a decreased need for sleep, awakening several hours earlier than usual, or may go for days without sleep, yet not feel tired (APA 1994). Manic individuals may talk nonstop for hours; excessively overproduce; simultaneously engage in multiple conversations (say on the phone and in person); or call friends or strangers at any time of the day or night. Very few people are just manic; instead, many individuals cycle between depression and mania in a pattern that was once termed *manic-depression*, and is now termed *bipolar affective disorder* (APA 1994). About 80% of individuals who are manic or depressive could benefit from antimanic and antidepressive drugs, as well as from psychotherapy, but less than one-third of those who need help actually receive treatment (IOM 1985).

Alcohol abuse affects approximately 10 million U.S. adults (IOM 1985). Although many people consume alcohol, and the beneficial effects of light to moderate alcohol consumption are lauded, excessive alcohol consumption contributes to increased mortality risks. Ten percent of drinkers can be considered problem drinkers or abusers of alcohol (IOM 1985). In this chapter, we focus on those individuals who have been identified as abusing alcohol, which is a select population. Chapter 14 provides a more in-depth examination of the relations between alcohol consumption at all levels and mortality.

Alcohol abuse contributes to problems at home, at school, at work, and in the community due to the after-effects of drinking and to intoxication. Physical symptoms of intoxication include slurred speech, unsteady gait, clouded memory, or in more extreme form, coma. Intoxicated individuals are more likely to be arrested, to use impaired judgment, to engage in inappropriate sexual actions, and to behave aggressively. Excessive alcohol consumption can contribute to physical problems with the liver, pancreas, heart, kidney, lungs, and brain. By definition, alcohol abuse is not stipulated if the symptoms are due to other medical conditions (APA 1994).

Substance abuse represents abuse of five major categories of psychoactive drugs: opiates, hallucinogens, marijuana, psychostimulants, and sedative-hypnotics. In 1985 in the United States, there were an estimated 500,000 heroin addicts, 5 million cocaine users, and 7 million users of prescription drugs without medical supervision (IOM 1985). Over time, the use of hallucinogens has become less popular, while the use of cocaine has increased; use of other illegal substances has remained relatively stable (Butz and Elder 1996). Many of these drugs can affect blood pressure, respiration, and appetite (IOM 1985). They may cloud judgment and can contribute to higher risk of infections, including increased risk of hepatitis B and HIV among intravenous drug users, and accidents, suicides, and homicides. Furthermore, users of illegal drugs are exposed to greater risk of death related to illegal behaviors to finance and purchase the drugs, as well as violent deaths associated with botched drug deals (Butz and Elder 1996). Substance abuse can lead to work absences, poor school performance, neglect of children, and such physically hazardous behaviors as driving under the influence of drugs (APA 1994). Nicotine in tobacco, which is examined in Chapter 13, is also considered addictive, but is not included in the category of drug abuse (APA 1994).

This review underscores the magnitude and diversity of mental and addictive disorders. Some mental and addictive disorders have declined dramatically in prevalence over time, in part, because of improved drug and psychosocial therapies. Even though the prevalence rates may be declining due to better treatment, the root causes and the disorders themselves may remain. Moreover, mental disorders continue to affect large numbers of individuals and may affect both social relations and health.

THE EFFECTS OF MENTAL AND ADDICTIVE DISORDERS

MENTAL AND ADDICTIVE DISORDERS AND SOCIAL FUNCTIONING

Some mental disorders may indirectly increase a person's risk of death by weakening social ties and curtailing health-promoting behavior. Individuals with mental illness may have difficulty attaining high levels of education, landing a job, maintaining continuous employment, building and sustaining social relations, maintaining a healthy diet, sleeping well, avoiding industrial and automobile accidents, and refraining from alcohol, tobacco, and drug abuse. For example, schizophrenia can decrease a person's ability to function socially. And alcohol may lead to alcohol-violence syndrome, which can increase the risk of homicide and disrupt family and other social relationships (IOM 1985).

MENTAL AND ADDICTIVE DISORDERS
AND PHYSICAL FUNCTIONING

There is a vast literature on the functional ability of individuals and how functional limitations predispose individuals to higher mortality. Various Instrumental Activities of Daily Living (IADL) scales that assess the ability to engage in basic activities around the house and in the community, such as the ability to manage money, shop for oneself, and get around outside the home are often assumed to depend on physical abilities. But some physical limitations may be a result of mental and addictive disorders. Individuals with mental disorders may have difficulty in completing basic tasks, in getting outside the home, and in working. For example, schizophrenics may have trouble preparing meals or in dressing: they may "wear multiple overcoats, scarves, and gloves on a hot day" (APA 1994:276). Moreover, even for physically able individuals, mental limitations—such as paranoia or depression—may prevent the person from, say, venturing outside the home.

MENTAL AND ADDICTIVE DISORDERS AND
EFFECTS ON OTHER FAMILY MEMBERS

Individuals with mental disorders may place other related and unrelated individuals at increased risk of death. For instance, alcoholics and drug addicts are more likely to place themselves at greater risk of death. But they may also kill close family members, friends, and unrelated individuals while under the influence of alcohol and/or drugs. Friends and family members affect and are affected by mental disorders. Family members may experience additional emotional, interpersonal, and financial stress and strain related to living and sometimes caring for a person with mental disorders.

MENTAL AND ADDICTIVE DISORDERS
AND THE RISK OF DEATH

Mental disorders increase the risk of death directly through specific diseases and indirectly by compromising beneficial social and physical buffering effects (see Eastwood et al. 1982; IOM 1985; Markush et al. 1977; Vogt et al. 1994). Mental and addictive disorders can heighten the risk of death from various causes, including accidents, homicides, circulatory diseases, cirrhosis of the liver, hyperimmune diseases, and medical complications, but especially suicides. Suicides may result from depression, schizophrenia, alcoholism, and drug abuse. Drug addicts experience very high rates of suicide; compared to the general male population, male heroin addicts are 20 times more likely to commit suicide (Lipsedge 1996). Many motor vehicle, industrial, and recreational accidents are caused by alcohol and drug abuse. About half of all deaths from cirrhosis of the liver are due to alcohol abuse. Depression contributes to hypertension, which in turn contributes to circulatory disease mortality. And some medical complications result from drug and alcohol abuse. For instance, alcohol can impede the body's ability to recover from injury (see Eastwood et al. 1982; IOM 1985; Vogt et al. 1994). Thus, mental and addictive disorders can increase the risk of death due to social pathologies and to degenerative causes of death. Nevertheless, few studies have examined the association between mental and addictive disorders and mortality, and the overwhelming majority of the studies have restricted their analyses to the clinical and institutionalized populations (see, for example, Felker et al. 1996).

Roberts et al. (1990), in one of the few studies that is based on a noninstutionalized population, examined the effects of depression on the risk of mortality using the Alameda County (California) study data. They found that compared to those individuals with no depression over the follow-up period, those with marked depression were twice as likely to die when only sociodemographic factors were applied, 56% were more likely to die when additional controls for health conditions (high blood pressure, heart disease, diabetes, cancer, chest pains, and shortness of breath) were considered, 28% were more likely to die when further controls for disability were introduced, and 7% were more likely to die when yet another control for perceived health status was included. They then remark that the depression/mortality relationship is spurious: depression is not directly associated with mortality because it is a result of chronic diseases and/or disability. Nevertheless, they concede that they "cannot say with certainty whether the illness/disability preceded the depression change or vice versa" (Roberts et al. 1990:532). Thus, there is some debate in the literature about whether the relationship between depression and mortality is direct, indirect, or spurious.

Zheng and associates (1997), in another study that is based on a non-institutionalized population, examined the effects of major depression on the risk of all-cause mortality using the National Health Initerview Survey Mental Health Supplement (NHIS-MH), the same data set we employ, but linked to follow-up death data only through the year 1991. Compared to their counterparts without a major depression in the previous year, depressed males were 3.1 times more likely to die, and depressed females were 1.7 times more likely to die, controlling for age, education, marital status, and body mass. Their results did not change substantially with self-reported health information, or for those who reported a doctor's diagnosis of major depression (Zheng et al. 1997). Bruce and Leaf (1989) obtained similar results for adults aged 55 and over in the New Haven Epidemiologic Catchment Area (ECA) project.

We expand previous results by examining adults aged 18 and over instead of ages 25 or 55 and over; adjusting for functional, instrumental, and social limitations due to the disorder; determining the effects of family members possessing mental disorders, and presenting results for overall and cause-specific mortality. Moreover, we can test whether the relationship between mental disorders and mortality is direct, indirect, or spurious, since we have questions that ascertain whether mental disorders have caused limitations in work, maintaining instrumental activities, and interpersonal relationships.

DATA AND METHODS

One clear reason for the paucity of studies on the relationship between mental and addictive disorders and mortality has been the lack of relevant data. Fortunately, in 1989 the National Center for Health Statistics (NCHS) fielded the NHIS-MH, which collected information on mental and addictive disorders for a total of 116,929 individuals, including 84,572 adults aged 18 and over (NCHS 1992a). The questions, which revolve around specific disorders, addictions, limitations, and treatments, are especially well suited for our purposes. Linked to National Death Index (NDI) data through 1995, this analysis includes 539,004 person years and 5,155 deaths.

The NHIS is based on the noninstitutionalized adult population of the United States. Because it excludes individuals who are in mental institutions, long-term care institutions, prisons, and nursing homes, it will tend to lower estimates of mental illness more than do clinical studies or estimates from national studies that include the institutionalized population. Moreover, two major differences between the institutionalized and noninstitutionalized population are likely to be the severity and the control of their mental condition; individuals with severe mental and addictive disorders who cannot control their condition are more likely to require institutionalization.

Respondents were asked whether they had had a mental and/or addictive disorder during the previous 12 months. Because the questionnaire asked about previous bouts, and because individuals may perceive a stigma attached to admitting that they have a mental health problem, this survey may underestimate the prevalence of mental disorders. On the other hand, the survey could overestimate the prevalence of mental disorders if respondents report disorders that occurred in the previous rather than the current reporting year, or if they disclose what they term a mental and/or addictive disorder that would not be clinically so defined. Nevertheless, we believe that the advantages of a population-based study—the large, national, representative character of the data—outweigh the potential disadvantages. Furthermore, individuals are quite willing to report their mental and/or addictive disorders in community surveys, so there is a relatively high level of accuracy in self-reported disorders (see Mirowsky and Ross 1989b).

The first question we address is whether the individual reported a mental and/or addictive disorder in the last 12 months. The disorders we include are schizophrenia, paranoia, manic episodes, manic depression, major depression, alcohol abuse, and drug abuse. If a respondent answered yes to having any of those disorders during the past 12 months, the person was included as possessing a mental or addictive disorder. Thus, we include a summary measure of mental and addictive disorders, along with an examination of the effects of specific disorders on mortality. We devote this chapter to disorders and addictions that individuals could acquire (and could recover from) during their lifetime.

We exclude from the analysis individuals who claimed to have a personality disorder, senility, or mental retardation. Because many individuals are born with and have low probability of recovering from mental retardation, we drop the 248 individuals who mentioned that they were mentally retarded. We also dropped the 201 individuals who mentioned that they possessed a personality disorder, such as being antisocial or obsessive-compulsive. Personality disorders are difficult to define (e.g., excessive cleanliness or neatness), and while important from a social perspective, will most likely have a weak relation with mortality. Last, we excluded 112 individuals who mentioned that they were senile. Senility disproportionately affected older adults, while this study is devoted to adults of all ages. Clearly, future studies could examine the effects of senility on mortality among the elderly.

The respondents are asked to mention any family member who may have had the disorder in the past year. Thus, these responses are self-reported and may not correspond to clinical assessments of the same individuals. But some individuals in the community who have successfully hidden their addiction might better know that they have, say, a drug abuse disorder than would health care personnel who have never dealt with the person. Thus, these data are suitable for our purposes: to examine the effects of self-reported mental disorders on mortality for the U.S. adult noninstitutionalized population.

Some NHIS supplements are based on a sample person, where one person in the family is selected, and all of the questions pertain to and are answered by that sample person. Because information for the MH supplement was collected from everyone in the family, one respondent may have answered for others in the family. Proxy responses may not be as accurate as individual responses. There was a substantial number of individuals who did not know whether the family member had a mental disorder over the last year ($N = 3,702$ or 3% of the total sample). Because there was a consistent unknown response for most all of the mental health questions, we deleted these records from subsequent analysis (including such individuals as not having a mental disorder would artificially bias the sample to represent proportionately fewer individuals with mental disorders than would actually be the case). Some of the unknown responses could be polite refusals, but we doubt that this is the case, because most all of the unknown responses are from proxies, who would not be expected to know about some disorders. There was little refusal to answer questions about mental disorders. For every question, less than a handful of respondents refused to answer (we dropped these few cases). Thus, most individuals are quite forthcoming with answers to questions about mental disorders.

Mental disorders can affect mortality directly and indirectly. For example, mental disorders may impair a person's ability to get outside the house or to maintain independence, and may thereby increase the risk of death. We specifically examine whether the mental disorder prevents a respondent from working, from managing money, from doing everyday household chores, from shopping, or from getting around outside the home.

The focus of the data set on mental and addictive disorders affected how the questions were asked. For example, questions about functional limitations were asked only of those who first responded that they had a mental disorder. Those respondents who did were then asked if they could, on their own and without help, adequately handle "routine matters such as managing money," "doing everyday household chores," "shopping," and "getting around outside the home." Thus, the data set does not capture those who are functionally limited but do not report a mental disorder. Moreover, the limitation may be coincidental to the mental disorder. To measure these relations, we created a set of dummy variables. The referent is those who have no mental disorder (recall that those with no mental disorder were not asked if they had a functional limitation). The other categories are those with a disorder who are not functionally limited, those with a disorder who are limited because of the disorder, and those with a disorder who are limited but not because of the disorder.

We applied similar coding strategies for those who had difficulty forming friendships, keeping friendships, concentrating, and coping with stress. The referent in each of these comparisons is those who do not have a mental disorder. Keep in mind, however, that some of the individuals with no mental disorder may still have difficulty in these realms. The categories are no difficulty, some difficulty, a lot of difficulty, and completely unable.

NHIS-MH asks for the number of family members in the household with a known mental disorder, with a range from none to five members. The effects on mortality should vary depending on whether the sample person or other family members have the disorder and on the total number of household members who have disorders. Therefore, we distinguish among families where (a) no one in the family has a mental disorder (the referent); (b) one person in the family has a mental disorder but is not the sample person; (c) one person in the family has a disorder and is the sample person; (d) two or more family members have the disorder but neither is the sample person; and (e) two or more family members have the disorder and one of them is the sample person.

We generally use the same cause-of-death coding scheme applied to the other chapters and discussed in Chapter 2. But in this chapter, we separate suicide (ICD E950-E959) from other social pathologies. Because mental and addictive disorders are directly linked to suicide (see, for example, Brown and Birthwhistle 1996; Lipsedge 1996), there are compelling reasons to separately examine this particular cause. Overall, this data set includes 2,152 deaths due to circulatory diseases, 1,458 to cancer, 462 to respiratory diseases, 279 to social pathologies not including suicides, 77 to suicides, and 727 to other causes.

RESULTS

Table 12.1 presents the percentages of individuals in the survey who survived and died during the period, who acknowledged having mental disorders. About 2% of the sample reported that they had a mental disorder. The prevalence rates in the sample are similar to those reported in other studies and general population estimates. For example, in calculations not

TABLE 12.1   Percentages of U.S. Adults with Mental and Addictive Disorders Who Survived or Who Died during the Period 1989–1995

Disorder reported	Alive (%)	Dead (%)
Mental and/or addictive disorders	1.7	2.4
Schizophrenia/paranoid-delusional	0.3	0.7
Manic episodes and depression	1.2	1.8
Alcohol abuse	0.4	0.5
Drug abuse	0.2	0.1
Unweighted person year totals	539,004	5,096

Sources: NCHS 1992a, 1997b.

shown, the prevalence rate in the sample for schizophrenia is .2%, compared to reported rates of .15% (see Kahn and Fawcett 1993). Manic depression is listed at .2%, compared to a maximum of .4% (see APA 1994). Note that because some individuals report multiple disorders, the overall percentage of mental and/or addictive disorders is smaller than the sum of individual disorder percentages.

Table 12.2 shows the risk of death for those with mental and addictive disorders. In Model 1, which controls for the basic demographic variables, individuals who reported a mental disorder are 2.3 times more likely to die than those with no mental disorder. Individuals are more likely to be psychologically distressed if they are unmarried, less educated, and poorer (Mirowsky and Ross 1989b). Models that control for marital status (Model 2), education (Model 3), and income (Model 4) diminish but do not eradicate the relationship between mental illness and mortality. Indeed, Model 4 shows that even if all three of these factors are controlled, compared to those with no mental illness, those with a mental illness are twice as likely to die in the follow-up period.

TABLE 12.2   Odds Ratios of Mental Disorder Reported and Mortality, U.S. Adults, 1989–1995[a]

	Model 1	Model 2	Model 3	Model 4	Model 5
Disorder reported	2.29*	2.16*	2.12*	2.02*	1.39*
Sociodemographic status					
Age (single years)	1.08*	1.08*	1.08*	1.08*	1.08*
Sex (1 = male)	1.69*	1.83*	1.82*	1.86*	1.85*
Race (1 = black)	1.75*	1.67*	1.58*	1.49*	1.36*
Marital status					
Currently married		ref	ref	ref	ref
Previously married		1.28*	1.26*	1.21*	1.24*
Never married		1.63*	1.64*	1.53*	1.61*
Socioeconomic status					
Education					
Less than 12 years education			1.41*	1.19*	1.01
High school graduate			1.19*	1.09+	1.02
Some college			ref	ref	ref
Income equivalence				0.85*	0.92*
Health status (continuous)					1.44*
−2*Log-likelihood	41,818.90	41,727.44	41,660.14	41,580.93	40,889.73

Sources: NCHS 1992a, 1997b.
[a] Mental disorders reported include mentions of schizophrenia, paranoia, manic episodes, manic depression, major depression, alcohol abuse, or drug abuse.
$+p \le .10$, $*p \le .05$.

Model 5 includes a control for health status. Since mental health is one of several dimensions that comprise health status, it is questionable whether these two measures should be included in the same model. We include both here to determine the degree to which these two variables are interrelated. Once health status is controlled, the risk of death associated with mental disorders is further attenuated. This suggests that individuals who report a compromised health status may do so because of known mental problems, in addition to known physical problems. Because mental disorders and health status are interrelated, and because this chapter's focus is on mental disorders, we do not include health status in subsequent tables (for more detail regarding perceived health status, refer to Chapter 10).

Mental disorders include a variety of maladies, which may act differently to affect mortality. Table 12.3 examines the effects of specific disorder categories on mortality. Generally, the presence of a mental disorder increases

TABLE 12.3 Odds Ratios of Specific Mental and Addictive Disorders and Mortality, U.S. Adults, 1989–1995[a]

	Model 1	Model 2	Model 3	Model 4
Mental and/or addictive disorders				
Cognitive disorders	2.33*			
Affective disorders		2.18*		
Alcohol abuse			2.17*	
Drug abuse				2.14
Sociodemographic status				
Age (single years)	1.08*	1.08*	1.08*	1.08*
Sex (1 = male)	1.86*	1.86*	1.85*	1.86*
Race (1 = black)	1.47*	1.49*	1.47*	1.47*
Marital status				
Currently married	ref	ref	ref	ref
Previously married	1.21*	1.21*	1.21*	1.22*
Never married	1.53*	1.54*	1.55*	1.54*
Socioeconomic status				
Education				
Less than 12 years education	1.19*	1.19*	1.19*	1.19*
High school graduate	1.09+	1.09+	1.09+	1.09+
Some college	ref	ref	rcf	ref
Income equivalence	0.85*	0.85*	0.85*	0.85*
−2*Log-likelihood	41,608.92	41,590.93	41,612.79	41,619.71

Sources: NCHS 1992a, 1997b.

[a] Cognitive disorders include mentions of schizophrenia or paranoia. Affective disorders include mentions of manic episodes, manic depression, or major depression.

$+p \leq .10$, $*p \leq .05$.

the risk of death more than twofold (see also Figure 12.1). For example, compared to individuals with no cognitive disorders, individuals with cognitive disorders (e.g., schizophrenia or paranoia) are 2.3 times more likely to die (Model 1). Similarly, compared to those with no affective disorders, those with affective disorders (e.g., manic-depressives) are 2.2 times more likely to die (Model 2). Abusers of alcohol and drugs also experience heightened mortality risks. For instance, compared to those who do not report drug abuse, those who report abusing drugs are 2.1 times more likely to die (Model 4).

One of the avenues through which mental disorders may operate to increase the risk of death is limitation in usual daily activities. Of central importance is the ability to work regularly. In Table 12.4, Model 1 shows that compared to individuals who can work, individuals who cannot work because of a mental disorder are 2.6 times more likely to die. Even if education and income are controlled, individuals who are prevented from working because of mental disorders are over twice as likely to die (Model 2).

Often, it is not only the ability to work, but the ability to perform a myriad of other day-to-day functions that increases longevity. This is confirmed with the data in Table 12.5. Some individuals have difficulty taking care of routine money matters, everyday household chores, shopping, and getting around outside of their homes. These limitations may or may not be due to the disorders. Recall that only those individuals who had mental disorders

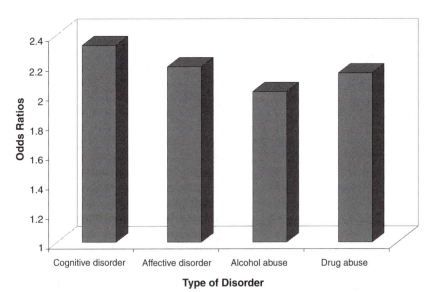

FIGURE 12.1   Odds ratios of dying by specific mental and addictive disorders, U.S. adults, 1989–1995. Cognitive disorders reported include mention of schizophrenia or paranoia. Affective disorders include mention of manic episodes, manic depression, or major depression. Note: Referent for each disorder is those without the disorder.

TABLE 12.4   Odds Ratios of Mental Disorder Limitations and Mortality, U.S. Adults, 1989–1995

	Model 1	Model 2
Work limitations due to disorder		
Prevent from working	2.64*	2.30*
Sociodemographic status		
Age (single years)	1.08*	1.08*
Sex (1 = male)	1.82*	1.86*
Race (1 = black)	1.66*	1.48*
Marital status		
Currently married	ref	ref
Previously married	1.28*	1.21*
Never married	1.64*	1.54*
Socioeconomic status		
Education		
Less than 12 years education		1.19*
High school graduate		1.09+
Some college		ref
Income equivalence		0.85*
−2*Log-likelihood	41,752.72	41,604.29

Sources: NCHS 1992a, 1997b.
$+p \leq .10$, $*p \leq .05$.

were asked if they also had limitations, so the persons reporting limitations are not representative of the entire sample. Even within this scheme, however, individuals may have a mental disorder but no limitation, may have a mental disorder and a limitation that is caused by the disorder, or may have a mental disorder and a limitation that is not caused by the disorder. There is a general mortality gradient from low mortality for those with no mental disorders to increasingly higher mortality first for those who are mentally impaired but not limited; next for those who are functionally limited because of the disorder; and last for those who are mentally impaired and limited, but not limited because of the mental disorder (see Figure 12.2). For example, compared to those with no mental disorders, those with a mental disorder but no limitation in getting around outside are 44% more likely to die, those with a mental disorder who cannot get outside because of the mental disorder are 3.2 times more likely to die, and those with mental disorders who cannot get around outside the home because of other limitations not caused by the disorders are 4.8 times more likely to die (Model 4). We posit that people in the latter group may have multiple mental and physical problems caused by multiple factors, which may exacerbate any problem and may complicate any treatment.

TABLE 12.5   Odds Ratios of Mental Disorders, Level of Independence, and Mortality, U.S. Adults, 1989–1995

	Model 1	Model 2	Model 3	Model 4
Mental disorder and level of independence				
Can adequately handle:				
Managing money				
No disorder	ref			
Disorder, not limited	1.81*			
Disorder, limited	2.77*			
Limited, not due to disorder	2.26+			
Everyday household chores				
No disorder		ref		
Disorder, not limited		1.32+		
Disorder, limited		4.31*		
Limited, not due to disorder		4.18*		
Shopping				
No disorder			ref	
Disorder, not limited			1.31	
Disorder, limited			2.84*	
Limited, not due to disorder			5.01*	
Getting around outside the home				
No disorder				ref
Disorder, not limited				1.44*
Disorder, limited				3.25*
Limited, not due to disorder				4.82*
Sociodemographic status				
Age (single years)	1.08*	1.08*	1.08*	1.08*
Sex (1 = male)	1.86*	1.87*	1.86*	1.88*
Race (1 = black)	1.49*	1.48*	1.49*	1.22*
Marital status				
Currently married	ref	ref	ref	ref
Previously married	1.21*	1.21*	1.21*	1.20*
Never married	1.53*	1.53*	1.53*	1.42*
Socioeconomic status				
Education				
Less than 12 years education	1.18*	1.19*	1.19*	1.19*
High school graduate	1.09+	1.09+	1.09+	1.06
Some college	ref	ref	ref	ref
Income equivalence	0.85*	0.85*	0.85*	0.84*
−2*Log-likelihood	41,579.52	41,566.09	41,569.31	47,722.88

Source: NCHS 1992a, 1997b.
+$p \leq .10$, *$p \leq .05$.

Mental disorders can also affect the ability to socialize and to deal with general daily issues. Table 12.6 shows that there is a mortality gradient for the ability to form and keep friendships (see also Figure 12.3). Compared to individuals with no known mental disorders, those with a disorder who

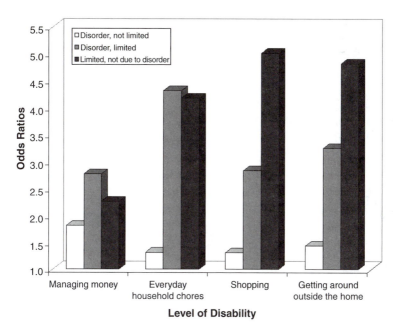

FIGURE 12.2   Odds ratios of dying by mental disorder and level of independence, U.S. adults, 1989–1995. Note: Referent is no disorder reported.

have no difficulty forming friendships are about 70% more likely to die, those who have a some difficulty are twice as likely to die, and those who have a lot of difficulty forming friendships are three times more likely to die (Model 1). Similar results for those with trouble keeping friendships are obtained for Model 2. Furthermore, individuals who have trouble concentrating and who have difficulty coping with stress because of a mental disorder show similarly high risks (Models 3 and 4).

Mental disorders are also more life threatening if they afflict both the respondent and others in the family. In Table 12.7, Model 2 shows that compared to those with no mental disorders in the family, those individuals who do not themselves have a mental disorder but who have one or more family members with a mental disorder do not have significantly higher mortality. But individuals who do have a mental disorder have lower mortality if they are the only person in the family to have the disorder. Compared to those with no disorder, those who have a mental disorder and are the only person in the family to experience a mental disorder have 92% higher mortality, but those who have a mental disorder and also have other family members who have a disorder are over three times more likely to die (Model 2).

Finally, mental disorders increase the risk of death from most causes of death (see Table 12.8). Indeed, compared to those with no mental disor-

TABLE 12.6   Odds Ratios of Mental Disorders, Related Difficulties, and Mortality, U.S. Adults, 1989–1995[a]

	Model 1	Model 2	Model 3	Model 4
Mental disorders and related social difficulties				
Forming friendships				
No known disorder	ref			
No difficulty	1.69*			
Some difficulty	2.04*			
A lot of difficulty	3.20*			
Completely unable	2.04+			
Keeping friendships				
No known disorder		ref		
No difficulty		1.62*		
Some difficulty		2.39*		
A lot of difficulty		3.35*		
Completely unable		2.11+		
Concentrating				
No known disorder			ref	
No difficulty			1.68*	
Some difficulty			2.23*	
A lot of difficulty			2.13*	
Completely unable			2.47+	
Coping with stress				
No known disorder				ref
No difficulty				1.21*
Some difficulty				2.46*
A lot of difficulty				2.10*
Completely unable				2.82*
Sociodemographic status				
Age (single years)	1.08*	1.08*	1.08*	1.08*
Sex (1 = male)	1.86*	1.86*	1.86*	1.87*
Race (1 = black)	1.48*	1.48*	1.49*	1.49*
Marital status				
Currently married	ref	ref	ref	ref
Previously married	1.21*	1.21*	1.21*	1.21*
Never married	1.52*	1.53*	1.53*	1.53*
Socioeconomic status				
Education				
Less than 12 years education	1.19*	1.19*	1.19*	1.19*
High school graduate	1.09+	1.09+	1.09+	1.06
Some college	ref	ref	ref	ref
Income equivalence	0.85*	0.85*	0.85*	0.85*
−2*Log-likelihood	41,579.93	41,580.08	41,585.93	41,577.66

Sources: NCHS 1992a, 1997b.

[a] Mental disorders reported include mentions of schizophrenia, paranoia, manic episodes, manic depression, major depression, alcohol abuse, or drug abuse.

$+p \leq .10$, $*p \leq .05$.

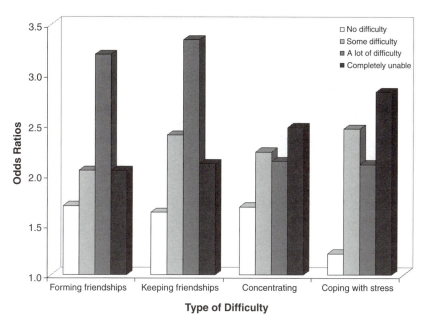

FIGURE 12.3 Odds ratios of dying by mental disorders and related difficulties, U.S. adults, 1989–1995. Mental disorders reported include mention of schizophrenia, paranoia, manic episodes, manic depression, major depression, alcohol abuse, or drug abuse. Note: Referent is no disorder reported.

ders, those with mental disorders are about 70% more likely to die from circulatory diseases, four times more likely to die from respiratory diseases, three times more likely to die from residual causes, and over three times more likely to die from suicide (note that the relation between mental disorders and social pathologies that do not include suicide is low but not significant). The high risk of suicide is consistent with the notion that individuals who are depressed, paranoid, or have problems with other mental and addictive disorders are more likely to take their own lives.

CONCLUSION

Few previous studies have examined the effects of mental and addictive disorders on mortality, especially within the noninstitutionalized population. NCHS was prescient in providing such important data. Our findings highlight the importance of mental and addictive disorders on the risk of death.

Compared to individuals without mental disorders, those with mental disorders have more difficulty in maintaining functional independence (in

TABLE 12.7   Odds Ratios of Mental Disorders among Family Members and Mortality, U.S. Adults, 1989–1995[a]

	Model 1	Model 2
Number of family members with mental disorder		
None	ref	ref
1 member, not self	1.31+	1.25
1 member, is self	2.05*	1.92*
2+ members, not self	0.67	0.64
2+ members, 1 is self	3.54*	3.19*
Sociodemographic status		
Age (single years)	1.08*	1.08*
Sex (1 = male)	1.83*	1.86*
Race (1 = black)	1.67*	1.49*
Marital status		
Currently married	ref	ref
Previously married	1.29*	1.21*
Never married	1.64*	1.54*
Socioeconomic status		
Education		
Less than 12 years education		1.19*
High school graduate		1.09+
Some college		ref
Income equivalence		0.85*
−2*Log-likelihood	41,718.07	41,573.72

Sources: NCHS 1992a, 1997b.
[a] Mental disorders reported include mentions of schizophrenia, paranoia, manic episodes, manic depression, major depression, alcohol abuse, or drug abuse.
$+p \leq .10$, $*p \leq .05$.

managing money, household chores, shopping, and getting around outside of the house), in social relations (forming and keeping friendships), and in mental processes (in concentrating and coping with stress). Thus, mental disorders directly affect mortality, and also indirectly affect mortality by limiting physical competence, social relations, and mental processing.

Some researchers have claimed that the relationship between mental disorders and mortality is spurious; that chronic conditions and disability produce depression and an increased risk of death (Roberts et al. 1990). But many such studies have not used data that allowed researchers to distinguish between the onset of a mental disorder and its social and health sequelae. The advantage of the NHIS-MH Supplement is that it directly ascertains whether the mental disorder leads to difficulty in working, managing money, engaging in everyday household chores, shopping, getting around outside the home, forming and keeping friendships, concentrating, and coping with stress. Thus, we assert that mental disorders do not appear

TABLE 12.8   Odds Ratios of Mental Disorder Reported and Cause of Death, U.S. Adults, 1989–1995[a]

	Cancer	Circulatory	Respiratory	Social pathology[b]	Suicide	Residual
Disorder reported	1.12	1.71*	4.39*	0.63	3.21*	3.19*
Sociodemographic status						
Age (single years)	1.08*	1.10*	1.10*	1.02*	1.02+	1.07*
Sex (1 = male)	1.61*	1.73*	2.81*	2.88*	4.48*	1.83*
Race (1 = black)	1.73*	1.54*	1.43*	0.93	0.95	1.68*
Marital status						
Currently married	ref	ref	ref	ref	ref	ref
Previously married	0.93	1.18*	1.28+	1.87*	1.91	1.27*
Never married	0.94	1.17	1.55+	2.67*	1.43	2.44*
Socioeconomic status						
Education						
Less than 12 years education	1.12	1.33*	1.21	1.05	0.43	0.95
High school graduate	1.07	1.13	1.07	1.27	0.96	1.11
Some college	ref	ref	ref	ref	ref	ref
Income equivalence	0.98	0.87*	0.72*	0.71*	1.09	0.77*
−2*Log-likelihood	13,978.91	18,285.13	47,53.28	39,62.63	12,95.71	8,217.92

Sources: NCHS 1992a, 1997b.
[a] Mental disorders reported include mentions of schizophrenia, paranoia, manic episodes, manic depression, major depression, alcohol abuse, or drug abuse.
[b] Social pathologies listed here do not include suicides.
$+p < .10, *p < .05.$

to be spuriously related to mortality; instead, they can directly contribute to mortality through, most notably suicide, and indirectly contribute to mortality through high blood pressure, heart disease, chest pains, shortness of breath, disability, poor perceived health status, exacerbated problems with diabetes and other chronic conditions through mismanagement, and risky behaviors, including excessive drinking, risky driving, and chronic smoking.

The mortality gap that we revealed is most likely artificially small because of the manner in which the questions were asked. For example, compared to those with no known mental disorders, those with a mental disorder who have difficulty keeping friendships are over twice as likely to die. But some individuals who have no known mental disorder have some or a lot of difficulty making and keeping friends, or are completely unable to keep friends. Thus, if we could have used as the referent those who were not mentally disabled *and* who had no difficulty keeping friendships, the mortality gap would probably be even larger.

Family relations affect mental disorders. Individuals who do not themselves have a mental disorder do not suffer higher mortality if they live with others who do. In fact, they most likely help the person(s) with the mental disorder. Other family members can act as role models and stabilizing forces. Moreover, family members can help individuals with mental illnesses by providing social support and social control. If necessary, family members can provide emotional, instrumental, and financial support. Family members may be able to help the mentally disabled individual to cope, to handle stress, and to maintain a regular regime, if needed, in taking psychotropic medication.

But if the respondent has a mental disorder and lives with other family members who also have mental disorders, much of this support may not be forthcoming. Role models may be lacking, and individuals in the family may experience the negative aspects of social control. Family members in general may experience more emotional turmoil, increased disruptive behavior, increased stress, and inappropriate coping strategies. And family members with alcohol and drug problems may encourage others to get involved in alcohol and drugs. Further, families with multiple members with mental disorders may be limited in the family income they can generate, which creates an economic disadvantage. Thus, multiple family members with mental and/or addictive disorders may interact to create additional problems, ultimately leading to higher risks of death for all members.

Mental disorders are linked to health status. Recall that health status is a summary measure that includes physical as well as mental conditions (see Chapter 10). Much previous research has not fully accounted for the power of health status in affecting mortality. Indeed, several researchers have stated that they were perplexed at how health status appeared to tap more than the clinical manifestation of disease (Idler and Benyamini 1997).

These results suggest that health status may also include an assessment of mental health, which we show to be strongly associated with mortality.

Although we have demonstrated a strong and persistent effect between mental disorders and mortality, we must remain mindful that the root causes and solutions to some disorders are social and environmental (Mirowsky and Ross 1989a). For example, Friedman (1998:xviii) remarks that "stress is increasingly recognized as a complex interaction of the person, the environment, the social support structure, and the culture." Environmental stresses—overcrowding, high crime rates, disorganized communities—along with social strains—difficult interpersonal relations with spouses, children, friends, or neighbors—can trigger mental disorders. While drug treatment and psychotherapy may control the mental disorders, they may not eradicate the root causes. The root problems may only be remedied through social intervention at the interpersonal level and through sociostructural change at the environmental level.

Mental disorders both directly and indirectly increase the risk of overall and cause specific mortality. Our results confirm previous studies, which demonstrate a heightened risk of death due to circulatory diseases, hyperimmune diseases, and suicides (see Eastwood et al. 1982; IOM 1985; Lipsedge 1996; Markush et al. 1977; Vogt et al. 1994). We found increased risk of respiratory diseases for those with mental and addictive disorders. It is possible that individuals with mental disorders are more likely to smoke cigarettes, which contributes to the increased risk of cancer and respiratory diseases. We also found that compared to those with no mental disorder, individuals with mental disorders are 3.2 times more likely to die from suicide. The increased risk of suicide may result from depression, schizophrenia, paranoia, and alcohol and drug abuse.

This chapter highlights the importance of examining the relation between mental and addictive disorders and mortality. Although this chapter provides a strong summary for the major effects of mental and addictive disorders on mortality, it also serves as a call for further research. Future research projects could examine the same relations reported here, but stratified by age, by sex, or by ethnicity (Mirowsky and Ross 1992; Zheng et al. 1997). Mentally ill individuals may have trouble in forming and keeping friendships, in coping with stress, in finding and keeping employment, in dealing with other family members, and ultimately, in ensuring a long life.

13

CIGARETTE SMOKING
AND MORTALITY

Considerable attention has been devoted in recent years to the morbid and mortal consequences of cigarette smoking. In 1964 the Surgeon General of the United States, reacting to a report from an expert advisory committee (U.S. Surgeon General's Advisory Committee on Smoking and Health 1964), announced that adequate research had been conducted to show that smoking was critically related to the risk of survival and he mandated that the statement "Cigarette smoking may be injurious to your health" be placed on cigarette packages. By that time the smoking prevalence rate for men had already begun to decline slightly from its earlier peak of about 54%, but the rate for women had risen to over 30% (Nam et al. 1996). In subsequent years, the proportion of smokers in the general population registered a sustained decline as the Surgeon General's caution was translated into various forms of publicity about the negative effects of smoking and into restrictions on smoking advertising as well as on smoking in public (and some private) places. By 1990 smoking prevalence rates for both men and women had fallen to about 25%. Since then, however, those rates have either stabilized or risen slightly (especially among the younger cohorts) (Nam et al. 1996).

While most persons accepted the Surgeon General's finding about the ill effects of smoking, a substantial minority were skeptical about the contribution smoking made to the risks of dying. The research on which the government's finding was based was scientifically sound, but there were limitations to the study that involved the nature of the populations being analyzed, the generalizability of the findings to all segments of the population, and the role of other variables not specified. The large volume of research conducted since the 1960s, and especially since the 1980s, on smoking and its health and mortality consequences has answered many of the skeptics' questions and has reinforced the initial findings (Friend et al. 1993; Hummer et al. 1998a; Nam et al. 1994; Peto et al. 1995). Yet there are those who still remain unconvinced about the mortal effects of smoking and who point to persisting limitations in the social science and epidemiologic research on the topic.

PAST STUDIES OF CIGARETTE SMOKING AND MORTALITY

Our own earlier research (summarized below) demonstrated that cigarette smoking, particularly heavy smoking, was highly related to greater mortality risks, even when a range of other variables were taken into account. This research augmented a growing body of similar findings from analysts in epidemiology, public health, medicine, and social and economic sciences.

Because prior research on the subject either used indirect methods for estimating smoking patterns or used direct information on smoking behavior but tied it to a limited number of explanatory variables or to restricted geographic areas or limited population categories, we focused our earlier research on a highly reliable, national database that derived from linked records and encompassed a broad range of meaningful analytical variables. We merged three data sets: the 1985 National Health Interview Survey (NHIS)—Health Promotion and Disease Prevention Supplement; the 1987 NHIS—Cancer Risk Factor Supplement, Epidemiology Study; and the 1986 National Mortality Followback Survey (NMFS). The merged database provided us with a large sample of the general U.S. adult population and of decedents circa 1986. The 1985 and 1987 NHIS bracketed the 1986 NMFS and gave us a basis for estimating death rates related to smoking for various population categories.

The overall study confirmed, once again, the negative effects of cigarette smoking on mortality risks and specified the relationships for different subgroups of the population. People who were heavy smokers, and those who quit smoking but at a late stage, were at a significantly higher risk of premature death than those who never smoked, quit early, or smoked only lightly (Hummer et al. 1998a; Nam et al. 1994). Even after controls were instituted for demographic, socioeconomic, and other behavioral factors, the negative survival effects of heavy smoking and late quitting remained (Hummer et al. 1995). From a life expectancy perspective, as of 1986, among those who had lived to age 25, persons who never smoked averaged 81 total years of life, whereas those who smoked heavily to the end of their lives died at an average age of 63 (a gap of 18 years). Those who smoked lightly, and those who quit smoking along the way, died at later average ages than continuing heavy smokers but earlier than never smokers (Nam et al. 1994; also see Rogers and Powell-Griner 1991).

By the 1990s, one-fourth of U.S. adults were currently smoking and another one-fourth had once smoked but had quit. Smoking prevalence was lowest among the youngest and oldest adults. Compared to men, women were more likely to have never started smoking and more likely (if smoking) to be smoking smaller numbers of cigarettes (Nam et al. 1996). Non-Hispanic Caucasian Americans were more likely than Blacks or Mexican-Americans to have ever smoked and to have smoked large quantities of cigarettes. Compared to other ethnic groups, Asian-Americans had low mortality, in part because of low rates of cigarette smoking. Persons with less education and lower incomes were more apt to be smokers and less likely to have quit. Smoking patterns varied by combined characteristics; for example, Mexican-American females were least likely to smoke and non-Hispanic White males were most likely to smoke. Also, Black males and females had higher rates of light smoking than non-Hispanic Whites, but only in the middle age ranges (Rogers et al. 1995).

Recognizing that other behavioral variables could contribute to the mortality effect, we looked at the extent to which high-risk categories of alcohol drinking and relative weight were related to high-risk categories of cigarette smoking among adults. We found, however, that high-risk smokers were not very likely to be simultaneously high-risk drinkers and abnormally overweight, and this finding was largely invariant with regard to age, sex, and education. Moreover, allowing for variability in alcohol consumption and in weight, and controlling for demographic and socioeconomic factors, the negative survival effects of heavy smoking and late quitting persisted (Hummer et al. 1995).

Analysis by medical cause of death was highlighted because publicity about smoking hazards had drawn particular attention to lung cancer deaths resulting from smoking. We found that some form of circulatory disease (heart-related illness or stroke) was by far the disproportionate underlying cause of death associated with smoking. Lung cancer was the underlying cause for only a small percentage of smoking-related deaths. Heavy smokers and late quitters (those who were most likely to have had a serious illness before they stopped smoking) had a great likelihood of dying from lung cancer, but more of them had a risk of dying from a circulatory disease. Since most deaths are tied to more than one medical condition, the relationship of smoking patterns to multiple or combined causes was of interest. Our research showed that smokers are more likely than nonsmokers to have had multiple causes of death. Circulatory diseases dominated multiple causes as well. For example, many of those who had lung cancer at the time of death also had been diagnosed with a circulatory disease. These findings were largely independent of age and sex (Nam et al.

1994; Hummer et al. 1998a). Additional analysis showed that disability was also linked to cigarette smoking. Continuing smokers were 30% more likely than never smokers to have experienced restricted physical activity at work or at home. Even persons who quit smoking were 23% more likely than never smokers to have had such physical activity limitations (Rogers et al. 1994).

Because smoking had once been practiced by a majority of the male population and was still practiced by a substantial minority, and given that smoking was currently leveling off or rising despite attempts to eliminate it entirely, we developed scenarios of future smoking patterns for adults in the United States and modeled their consequences for future mortality trends (Nam et al. 1996). Our projections were based on four alternative smoking patterns (basically, some increase in smoking prevalence, stability, gradual decline, or more rapid decline). We assumed that the links we had previously found between smoking and other variables, including mortality, would continue to hold. We discovered that 2.5 million "excess" deaths would take place in the 2020s alone if prevalence returned to 1983 levels, as opposed to smoking being eliminated by 2020. On a more conservative comparison, 1 million "excess" deaths would be generated in the 2020s if smoking prevalence remained constant at 1992 levels, as opposed to declining moderately (at the 1983–1992 rate of decline). This conservative comparison suggests an "excess" of 5.5 million deaths over the first half of the 21st century. In light of some rise in smoking prevalence among teens and young adults in recent years, we seem to be on course for a very substantial number of "excess" deaths in the years to come.

NEWER ANALYSIS AND ITS SIGNIFICANCE

Although it appears to many that we know most all that needs to be known about the relationship of cigarette smoking and mortality in the U.S. adult population, the data set on which this book's analysis is based can provide superior results in two respects. First, deaths and populations from which they derive are drawn from the same universe and represent a cohort of persons, some of whom smoke and some of whom do not, with risks of mortality that can be differentiated over the follow-up period. Second, some variables not heretofore included in analysis of smoking and mortality are incorporated into the models. While more inclusive statistical models still cannot "prove" the fatal effects of smoking, it strengthens the inference still further in associating cigarette smoking with the risks of dying from it.

In this analysis, we relate smoking status (by amount smoked for former and current smokers) to mortality risk while controlling for age, sex, race, marital status, education, income equivalence, and health status. The analysis is repeated for major causes of death, and some simple interactions between smoking and sex are examined.

MEASUREMENT AND METHODS

The data are drawn from both the 1987 and the 1990 NHIS (which included questions on smoking habits) and related death records from the Multiple Cause of Death (MCD) file through the end of 1995. The 1987 NHIS incorporated a Cancer Risk Factor Supplement (CRFS) for which 22,080 adults in the noninstitutionalized population were interviewed. After some case deletions for missing variables, 1,942 of these individuals were recorded as deceased by the end of 1995. For the 1990 NHIS, we used the Health Promotion and Disease Prevention (HPDP) supplement linked to the MCD through the end of 1995. The 1990 NHIS-HPDP provided a cohort of 41,104 adults for analysis; by the end of 1995, 2,388 of these individuals had died. Both the 1987 NHIS-CRFS and the 1990 NHIS-HPDP contain smoking information. However, only the 1990 data permit the additional examination of a number of other health behaviors critical for mortality risk. Thus, some of the detailed modeling relies only on the 1990 data, while much of the analysis relies on the combined 1987 and 1990 baseline data sets.

Our multivariate analysis relates mortality risks to cigarette smoking and a host of other variables. The dependent variable measures whether persons interviewed in the survey year died between then and the end of 1995. The smoking variable is derived from several questions asked in the surveys. These include a smoking status recode (Never, Former, Current, and Unknown), and the number of cigarettes usually smoked per day (specific number up to 98+, Unknown).

The smoking status classification used in our analysis consists of the following:

Never smoked
Former smoker
  Less than a pack per day
  1 to less than 2 packs per day
  2 to less than 3 packs per day
  3 or more packs per day
Current smoker
  Less than a pack per day
  1 pack or more per day

Never smokers are those who had smoked no cigarettes, or fewer than 100 in their lifetime. Former smokers are those who had smoked at least 100 cigarettes in their lifetime but were no longer smoking at the time of

the survey. Current smokers are those who had smoked 100 or more cigarettes in their lifetime and were still smoking at the time of the survey. A
pack normally contains 20 cigarettes. In some of the analysis, this detailed
classification was collapsed because of inadequate cell frequencies in some
of the categories. For example, relatively few female former or current
smokers smoked 2 or more packs per day; thus, we combined the former
and current smoking categories for that portion of the analysis.

Note also that some aspects of smoking status are not captured in this
classification—for example, age at initiation of smoking, age at time of quitting, type of cigarettes smoked, extent of inhaling, and other forms of tobacco use.

Demographic variables included Age (in single years), Sex (male or female), and Race (Black and other). Marital status was distinguished as Currently married, Previously married, and Never married. Socioeconomic
variables included Education (0–11 years, High school graduate, Some college), and Income equivalence (a continuous measure of family income adjusted for family size). (See Chapter 6 for a detailed discussion of this variable.)

Exercise is differentiated according to regular and not regular. Body
mass index (which is measured as weight in grams divided by height in me-
ters squared) is classified into five categories—top 10%; 80th to 90th percentile; middle 60%; 10th to 20th percentile; and bottom 10%. Alcohol use
is classified into six categories—abstainer or very infrequent drinker; former drinker; current drinker, fewer than three drinks per day and drinks
fewer than three days per week; current drinker, fewer than three drinks
per day and drinks three or more days per week; current drinker, three or
more drinks per day and drinks fewer than three days per week; and current drinker, three or more drinks per day and drinks three or more days
per week.

A general question on health status distinguished among those who regarded their health status as excellent, very good, good, fair, or poor (see
Chapter 10). These responses were treated as a linear scale with excellent
equal to 1 and poor equal to 5. The analysis is repeated for selected underlying causes of death generally regarded as linked to smoking habits (using
1987 and 1990 base samples combined in order to increase sample size)—
circulatory diseases, cancers, respiratory diseases, social pathologies, and a
residual cause-of-death category.

RESULTS

Tables 13.1 through 13.4 rely on data from the 1990 cohort of individuals surveyed in the NHIS-HPDP. Table 13.1 provides the frequency distributions for smoking status according to whether the survey respondent re-

TABLE 13.1   Frequency Distribution of Smoking Status
by Survival, U.S. Adults, 1991–1995

Smoking status	Alive (%)	Dead (%)
Never smoked	49.3	40.2
Former smoker		
Less than 1 pack	8.5	9.9
1 to less than 2 packs	8.8	11.5
2 to less than 3 packs	3.1	5.7
3 or more packs	1.3	3.2
Current smoker		
Less than 1 pack	12.6	11.3
One pack or more	16.3	18.3

Sources: Derived from NCHS 1993c, 1997b.

mained alive or died during follow-up. We note, first of all, that survivors were more likely never to have smoked and, if current smokers, they were more likely to be smoking less than a pack a day at the time of the interview. Former smokers, particularly those who at one time averaged smoking 2 or more packs per day, were also over-represented among the deaths.

The multivariate analysis presented in Table 13.2 summarizes the effects of several variables on the odds of death during the 1990–1995 interval and reveals how robust the smoking effect is by introducing other variables sequentially (see also Figure 13.1). In this table, the categories of former smoking have been collapsed into heavy (20+ per day, on average) and light (<20 per day, on average) for reasons of cell sizes and parsimony. Starting with Model 1, where only age is controlled, we see that, compared to never smokers, all smoking categories have significantly higher odds of dying, with the odds being highest for current heavy smokers. For example, compared to never smokers, current heavy smokers experience 2.8 times the risk of death over the follow-up period. In Model 2, the introduction of sex as a control (in addition to age) serves to reduce the odds ratios of smoking somewhat, but the current and former heavy smokers and the current light smokers continue to have higher odds of dying than never smokers. In Model 3, the further introduction of race as a control has a negligible effect on the effects of smoking. The addition of marital status as a control in Model 4 likewise has little effect on the smoking variables. The next two models introduce socioeconomic factors. In Model 5, the inclusion of education as a control does not change the pattern of odds ratios perceptibly, and in Model 6, the inclusion of income also fails to alter the odds ratios of smoking.

The next three models bring in other behavioral factors. In Model 7 the inclusion of exercise has very little impact on the smoking patterns of mortality. In Model 8 incorporating body mass dampens the odds ratios of

TABLE 13.2 Odds Ratios of Death for Cigarette Smoking and Other Covariates, U.S. Adults 1990–1995

	Model 1	Model 2	Model 3	Model 4	Model 5	Model 6	Model 7	Model 8	Model 9	Model 10
Cigarette smoking										
Currently heavy	2.83*	2.52*	2.59*	2.58*	2.48*	2.46*	2.39*	2.34*	2.35*	2.11*
Currently light	2.44*	2.29*	2.22*	2.21*	2.16*	2.14*	2.13*	2.08*	2.11*	1.98*
Former heavy	1.81*	1.51*	1.56*	1.59*	1.59*	1.59*	1.60*	1.59*	1.59*	1.49*
Former light	1.22*	1.10	1.11	1.12	1.15+	1.15+	1.18*	1.17*	1.18*	1.15+
Never	ref	ref	ref	ref	ref	ref	ref	ref	ref	ref
Age (continuous)	1.09*	1.09*	1.09*	1.09*	1.09*	1.09*	1.08*	1.08*	1.08*	1.08*
Sex										
Male		1.50*	1.50*	1.87*	1.59*	1.61*	1.64*	1.62*	1.62*	1.66*
Female		ref	ref	ref	ref	ref	ref	ref	ref	ref
Race										
Black			1.56*	1.50*	1.40*	1.34*	1.33*	1.31*	1.30*	1.23*
Non-black			ref	ref	ref	ref	ref	ref	ref	ref
Marital status										
Never married				1.44*	1.44*	1.38*	1.38*	1.33*	1.32*	1.43*
Formerly married				1.20*	1.18*	1.14*	1.15*	1.15*	1.15*	1.18*
Married				ref	ref	ref	ref	ref	ref	ref
Education										
<12 years					1.54*	1.35*	1.29*	1.29*	1.26*	1.10
12 years					1.26*	1.17*	1.14*	1.14*	1.13*	1.08*
13+ years					ref	ref	ref	ref	ref	ref
Income equivalence (continuous)						0.88*	0.89*	0.89*	0.90*	0.96+

Exercise										
Not regular							1.38*	1.37*	1.36*	1.24*
Regular							ref	ref	ref	ref
Body mass index										
Top 10%								1.27*	1.25*	1.12+
80th to 90th percentile								1.01	1.01	0.93
10th to 20th percentile								1.17*	1.17*	1.16+
Bottom 10%								1.36*	1.36*	1.25*
Middle 60%								ref	ref	ref
Alcohol use										
Current, 3+ drinks per day, 3+ days per week									1.11	1.17
Current, 3+ drinks per day, 2 or fewer days per week									0.79+	0.86
Current, <3 drinks per day, 3+ days per week									0.85+	0.93
Current, <3 drinks per day, 2 or fewer days per week									0.90+	0.94
Former									1.14*	1.07
Abstain or drink very infrequently									ref	ref
Health status (continuous)										1.43*
−2*Log-likelihood	21,571.8	21,492.6	21,451.1	21,424.4	21,280.4	21,252.4	21,207.0	21,056.8	21,034.3	20,683.4

Sources: Derived from NCHS 1993e, 1997b.

$+p \leq .10$; $*p \leq .05$.

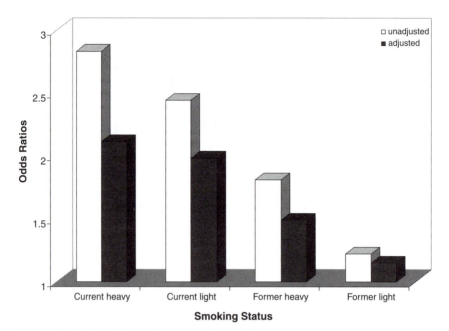

FIGURE 13.1   Odds ratios of dying by smoking status, U.S. adults, 1990–1995. Note: Referent is never smokers.

smoking only slightly, and in Model 9 adding alcohol use to the analysis makes little difference. Last, in Model 10, we introduce health status along with all of the other variables. Because health selection does influence the mortality prospects of people in differing smoking categories, we note some reduction in the odds ratios of dying for the different smoking categories. However, the resulting odds ratios of death for each of the smoking categories remain significantly high relative to never smokers. For both heavy and light current smokers, the odds of dying (after all controls) is about twice that of never smokers. For former heavy smokers, the odds ratio of death is 49% higher than never smokers, and for former light smokers, the odds ratio of death is slightly (15%), but significantly, higher than never smokers. Thus, the robustness of the smoking effect is once again confirmed, even with a large number of control variables included in the model.

SEX DIFFERENCES

Because American women started smoking in substantial numbers much later than American men and continue to have lower smoking prevalence rates, we compared the sexes with regard to the various smoking effects summarized for the total adult population (again based on the 1990 NHIS-HPDP and deaths through the end of 1995). In Table 13.3, note that almost

TABLE 13.3 Frequency Distribution of Smoking by
Sex, U.S. Adults, 1990

Smoking status	Female (%)	Male (%)
Never smoked	56.9	41.0
Former smoker		
Less than two packs	16.9	22.9
Two or more packs	2.4	7.1
Current smoker	23.9	29.0
TOTAL	100.0	100.0

Source: Derived from NCHS 1993c.

57% of women had never smoked, as compared to 41% of men. A smaller
percentage of women were current smokers at the time of the survey, and,
among former smokers, men on average smoked larger numbers of cigarettes.

Since there were differences in smoking patterns between the sexes, we
examined the effect of interactions between smoking and sex on mortality
risk (Table 13.4). Compared to female never smokers, female smokers had
a much greater chance of dying in the follow-up interval. For example, female former heavy smokers exhibited 2.35 times the risk of death over the
follow-up period compared to female never smokers. Further, both male
never smokers as well as male smokers showed greater risk of dying over
the follow-up period compared to female never smokers. Indeed, the fatal
effects of smoking are most pronounced for men who were current smokers at the time of the survey. For example, compared to women who never
smoked, male current smokers were 3.7 times more likely to die during the
follow-up period. These differing patterns of current smoking-related mor-

TABLE 13.4 Smoking Status Differences in Mortality
by Sex, U.S. Adults, 1990–1995[a]

Smoking status	Odds ratios	
	Female	Male
Never smoked	ref	1.88*
Former smoker		
Less than two packs	1.36*	2.03*
Two or more packs	2.35*	2.43*
Current smoker	2.20*	3.68*

Source: Derived from NCHS 1993c.
[a]Controls for age, race, marital status, education, income,
and health status.
$+p \leq .10$; $*p \leq .05$.

tality by sex most likely reflect the unique smoking histories of men and women in the United States (Nam et al. 1996).

CAUSES OF DEATH

Table 13.5 displays the odds ratios of dying for smoking categories by major cause of death categories. These data are based on the combined 1987 NHIS-CRFS and 1990 NHIS-HPDP data described above. This enables us to analyze a larger number of deaths for cause-of-death model-

TABLE 13.5   Odds Ratios of Cigarette Smoking, Other Covariates, and Cause-Specific Mortality, U.S. Adults, 1990–1995

	Circulatory	Cancer	Respiratory	Social pathology	Residual
Smoking status					
Never smoked	ref	ref	ref	ref	ref
Former smoker					
Less than 1 pack	1.05*	1.34*	1.95*	1.06	1.11+
1 to less than 2 packs	1.29*	1.76*	2.55*	.76*	.96
2 to less than 3 packs	1.46*	2.15*	3.36*	1.00	1.04
3 packs or more	1.86*	2.18*	4.35*	.91	1.69*
Current smoker					
Less than 1 pack	1.75*	1.95*	2.78*	1.24*	1.47*
1 pack or more	2.07*	3.61*	3.68*	1.61*	1.59*
Demographic factors					
Age (continuous)	1.66*	1.48*	1.65*	1.05*	1.41*
Sex (1 = male)	1.74*	1.51*	1.81*	4.00*	1.91*
Race (1 = black)	1.11*	1.34*	.70*	1.00	1.45*
Social and economic factors					
Marital status					
Currently married	ref	ref	ref	ref	ref
Previously married	1.36*	1.02	1.16*	1.62*	1.77*
Never married	1.50*	1.02	1.09	1.63*	2.55*
Education					
<12 years	1.27*	1.04	.66*	1.50*	.78*
12 years	1.27*	1.06	.69*	.85*	.86*
13+ years	ref	ref	ref	ref	ref
Income equivalence (continuous)	.90*	.94*	.77*	.82*	.78*
Health factors					
Health status (continuous)	1.46*	1.30*	1.84*	1.25*	1.44*
−2*Log-likelihood = 192,921.0					

Sources: Derived from NCHS 1989c, 1993c, 1997b.
+$p \leq .10$; *$p \leq .05$.

ing. Because the 1987 survey lacked the comprehensive coverage of behavioral variables used in the earlier portion of this chapter, we lack those controls, but maintain controls for demographic, socioeconomic, and health status variables in this portion of the analysis. In this table, never smokers are the reference group for each of the cause categories. We determine the odds of dying from each cause, while excluding those dying from other causes.

Note first the high odds ratios of dying from respiratory diseases and cancer among current and former heavy smokers (see also Figure 13.2). The odds are also high for circulatory diseases and residual causes among heavy smokers. There is also a fairly high odds of dying from social pathologies and residual causes among current smokers, probably linked to accidents and fires among the social pathologies as well as to diabetes among the residual causes.

We further call attention to a distinction between the causes with the highest odds of dying from smoking and the causes with the greatest numbers of persons dying from smoking. For example, although the odds ratios of dying are not as great for circulatory diseases as for respiratory diseases or cancer, the number of smoking-related deaths is highest for circulatory disease because many more persons die of circulatory diseases in the general population.

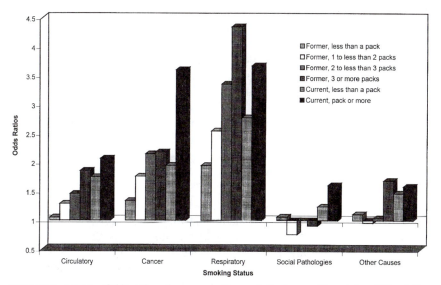

FIGURE 13.2   Odds ratios of cause-specific mortality by smoking status, U.S. adults, 1987–1995. Note: Referent is never smokers.

CONCLUSION

These results show clearly that, even after accounting for several demo-graphic, socioeconomic, health, and behavioral variables, persons who for-merly smoked or currently smoke cigarettes at the time of the interview have an increased prospect of dying over the follow-up period compared to never smokers. This prospect is magnified greatly for persons who smoke large numbers of cigarettes daily. Risks of death are moderate for persons who smoke fewer numbers of cigarettes daily. For former smokers, mortal-ity prospects depend on the volume of their previous smoking and, not shown here, whether they quit before or after contracting a serious illness (Nam et al. 1994). Indeed, many illnesses are linked with cigarette smoking. Because the data examined here are crosssectional, we cannot determine whether smoking causes the morbid conditions that ultimately result in death. But previous literature and the strong associations persuasively sug-gest causal ordering.

The bodily effects of smoking are pervasive. The public links smoking primarily to lung cancer, whereas studies show the extensive effects of smoking on a broad range of diseases and causes of death, including car-diovascular disease and stroke, emphysema, other forms of cancer, dia-betes, and other ailments. In addition, smokers are more likely to have mul-tiple causes of illness and death (Nam et al. 1994). Thus, it is important to balance risk of dying from a specific cause with the increased risk con-tributed by smoking. For example, while there are fewer deaths due to res-piratory causes than to circulatory causes among smokers, the fatality rate due to heavy smoking is much greater for people ill with a respiratory dis-ease than with a circulatory disease.

The interactions between sex and smoking provide additional insight into the sex gap in mortality. The sex difference in mortality was small at the turn of the century, consistently widened until the 1980s, and has since slowly narrowed. Our results—more thoroughly discussed in Chapter 3—suggest that smoking contributes to a substantial part of the current sex gap in mortality. High male prevalence of cigarette smoking through the 1980s coincides with a large sex gap in mortality; reductions in prevalence for males since the 1980s, and increases for females, correspond with a nar-rowing sex difference in mortality.

This indictment of cigarette smoking as a form of behavior that puts peo-ple at great risk of early death has been strongly advanced by the medical profession, the mass media, various health organizations, and governmen-tal agencies. At the same time, the message often overgeneralizes existing research findings. For example, smoking in general is identified as a death risk without consideration of the volume of cigarettes smoked, whereas this and other research shows clearly that the highest mortality risks are associ-ated with heavy smoking while mortality risks for light smokers are not a great deal higher than for never smokers. It is difficult to translate this finding into policy imperatives because some smokers may have trouble controlling their volume of smoking. To the extent that they can, significantly reducing the volume of smoking may be almost as beneficial as quitting smoking altogether.

These findings about the deleterious effect of smoking have received great attention in recent years; however, similar findings of researchers have been presented for a long time without appropriate attention. For example, in 1938, the social biologist Raymond Pearl analyzed medical records that had been amassed at Johns Hopkins University School of Hygiene and Public Health on tobacco use and longevity and reached the following conclusion: "In this sizable material the smoking of tobacco was statistically associated with an impairment of life duration, and the amount or degree of the impairment increased as the habitual amount of smoking increased" (Pearl 1938: 217).

Cigarette smoking, while a critical variable in the risk of death, is of course not the only major risk to survival. The purpose of our overall analysis of the health, behavioral, and social forces affecting mortality is to stress that a battery of factors act both separately and synergistically to determine the time and cause of an individual's death. Smoking exerts a profound effect on that outcome, yet there are other forces acting on the body at the same time. Some of those forces add to the negative effects of smoking, while others serve to counter those negative effects. The complete elimination of smoking from the behavioral patterns of American adults would not extend life expectancy greatly if other deleterious behaviors and biological and social conditions took its place. Efforts to improve health and life expectancy must consider a panoply of policies and programs for health protection and disease avoidance to enable individuals to achieve a higher quality of life. Our analysis shows that moderating or eliminating cigarette smoking is definitely one of those steps.

14

ALCOHOL CONSUMPTION AND MORTALITY

Fermented drinks date back thousands of years, and the consumption of both fermented and distilled beverages has been recorded in virtually all cultures since that time. The alcoholic content of these drinks has had a euphoric effect on individuals and has become associated with festivities, such as birth, death, marriage, migration, and other rituals and important social events (Sournia 1990: 3).

For some persons, drinking alcohol has become a routine not sanctioned by particular festivities, such as the before-dinner cocktail and brews imbibed while watching television shows. For others, drinking has become a means of "drowning one's sorrows" or "escaping from unhappiness."

Traditions of drinking strong liquors, beers, ales, and wines in Europe during the 18th and 19th centuries were brought to the United States with each succeeding wave of immigration. Distilled drinks augmented fermented ones, and excessive drinking of these often led to both private and public drunkenness and loss of inhibition or improper behavior (Sournia: 1990: 27–33).

Alcoholic abuse has had a morbid and mortal impact on both the individual drinker and the community at large. Heavy drinking has been associated principally with such illnesses and causes of death as cirrhosis of the liver, alcoholic psychoses, and suicide, which account for a significant number of deaths, as well as cancers of the mouth, esophagus, pharynx, and larynx. People under the influence of alcohol are likewise prone to automobile and other accidents and various forms of violence, which can result in deaths to both the drinker and innocent others (Thun et al. 1997).

Of course, not all alcohol consumption is deleterious to one's health.

Intake of moderate amounts of alcohol, especially of beers and wines, has been tied to healthier conditions of individuals (Marmot et al. 1981). Limited drinking is believed to result in improved digestion of food, to stimulation of blood and other bodily processes, to an increase in cholesterol-reducing lipids, and to a calming effect on persons' nerves.

Our aim in this chapter is to examine the linkages between alcohol consumption and mortality among adults in the United States during the early 1990s and to determine some factors that may be related to them.

PREVIOUS STUDIES OF DRINKING BEHAVIOR

Based on the 1984 National Alcohol Survey of persons 18 and over, 76% of men and 64% of women drank alcoholic beverages at least once a year. Daily drinkers included 12% of men and 4% of women; an additional 37% of men and 21% of women drank liquor, beer, or wine at least weekly (Hilton 1991a: 75). Drunkenness is usually associated with binge drinking. As many as 24% of men and 6% of women had such drinking bouts at least monthly. Both the incidence of drinking, generally, and the habit of binge drinking, specifically, were greatest for younger adults, slightly higher for white than black adults, and greater for those never married as opposed to those in other marital states. They were also greater among higher educational and income categories of people.

A comparison of drinking patterns between 1967 and 1984 shows a general increase in alcohol consumption, from 38 drinks per month in 1967 to 41 drinks per month in 1984. However, the trend differed among types of drinks, going up for wine and beer and down for distilled liquors (Hilton and Clark, 1991). More detailed analysis indicated that there was an upward trend in heavy drinking, especially among younger adults. The percentage of both men and women who had five or more drinks per sitting as often as once per week went up, as did extremely heavy drinking by men. In both cases, the inclines were greatest for the 21–34 age group (Hilton 1991b).

Midanik and Clark (1994) observed a downward turn in alcohol use between 1984 and 1990, suggesting that drinking habits remain variable over time and may be tied to particular societal stages and events. They found no change in the correlates of alcohol use between 1984 and 1990.

The 1984 National Alcohol Survey was also examined more extensively among Hispanics, blacks, and whites. Among men, frequent heavy drinking was similar for the three groups (though slightly higher for whites), but age patterns of drinking varied. Peak consumption percentages for whites occurred during the 20s, for Hispanics in the 30–39 age group, and for blacks in the 50–59 age category. Among women, frequent heavy drinking was low for all groups, but drinking overall was higher among white than black or

Hispanic women. Among Hispanics, Mexican Americans reported more drinking than did Puerto Rican or Cuban Americans (Caetano, 1991). But among the three groups, Mexican Americans are more likely to drink beer, while Cuban Americans are more likely to drink wine and liquor (Rogers, 1991b).

PREVIOUS STUDIES OF DRINKING AND MORTALITY

Alcohol consumption alone has been tied to mortality risks. Camacho et al. (1987) found that men who were heavy drinkers were at significantly greater risk of death from all causes than were light drinkers, even with eleven covariates controlled. Gordon and Doyle (1988) discovered a strong linkage between alcohol use and mortality from several causes for middle-age men. Klatsky and associates (1992) uncovered similar findings, but found heavier drinking more related to noncardiovascular causes and lighter drinking more related to cardiovascular disease, as had Marmot et al. (1981).

Inconsistent findings have arisen with regard to the shape of the drinking-mortality relationship. According to Blackwelder et al. (1980), the relationship between alcohol use and mortality is U-shaped, even after controls for age, race, height, education, and physical activity, with moderate drinkers having the lowest mortality risks (see also Marmot et al. 1981; Shaper et al. 1988). Shaper (1990) added that 70% of nondrinkers were ex-drinkers, and that they have higher rates of specific illnesses.

Marmot and Brunner (1991) found that having two drinks per day was associated with no cardiovascular harm and may be protective against coronary heart disease. DeLabry et al. (1992) discovered that the incidence rate for overall mortality was lowest for moderate drinkers in each of three age groups, even after prescreening for absence of serious or chronic disease. Groenbaek et al. (1994) found the U-shaped relationship with a nadir at 1–6 alcoholic beverages a week, after controls for age, sex, body mass index, and smoking, and this relationship remained stable over 12 years in a cohort study in Denmark.

Hummer et al. (1995), using data from the National Health Interview Surveys for 1985 and 1987 and the National Mortality Followback Survey of 1986, found that heavy drinkers (those having three or more drinks per day, on average) had substantially higher odds of mortality than never or light drinkers, while moderate drinkers (one or two drinks per day, on average) enjoyed slightly lower mortality risks than never or light drinkers.

More recently, Thun and colleagues examined the link between alcohol consumption and mortality among middle-aged and elderly U.S. adults. They found that moderate alcohol consumption slightly reduced overall mortality, but the benefit depended in part on age and background cardiovascular risk and was far smaller than the large increase in risk produced by tobacco (Thun et al. 1997).

DATA AND METHODS

To determine the relationship of drinking and mortality and the association of other variables with it, we used the 1990 National Health Interview Survey—Health Promotion and Disease Prevention Supplement (NHIS-HPDP), which contains most of the variables in which we are interested, and the linked records of death from the Multiple Cause of Death (MCD) file through 1995. There were 41,104 people in the NHIS-HPDP data set, resulting in 234,921 person-years for analysis. After case deletions for a small amount of missing data, the analysis is based on 2,328 deaths occurring during the 1990–1995 follow-up period.

The NHIS-HPDP contained several items related to drinking behavior. We made use of four of them. "Drinking Status" was categorized into Abstainer, Lifetime infrequent drinker, Former drinker, and Current drinker. For those not currently drinking, "Main Reason for Not Drinking" included No need/not necessary, Don't care for/dislike it, Medical/health reasons, Religious/moral reasons, Brought up not to drink, Costs too much, Family member an alcoholic, Infrequent drinker, Recovering alcoholic, and Other or Unknown. For drinkers, the "Average Number of Drinks Per Day on Days You Drank" encompassed a series from 1 to 12 or more. Information was also available on the "Number of Days Drank Any Alcoholic Beverage in Past Two Weeks" and the responses formed a series from None/never to 14/every day.

In the analysis, the basic drinking variable includes six categories— Abstainer or Very Infrequent Drinker, Former Drinker, Current Drinker of less than three drinks per day (separated into those drinking two or fewer days per week and those drinking three or more days per week), and Current Drinker of three or more drinks per day (separated as in the prior category). In some versions of the drinking variable, those who were Abstainers or Very Infrequent Drinkers and Former Drinkers were classified by their reason for not drinking or not drinking more.

As is conventional in alcohol use surveys of this kind, drinking includes the reported consumption of either beer, wine, or liquor. Each is an alcoholic beverage, but each typically contains different amounts of alcohol. Modern beers usually have an alcoholic content of from 2 to 6%. Most of the wines consumed by Americans (including European and domestic wines) have an alcoholic content of 14% or less. Aromatized wines (such as vermouth) and fortified wines (such as Malaga, port, sherry, and muscatel) may have as much alcoholic content as 15 to 21%. The alcoholic content of brandies, whiskeys, and gin ranges from 40 to 55% (The 1998 World Book Multimedia Encyclopedia 1998). Thus, different individuals drinking the same amount of alcoholic beverages may be consuming quite different levels of alcohol.

Our analysis is based on a series of statistical tables which show drinking behavior and mortality while controlling for several other variables related to both alcohol use and mortality. Table 14.1 describes the distribution of drinking behavior in this sample. Table 14.2 presents odds ratios of dying by drinking category, with successive models allowing for the effects of demographic, social, and health factors. Table 14.3 incorporates the reasons for not drinking. Table 14.4 takes account of smoking behavior in an attempt to see if mortality variations by drinking are accounted for by smoking status. Table 14.5 builds on Table 14.4 by examining the effects of alcohol use on mortality separately by broad categories of underlying cause of death.

RESULTS

The data in Table 14.1 reveal that American adults generally do not drink to excess. In 1990, almost 40% of adults were never or infrequent drinkers or had stopped drinking. The majority of those (both survivors and those who died since the survey) did not drink for general reasons. Another 45% did drink but fewer than three drinks per day, and most of those drank only one or two days in the week. Of the 16% who had three or more

TABLE 14.1   Percentages for Drinking among U.S. Adults Who Survived and Who Died, 1990–1995

Drinking	Alive (%)	Dead (%)
Abstainer or very infrequent drinker		
Don't drink for general reasons	23.4	28.2
Don't drink for health/medical reasons	3.0	4.0
Don't drink for religious reasons	3.2	3.4
Former drinker		
Don't drink for general reasons	6.0	11.7
Don't drink for health/medical reasons	2.2	7.3
Don't drink for religious reasons	1.1	1.4
Current drinker, <3 drinks per day		
Drink two or fewer days per week	35.9	26.3
Drink three or more days per week	9.1	9.2
Current drinker, 3+ drinks per day		
Drink two or fewer days per week	10.7	3.5
Drink three or more days per week	5.5	5.0
Total	100.0	100.0
Person years and deaths	234,921	2,328

Sources: Derived from NCHS 1993c, 1997b.

drinks per day, two-thirds of these consumed them on one or two days of the week and one-third drank that much three or more days a week. Thus, a small minority of U.S. adults would be considered heavy drinkers.

Those in the 1990 sample who died during the following 5 years were much more likely to have stopped drinking at some point, but many of these may have already incurred a serious illness from alcohol or had another morbid condition aggravated by the use of alcohol.

The mortality risks of alcohol are brought out more clearly in Table 14.2. In Model 1, adjusting for the demographic factors of age, sex, and race, cur-

TABLE 14.2   Adjusted Odds Ratios for the Association between Drinking and Mortality, U.S. Adults, 1990–1995

	Model 1	Model 2	Model 3	Model 4
Drinking				
Abstainer or very infrequent drinker	ref	ref	ref	ref
Former drinker	1.35*	1.35*	1.23*	1.23*
Current drinker, <3 drinks per day	0.91+	1.04	1.09	
Drink 2 or fewer days per week				1.08
Drink 3 or more days per week				1.12
Current drinker, 3+ drinks per day	1.18+	1.24*	1.31*	
Drink 2 or fewer days per week				1.06
Drink 3 or more days per week				1.57*
Demographic factors				
Age (single years)	1.10*	1.09*	1.09*	1.09*
Sex				
Male	1.65*	1.80*	1.81*	1.80*
Female	ref	ref	ref	ref
Race				
Black	1.46*	1.25*	1.16*	1.16*
Other	ref	ref	ref	ref
Social factors				
Education				
<12 years		1.41*	1.17*	1.18*
12 years		1.24*	1.15*	1.16*
13+ years		ref	ref	ref
Income equivalence (continuous in $10,000s)		0.88*	0.94*	0.93*
Marital status				
Divorced or widowed		1.21*	1.25*	1.25*
Never married		1.28*	1.40*	1.40*
Married		ref	ref	ref
Health factors				
Self-reported health (continuous)			1.49*	1.49*
−2*Log-likelihood	21,820.2	21,611.5	21,156.9	21,148.4

Sources: Derived from NCHS 1993c, 1997b.
$+p \leq .10$; $*p \leq .05$.

rent heavy drinkers had higher levels of death than abstainers/very infrequent drinkers (the reference group) while current light drinkers had lower levels of death than the reference group. Excess mortality was especially severe for former drinkers, confirming the expectation from Table 14.1.

Putting social factors (education, income, and marital status) into the equation (Model 2) has little effect on the drinking-mortality relationship, except that the survival advantage of current light drinkers disappears. This reflects the better socioeconomic status of light drinkers. Adding a measure of self-reported health (Model 3) slightly reduces the odds ratio for former drinkers and slightly increases the odds ratio for heavy drinkers, but the mortality disadvantage remains high for both groups. Specifying the number of days per week the drinking takes place (Model 4), in conjunction with all of the other variables, serves to isolate the heaviest drinkers whose odds ratio of dying is half again as high as that for abstainers/very infrequent drinkers.

In Table 14.3, the drinking variable is expanded with the addition of reasons for not drinking or not drinking more. For abstainers/very infrequent drinkers, not drinking for health or medical reasons predominates (with demographic and social factors controlled as in Model 1). Among former drinkers, health or medical reasons are even more strongly associated with not drinking. This substantiates the earlier finding regarding stopping drinking. When the measure of self-reported health is included (Model 2), the odds ratios of dying linked to health and medical reasons are reduced, but those reasons are still dominant.

Because cigarette smoking has been shown to have such a major effect on survival prospects (see Chapter 13), we have incorporated that variable into the analysis of drinking effects in Table 14.4. Data limitations prevent us from detailing the smoking variable, as we did in the previous chapter, but we are able to differentiate among never smokers, former smokers, and current smokers.

The odds ratios for the drinking categories (with the smoking variable included) are modified somewhat (compared to the models shown in Table 14.2 which contains the same variables and categories without the smoking factor). This suggests the power of the smoking effect. Yet, even with the smoking variable included in the analysis, the excess mortality of heaviest drinkers persists. The relatively lower mortality of light drinkers is also observed (although not statistically significant). Likewise, the higher odds of dying for former drinkers is reduced by inclusion of the smoking factor, but there is still an 8% excess risk of mortality compared to never drinkers (though not statistically significant).

The set of variables used in Table 14.4 is applied to major causes of death in Table 14.5. These causes include circulatory diseases, cancers, social pathologies, and a residual category. The lower mortality of light drinkers is highlighted for those dying from circulatory disease. Among

TABLE 14.3   Adjusted Odds Ratios for the Association between Drinking and
Mortality, Focusing on Reasons Why Some Individuals Do Not Drink, U.S. Adults,
1990–1995

	Model 1	Model 2
Drinking		
Abstainer or very infrequent drinker		
Don't drink for general reasons	ref	ref
Don't drink for health/medical reasons	1.22+	1.15
Don't drink for religious reasons	0.90	0.86
Former drinker		
Don't drink for general reasons	1.25*	1.19*
Don't drink for health/medical reasons	1.70*	1.38*
Don't drink for religious reasons	1.07	1.00
Current drinker, <3 drinks per day	1.05	1.09
Current drinker, 3+ drinks per day	1.25*	1.31*
Demographic factors		
Age (single years)	1.09*	1.09*
Sex		
Male	1.79*	1.80*
Female	ref	ref
Race		
Black	1.24*	1.15*
Other	ref	ref
Social factors		
Education		
<12 years	1.41*	1.17*
12 years	1.24*	1.15*
13+ years	ref	ref
Income equivalence (continuous in $10,000s)	0.88*	0.93*
Marital status		
Divorced or widowed	1.22*	1.25*
Never married	1.29*	1.40*
Married	ref	ref
Health factors		
Self-reported health (continuous)		1.49*
−2*Log-likelihood	21,596.1	21,149.8

Sources: Derived from NCHS 1993c, 1997b.
$+p \leq .10$; $*p \leq .05$.

cancer victims, light drinking is associated with a higher mortality effect,
but this may occur because those with cancer who had quit their lethal
smoking had turned to drinking before death. Light drinking also seems not
to have provided an advantage for those dying from social pathologies. No
mortality effect is related to drinking for residual causes of death.

   Heavy drinking does not seem to be linked to excess mortality for those
dying from circulatory diseases or for residual causes of death, but it re-

TABLE 14.4   Adjusted Odds Ratios of Drinking,
Smoking, and Mortality, U.S. Adults, 1990–1995

Drinking	
Abstainer or infrequent	ref
Former	1.08
Current, <3 drinks/day	
2 or fewer days/week	0.95
3+ days/week	0.93
Current, 3+ drinks/day	
2 or fewer days/week	0.86
3+ days/week	1.21+
Smoking	
Never	ref
Former	1.36*
Current	2.05*
Demographic factors	
Age (single years)	1.09*
Sex	
Male	1.67*
Female	ref
Race	
Black	1.19*
Other	ref
Social factors	
Education	
<12 years	1.12+
12 years	1.11+
13+ years	ref
Income equivalence (continuous in $10,000s)	0.95*
Marital status	
Divorced or widowed	1.21*
Never married	1.47*
Married	ref
Health factors	
Self-reported health (continuous)	1.46*
−2*Log-likelihood	9,814.7

Sources: Derived from NCHS 1993c, 1997b.
+$p \le .10$; *$p \le .05$.

mains significantly linked for cancers and social pathologies. Unfortunately, we were not able to examine drinking effects on mortality for those
who died of accidents or injuries, separately from other social pathologies.
There was not a sufficient number of sample cases in those categories. Yet,
as noted earlier, excessive drinking has been linked to automobile and
other accidents. Sournia (1990: 162) points out that almost 45% of drivers
involved in a fatal automobile accident in France had blood alcohol levels

TABLE 14.5 Adjusted Odds Ratios of Drinking, and Cause-Specific Mortality, U.S. Adults, 1990–1995

	Circulatory	Cancer	Social pathologies	Residual
Drinking				
Abstainer or infrequent	ref	ref	ref	ref
Former	0.98	1.42*	0.83	0.98
Current, <3 drinks/day				
2 or fewer days/week	0.81*	1.22+	1.07	0.93
3+ days/week	0.73*	1.12	1.28	1.04
Current, 3+ drinks/day				
2 or fewer days/week	0.76	0.70	1.27	0.98
3+ days/week	0.99	1.49*	1.89*	1.08
Smoking				
Never	ref	ref	ref	ref
Former	1.23*	1.75*	0.45*	1.67*
Current	1.97*	2.64*	1.12	2.25*
Demographic factors				
Age (single years)	1.12*	1.09*	1.01*	1.10*
Sex				
Male	1.84*	1.22*	3.34*	1.67*
Female	ref	ref	ref	ref
Race				
Black	1.08	1.32*	0.87	1.42*
Other	ref	ref	ref	ref
Social factors				
Education				
<12 years	1.21*	1.02	1.57*	0.98
12 years	1.16	1.16	0.92	1.05
13+ years	ref	ref	ref	ref
Income equivalence (continuous)	0.93+	1.04	0.91	0.89*
Marital status				
Divorced or widowed	1.15+	0.90	1.55*	1.60*
Never married	1.30+	0.93	1.46+	2.11*
Married	ref	ref	ref	ref
Health factors				
Self-reported health (continuous)	1.46*	1.36*	1.30*	1.69*
−2*Log-likelihood	9,988.9	7,891.6	2,409.0	5,928.3

Sources: Derived from NCHS 1993c, 1997b.
$+p \leq .10$; $*p \leq .05$.

in excess of the legal limit. In the United States in 1995, 50% of all traffic fatalities among persons aged 15–34 were alcohol-related, meaning that either the driver, occupant, or outsider had a blood alcohol concentration of 0.01 grams per deciliter or greater. Between 1985 and 1995, the alcohol-related traffic fatality rate declined 32% for these young adults and fell also for those in older age groups (National Center for Health Statistics 1997a). The decline may be attributed to programs to control highway speeds, DUI roadway checks, and other safety requirements, including stricter use of car seat restraints.

CONCLUSION

While some individual behaviors are beneficial to one's health and survival and others are detrimental to them, drinking alcohol can be both beneficial and detrimental. The effects of drinking depend on a number of factors, including the amount of alcoholic consumption, the presence of other behaviors, and one's demographic and social characteristics. In this analysis, we have attempted to assess the mortality consequences of drinking in the context of some of these other factors. Particular attention has been paid to the association of variables such as age, sex, race, marital status, education, income, self-reported health, and smoking behavior as well as the amount and frequency of drinking alcohol and the reasons for stopping among those who quit or substantially reduced the behavior.

Drinking is not a universal habit among adult Americans. In our 1990 sample, more than one-third were abstainers or former drinkers, over one-third were moderate drinkers (1 or 2 drinks per day), and the vast majority of these drank only 1 or 2 days per week. About one-sixth of the sample were heavy drinkers (an average of 3 or more drinks per day) and a third of those imbibed alcohol on 3 or more days per week.

Taking into account only age, sex, and race as controls for the analysis, the familiar U-shaped curve of mortality by drinking status was observed. Light drinkers had a lower mortality risk than abstainers, and heavy drinkers had a higher risk. Former drinkers had an especially high risk, presumably due to the health problems of many of them that resulted from drinking (a factor borne out by subsequent attention to the reasons given for not drinking or having stopped drinking).

Inclusion of marital status, education, and income in the equation did not modify the mortality risks of the several drinking categories, except that the survival advantage of light drinkers was not sustained. This might reflect the disparity among socioeconomic groups in drinking behavior, with the lower SES categories drinking more heavily, or the drinking consequences of lower SES individuals imparting heavier penalties. The inclusion of self-reported health in the analysis did not change the picture.

Since we have already shown cigarette smoking to be so detrimental to one's survival, the question arises as to how that behavior relates to drinking alcohol in their impact on mortality. We discovered that incorporating smoking habits into the analysis does change the effect of drinking status somewhat. The high risk of former drinkers is seen to be mainly a consequence of many of them being former smokers as well. With smoking controlled, the high mortality risk of former drinkers is reduced greatly. Yet, the U-shaped pattern of drinking behavior remains even when smoking is considered. With all of the variables included in the analysis along with smoking, the heaviest drinkers still have relatively high odds of dying while moderate drinkers have odds that are less than for abstainers (although sample size limitations restrict the statistical significance of that finding).

Moreover, when the analysis is done separately for broad cause-of-death groupings, the U-shaped pattern is found only for those dying from circulatory diseases (heart ailments and stroke), while a relatively high mortality risk is observed for all nonabstainer drinking categories when deaths were due to cancers or social pathologies.

A recent large-scale study of alcohol consumption and mortality among middle-aged and elderly U.S. adults (Thun et al. 1997) led to results consistent with those found here. The large sample of persons 30 to 104 years of age were followed for 9 years to determine which ones died. For both men and women, averaging one drink per day resulted in lower risks of cardiovascular deaths than for abstainers. Heavy drinking did not provide that protection. The benefit of light drinking did not carry over to other cause-of-death categories; in fact, having one drink per day actually increased the chances of women having breast cancer.

Our analysis, and others found in the research literature, leads to the conclusion that moderate drinking can have a beneficial effect on forestalling death from circulatory diseases but not from other causes of death. Heavy drinking, on the other hand, can hasten death regardless of the cause. Furthermore, the effects of cigarette smoking are so great that they overshadow those of drinking. Some benefit of light drinking is observed even when smoking generally is taken into account, but heavy smoking will wipe out any benefit that accrues from moderate drinking.

We have not been able to focus our analysis on the impact of drinking on accidental deaths, but the evidence from other studies linking the two is substantial. Thus, when that fact is combined with the findings we are able to present about drinking behavior and mortality risks, it is clear that the admonition "Moderation in all things" applies equally to both smoking and drinking behaviors.

15

EXERCISE AND MORTALITY

Exercise is an important factor in improving health and reducing the risk of death. The beneficial effects of exercise continue into advanced ages, and work even for individuals who begin exercise programs late in life (Gunnarsson and Judge 1997; Paffenbarger et al. 1993). For these reasons and more, a central national objective is to increase the proportion of individuals who engage in regular physical activity (NCHS 1994c). The beneficial effects of exercise are many. Exercise can reduce the risk of contracting numerous diseases, enhance recovery from chronic conditions, combat obesity, and reduce the risk of limitations in activities of daily living (ADLs).

Exercise is one of a cluster of health behaviors known to influence mortality. Central healthy habits, commonly called the "Alameda 7," include engaging in regular physical activity, never smoking, drinking less than five drinks at one sitting, sleeping 7 to 8 hours a night, maintaining desirable body mass, avoiding snacks, and eating breakfast regularly (Schoenborn 1986). We address or have already addressed each of these behaviors in some detail: exercise, in this chapter; cigarette smoking in Chapter 13; drinking in Chapter 14; and body mass, appropriate sleep patterns, snacking, and eating breakfast regularly, in addition to other important health factors, in the next chapter, Chapter 16.

Most studies that have documented the inverse relationship between exercise and mortality are community-based behavioral risk-factor surveys. Paffenbarger et al. (1986) examined physical activity among Harvard alumni aged 35–74 from 1962 to 1978 and found that individuals who walked, climbed stairs, or played sports experienced lower mortality than those who did not exercise. Hakim et al. (1998) employed the Honolulu

Heart Program Study to examine the effects of walking on nonsmoking retired men aged 61 to 81 years of age. They found that compared to men who walked more than 2 miles per day, those who walked less than one mile were nearly twice as likely to die. Blair et al. (1989) divided a sample of Cooper Clinic patients in Dallas, Texas, into quintiles. Compared to the most-fit quintile, men who were least fit had a relative risk of death of 1.82; those in quintile 2 had a risk of 1.33; in quintile 3, a risk of 1.29; and in quintile 4, a risk of 1.06. Women exhibited a similar gradient. Kaplan et al. (1987) used the Alameda County (California) Study to examine individuals aged 38 and over in 1965. Compared to active individuals, physically inactive ones are 30 to 50% more likely to die.

Not only does exercise reduce the risk of overall mortality, it also reduces the risk of death from cardiovascular disease, cancer, diabetes, and respiratory disease (Blair et al. 1989; Donahue et al. 1988; Helmrich et al. 1991; Paffenbarger et al. 1986). These results are strong and do not appear to be due to selectivity or to other factors. In fact, the exercise gradient in mortality persists even net of hypertension, cigarette smoking, and cholesterol level (Blair et al. 1989; Hakim et al. 1998; Paffenbarger et al. 1986).

To reduce potential selectivity effects, Paffenbarger et al. (1986) excluded individuals who initially reported coronary heart disease; Blair et al. (1989) excluded individuals who at baseline had a history of heart attack, hypertension, stroke, or diabetes; and Hakim et al. (1998) excluded smokers, those still working (who would not have as much time for exercise), and those who were not initially physically capable of at least slight physical activity. These exclusions help to assuage concerns that ill health may confound the relation between exercise and mortality. A further test of selectivity was to examine effects of activity on mortality over successive follow-up intervals. The results remained consistent over each follow-up period, suggesting little confounding by illness; lack of exercise leads to poor health and subsequently to death (Paffenbarger et al. 1986; Blair et al. 1989).

The results of the Alameda County, Cooper Clinic, Harvard alumni, and Honolulu Heart studies are important, but may not be widely generalizable since they select highly educated, older, middle and upper class individuals who live in specific regions of the country. We endeavor to build on this study by updating the results and by using a national sample. This is a major strength of this analysis.

Regular physical activity can prevent and manage a host of chronic conditions, including coronary heart disease, hypertension, osteoporosis and osteoarthritis, obesity, and noninsulin-dependent diabetes mellitus (NIDDM). Physical activity helps prevent NIDDM and benefits individuals with NIDDM because it increases sensitivity to insulin. It is crucial to control if not prevent NIDDM because it contributes to death due to diabetes, kidney failure, and coronary heart disease (Helmrich et al. 1991). Continued physical activity maintains bone density among older athletes (Simonsick et al. 1993). Physical activity can also reduce mental health problems such as anxiety and depression (Gunnarsson and Judge 1997; NCHS 1994c). The added bonus of exercise is that as it reduces the effects of some chronic conditions, it alleviates the need for over-the-counter and prescribed medications. Thus, many individuals will be able to reduce the number of medications they take as they continue with their exercise programs.

Even as the beneficial effects of exercise are touted in the news, the number of individuals exercising remains flat. In 1991 in the United States, among persons aged 25 years of age and over, 30% of women and 25% of men were classified as sedentary, that is, not engaging in any leisure time physical activity during the previous 2 weeks (NCHS 1996b). Exercise is related to other social factors. Generally, those with more education are more likely to exercise (NCHS 1996b).

Exercise helps individuals maintain their ideal body weight. Even though individuals who exercise are less likely to be overweight, the proportion of individuals in the U.S. who are overweight has increased considerably over time. Between 1976 and 1980 and 1988 and 1991, the prevalence of overweight among individuals aged 20–74 increased from 24 to 32% for men, and from 27 to 34% for women (NCHS 1996b). Physical activity contributes not only to better health, but to longer lives.

MECHANISMS THROUGH WHICH EXERCISE REDUCES MORTALITY

PHYSICAL

Exercise reduces mortality for several reasons. Exercise improves strength and endurance. Aerobic exercise—walking, jogging, and aerobics—increases cardiovascular functioning. Exercise can increase blood circulation, improve lung functioning, and strengthen the heart. Individuals who exercise have better left ventricular function (Blair et al. 1989). Such improvements provide a person more stamina, more energy. With increased oxygenation, a person "feels" better. Better cardiovascular functioning reduces the chances of cardiovascular failure. And individuals who are fit are more likely to recover from heart attacks or strokes.

Anaerobic exercise can strengthen a person's muscles. Anaerobic exercise—for example, weight lifting—can increase muscles in the chest as well as the arms and legs. Some individuals who experience difficulty breathing have weak chest muscles. Once they begin an exercise regimen to strengthen their chest, they breathe easier.

Moreover, exercise improves balance, reduces the risk of physical impairments, and contributes to maintaining activities of daily living (ADL), all of which help to maintain or to regain independence (Simonsick et al. 1993). Some individuals who do not exercise do not have the strength to grasp objects, walk a quarter of a mile, carry a sack of groceries, or transfer from bed to chair. Exercise provides the needed strength to maintain these basic activities. Exercise can also make a person more limber; individuals who exercise may be more able to bend or squat to do light housework, to carry groceries, and to transfer from bed to chair. And exercise improves balance and gait and thereby reduces the chance of falls. Exercise programs implemented at any age improve physical functioning (Gunnarsson and Judge 1997). Thus, exercise can help individuals regain lost functioning. Some individuals in wheelchairs have been able to regain their ability to walk with weight training.

PSYCHOLOGICAL

Exercise can provide relaxation, work off stress, and contribute to a sense of worth. Individuals who garden may experience a sense of accomplishment in creating a particularly stunning garden; gardening can also be relaxing, and can even be a form of mediation. Individuals who engage in strenuous exercise can work off aggression, stress, and strain. Much exercise requires concentration, so that individuals shut out other distractions and problems. Exercise can reduce anxiety and depression. Moreover, exercise can improve the perceived quality of sleep and can help cure insomnia (Gunnarsson and Judge 1997).

SOCIAL

Exercise often indicates that individuals are socially engaged. Many forms of exercise are customarily performed in groups, and much exercise encourages people to be involved in the community or to get outdoors. Walking is a way for individuals to get outside and to see others within the neighborhood or community. Moreover, many people walk in groups and thus have others to talk with, to confide in, and to get instrumental support from. Moreover, group members have someone else to check on them if there are problems.

Some forms of exercise, like tennis, require other individuals and thus serve a social function. Exercise can be a way to meet new people. Many clubs offer group lessons or create tournaments, both of which bring people together.

Exercise also includes a comparative element and is related to age. Individuals may endeavor to maintain levels of exercise coincident with their peers. Certainly, levels of exercise experienced by individuals in their 20s are different from those experienced by individuals in their 80s. Thus, we expect that individuals who are more active than their peers will live longer than individuals who are less active. One way to adjust for this is to control for age. But a further elaboration is to control for activity levels for other individuals who are the same age.

CROSS TRAINING

Recent literature has lauded the advantages of cross training, or engaging in several forms of exercise. For example, it should help individuals to engage in both aerobic and anaerobic exercise to both increase lung and cardiovascular function and muscle strength. Rather than walk for longer periods of time, individuals might improve their health more if they walked and also lifted weights. Thus, we surmise that compared to individuals who engage in only one form of exercise, individuals who engage in more than one form of exercise will be healthier and can expect to live longer.

POTENTIAL CONFOUNDING EFFECTS

Some forms of exercise are indirect measures of wealth because they require expensive equipment or membership fees. Golf, for example, requires golf clubs, in addition to green fees and therefore indicates that an individual has discretionary money. In such cases, it is obviously important to control for the effects of income.

More importantly, individuals who do not exercise may want to exercise, but be prevented from doing so because of disabilities, chronic conditions, or poor health. In such cases, inactivity may affect mortality as a proxy for other health conditions and limitations. Individuals who are acutely ill or recovering from surgery may temporarily be unable to exercise; individuals with chronic respiratory conditions—asthma, emphysema, or bronchitis— may be permanently limited in the extent of exercise (especially aerobic exercise) they can tolerate, as may individuals with heart conditions. Furthermore, individuals who are disabled or in poor health may be limited in the forms of exercise they can do or in range of movement. Like individuals who are undergoing rehabilitation, they may be able to exercise only with personal assistance. For all of these reasons, it is important to control for the effects of health status on mortality.

DATA AND METHODS

For this analysis, we use the 1990 National Health Interview Survey (NHIS) Health Promotion and Disease Prevention (HPDP) Supplement, which includes 41,104 adults aged 18 and over (NCHS 1993c). Before asking individuals about exercise, the interviewer determined, from observation or from responses to previous questions, whether the respondent was physically handicapped. If so, the interviewer did not ask about exercise. Thus, we exclude from the analysis 1,197 individuals who were classified as physically handicapped.

Questions about exercise are based on a set of specific and more global questions. A general question asks whether the individual exercises or plays sports regularly. Individuals are also asked whether they are physically more active, less active, or about as active as other persons of the same age.

More specific questions pertain to the 2 weeks before the interview. Although this is a reasonable time frame, some individuals may exercise regularly but have not done so during the previous 2 weeks. Conversely, some individuals may exercise infrequently, but have happened to exercise in the previous 2 weeks.

Individuals are asked "In the past 2 weeks, beginning Monday (date), and ending this past Sunday (date), have you done any of the following exercise, sports, or physically active hobbies?" Respondents are then prompted with 22 different activities, ranging from walking to skiing. We have selected five activities—walking, gardening, aerobics or aerobic dancing, golf, and tennis—that are performed by a large number of people. Some activities, like yoga and skiing, had been performed by too few people over the last 2 weeks. Other activities were disproportionately performed by one sex—for example, football.

Most studies of exercise have taken a public health perspective, employing a medical model of health behaviors, disease, and mortality. Thus, several studies have converted type and duration of exercise into summary measures of kilocalories per kilogram per day (see, for example, Schoenborn 1986). Such a perspective assumes that exercise directly increases cardiovascular and respiratory functioning, strengthens muscles, and burns unneeded calories. While we agree that exercise provides clear and important physiological benefits, we suggest that it also provides social and psychological benefits. Exercise relaxes, reduces stress, contributes to a sense of worth, and encourages social involvement. Moreover, the amount of kilocalories per kilogram per day varies by sex and by age. For these reasons, we examine the actual types of exercise, rather than the amount of kilocalories expended.

RESULTS

Individuals who engage in exercise and sports and who are physically active are less likely to die than those who are inactive (see Table 15.1). Moreover, individuals who are active in specific forms of exercise derive benefits from the exercise. Compared to individuals who do not engage in the activities, individuals who walk, garden, practice aerobics, play golf, and play tennis are less likely to die. For example, fully 27% of the sample gar-

TABLE 15.1   Descriptive Statistics for Exercise for U.S. Adults Who Survived and Adults Who Died during the Period 1990–1995

	Alive (%)	Dead (%)
Exercise[a]		
Exercise or play sports regularly	41.3	26.1
Physical activity compared to others own age		
More active	32.4	30.1
About as active	46.9	47.6
Less active	20.7	22.3
Type of exercise[a]		
Walk	45.8	41.2
Garden	27.0	18.5
Aerobic	7.5	1.2
Golf	4.3	1.7
Tennis	2.6	0.3
Number of above exercises performed		
0	39.2	49.0
1	38.4	39.9
2	18.9	10.3
3 or more times	3.6	0.8

Source: NCHS 1993c, 1997b.
[a]Values do not sum to 100% because they are not totally inclusive.

dened, but among those who died within the time period, only 19% gardened. Individuals who engage in a variety of exercises are less likely to die than those who engage in few exercises. For instance, 22% of the sample participated in two or more kinds of exercise, whereas only 11% of the individuals who died during the period did so. To see how exercise is affected by other sociodemographic factors, we turn to Table 15.2.

Table 15.2 reveals the effects of exercise on mortality, net of other factors. Model 3 shows that compared to those who do not exercise, those who exercise or play sports regularly are 30% less likely to die, even when social, demographic, and economic factors are controlled. Controlling for health status in Model 4 slightly reduces the effect of exercise, suggesting that some individuals may want to exercise, but are limited because of poor health.

Table 15.3 shows a graded relationship between exercise and mortality. Compared to those who are about as active as others their age, those who are less active are 30% more likely to die, and those who are more active are 20% less likely to die. This exercise gap is even larger between the two extremes. Compared to those who are more active than others their same age, those who are less active are over 60% more likely to die $(1 - e^{[\ln(1.30) - \ln(.80)]})$. Thus, maintaining activity levels the same as or higher than one's peers can be important.

TABLE 15.2   Odds Ratios of Exercise and Mortality, U.S. Adults, 1990–1995

	Model 1	Model 2	Model 3	Model 4
Exercise				
Exercise or play sports regularly (yes = 1)			0.70*	0.76*
Sociodemographic				
Age (single years)	1.08*	1.08*	1.08*	1.08*
Sex (male = 1)	1.92*	1.96*	1.96*	1.98*
Race (black = 1)	1.25*	1.17+	1.23*	1.16+
Marital status				
Currently married	ref	ref	ref	ref
Previously married	1.21*	1.25*	1.22*	1.26*
Never married	1.30*	1.40*	1.30*	1.40*
Education				
Less than 12 years	1.42*	1.21*	1.35*	1.17*
12 years	1.25*	1.19*	1.21*	1.17*
Some college	ref	ref	ref	ref
Income equivalence	0.88*	0.94*	0.89*	0.94+
Health status		1.44*		1.42*
−2*Log-likelihood	18,434	18,154	18,389	18,128

Sources: Data derived from NCHS 1993c, 1997b.
$+p \le .10$; $*p \le .05$.

Table 15.4 examines the effects of five specific forms of exercise, both singly and in combination, on mortality. Singly, each form of exercise is significantly related to mortality (see Models 2–6). Model 2 shows that compared to those who do not walk for exercise, those who do are 10% less likely to die; walking increases life expectancy. The more active, aerobic forms of exercise appear to be more beneficial than the less active forms. For example, compared to those who do not exercise, those who walk are 10% less likely to die, but those who engage in aerobics are 45% less likely to die. Moreover, even when the different types of exercise are examined together in one model (Model 7), all confer higher survival and most remain significant. The odds ratios increase slightly, indicating some interrelations among the exercise variables.

Table 15.5 shows an exercise gradient in mortality. Those individuals who engage in multiple forms of exercise experience lower mortality than those who engage in single forms of exercise. Compared to those who do not exercise, those who engage in one form of exercise are 6% less likely to die, those who engage in two forms of exercise are 25% less likely to die, and those who engage in three or more forms of exercise are 55% less likely to die.

Table 15.6 examines the effect of physical activity on cause-specific mortality. Individuals who are more active than others their own age are significantly less likely to die from circulatory and respiratory diseases. For in-

TABLE 15.3 Odds Ratios of Physical Activity Compared to Others
Own Age and Mortality, U.S. Adults, 1990–1995

	Model 1	Model 2
Activity compared to others own age		
More active		0.80*
About as active		ref
Less active		1.30*
Sociodemographic		
Age (single years)	1.08*	1.08*
Sex (male = 1)	1.95*	1.99*
Race (black = 1)	1.16+	1.15+
Marital status		
Currently married	ref	ref
Previously married	1.26*	1.25*
Never married	1.42*	1.41*
Education		
Less than 12 years	1.19*	1.18*
12 years	1.16+	1.16+
Some college	ref	ref
Income equivalence	0.93*	0.94+
Health status	1.45*	1.39*
−2*Log-likelihood	17,609	17,564

Sources: Data derived from NCHS 1993c, 1997b.
$+p \leq .10; *p \leq .05$.

stance, compared to individuals who consider themselves about as active as others their own age, those who are more active are 23% less likely to die from circulatory and 48% less likely to die from respiratory diseases. Conversely, those who are less active than others are more likely to die from most causes of death, save cancer. The exercise gap in mortality would be even greater if the comparisons were between the exercise extremes. For example, compared to those who are more active, those who are less active than others their own age are 80% more likely to die from circulatory diseases $(1 - e^{[\ln 1.39 - \ln .77]})$ and almost three times more likely to die from respiratory diseases. Cancer does not show much of a difference by exercise.

CONCLUSION

Physically active individuals live longer than inactive ones. The form of exercise is less important than the fact that a person exercises; walking, gardening, aerobics, golf, and tennis all reduce a person's risk of death. Indeed, even low-intensity activity increases the chances of longevity (Hakim et al.

TABLE 15.4 Odds Ratios of Types of Exercise and Mortality, U.S. Adults, 1990–1995

	Model 1	Model 2	Model 3	Model 4	Model 5	Model 6	Model 7
Exercise							
Walk (yes = 1)		0.90*					0.92
Garden/yardwork (yes = 1)			0.87*				0.89
Aerobics/aerobic dancing (yes = 1)				0.55*			0.57*
Golf (yes = 1)					0.56*		0.58*
Tennis (yes = 1)						0.49+	0.53
Sociodemographic							
Age (single years)	1.08*	1.08*	1.07*	1.07*	1.08*	1.07*	1.07*
Sex (male = 1)	1.96*	1.96*	1.98*	1.94*	1.99*	1.96*	1.99*
Race (black = 1)	1.17+	1.16+	1.16+	1.17+	1.16+	1.16+	1.15+
Marital status							
Currently married	ref	ref	ref	ref	ref	ref	ref
Previously married	1.25*	1.26*	1.24*	1.26*	1.25*	1.26*	1.24*
Never married	1.40*	1.41*	1.37*	1.41*	1.39*	1.41*	1.38*
Education							
Less than 12 years	1.21*	1.20*	1.21*	1.20*	1.19*	1.20*	1.17*
12 years	1.19*	1.19*	1.19*	1.18*	1.18*	1.18*	1.16*
Some college	ref	ref	ref	ref	ref	ref	ref
Income equivalence	0.94*	0.94*	0.94*	0.94*	0.95+	0.94*	0.95+
Health status	1.44*	1.43*	1.43*	1.43*	1.43*	1.43*	1.42*
−2*Log-likelihood	18,434	18,154	18,389	18,128	18,139	18,149	18,121

Sources: Data derived from NCHS 1993c, 1997b.

+$p \leq$ .10; *$p \leq$ .05.

TABLE 15.5   Odds Ratios of Numbers of Types of Exercise^a and Mortality, U.S. Adults, 1990–1995

	Model 1	Model 2
Number of types of exercise		
No exercise		ref
One type		0.94*
Two types		0.75*
Three or more types		0.46*
Sociodemographic		
Age (single years)	1.08*	1.07*
Sex (male = 1)	1.96*	1.99*
Race (black = 1)	1.17+	1.16+
Marital status		
Currently married	ref	ref
Previously married	1.25*	1.24*
Never married	1.40*	1.37*
Education		
Less than 12 years	1.21*	1.18*
12 years	1.19*	1.17*
Some college	ref	ref
Income equivalence	0.94*	0.95*
Health status	1.44*	1.43*
−2*Log-likelihood	18,154	18,130

Sources: Data derived from NCHS 1993c, 1997b.
^{a} Types of exercise are walking, gardening or yard work, aerobics or aerobic dancing, golf, and tennis.
$+p \leq .10$; $*p \leq .05$.

1998). But some forms of exercise, especially those that are more active, appear more life prolonging than others. For example, compared to those who do not exercise, those who walk are 10% less likely to die, but those who do aerobics are 45% less likely to die.

Physical exertion, or kilocalories per kilogram, may be one of several dimensions that affect longevity. Gardening is not only less active than aerobics and golf, it also can be more socially isolating. Thus, we cannot fully parse out the physiological from the social or economic benefits of exercise. For instance, tennis and golf require individually purchased equipment and collectively financed facilities that are more likely to be available in affluent than in poor neighborhoods. These issues call for future research to sort out the physiological, psychological, economic, and social benefits to exercise in reducing the risk of death.

Similarly, maintaining higher activity levels than one's peers may reflect more than vigorous activity. It can also reflect a perceived relative advantage: individuals may develop a healthier outlook on life and on life's

TABLE 15.6   Odds Ratios of Physical Activity Compared to Others Own Age and
Cause-Specific Mortality, U.S. Adults, 1990–1995

	Circulatory diseases	Cancer	Respiratory diseases	Social pathologies	Residual
Activity compared to others own age					
More active	0.77*	0.87	0.52*	0.90	0.82
About as active	ref	ref	ref	ref	ref
Less active	1.39*	0.98	1.50*	1.30	1.89*
Sociodemographic					
Age (single years)	1.10*	1.08*	1.11*	1.01	1.08*
Sex (male = 1)	1.95*	1.68*	2.99*	3.77*	1.84*
Race (black = 1)	1.03	1.45*	0.39*	0.71	1.94*
Marital status					
Currently married	ref	ref	ref	ref	ref
Previously married	1.18*	0.97	1.41	1.58+	1.59*
Never married	1.25	0.94	0.65	1.49	2.73*
Education					
Less than 12 years	1.29*	1.10	0.86	1.69+	1.02
12 years	1.24*	1.23	0.99	0.90	1.16
Some college	ref	ref	ref	ref	ref
Income equivalence	0.95	1.07	0.85	0.93	0.85*
Health status	1.39*	1.35*	1.57*	1.15	1.46*
−2*Log-likelihood	8,008	6,609	1,979	1,910	3,227

Sources: Data derived from NCHS 1993c, 1997b.
$+p \leq .10$; $*p \leq .05$.

prospects if they perceive that they are faring well relative to their friends of the same age. Thus, it may tap into a positive assessment of their abilities, health status, and life fortune in addition to an empirical comparison of energy consumed during workouts.

Compared to those who engage in few exercise forms, those who engage in a variety of exercises experience lower risks of death. These results parallel the research findings about social roles: that individuals with more social roles enjoy longer lives than individuals with fewer roles. Additional forms of exercise indicate more complex, interrelated social, physiological, and psychological effects. Moreover, many forms of exercise are complementary, so that one form contributes to another, an effect termed cross-training. For example, aerobics classes may contribute to increased stamina and result in a more satisfying tennis game; or friends with whom one walks may also form the pool of golf partners.

Exercise promotes several beneficial health effects. It reduces such mental health problems as anxiety and depression (NCHS 1994c). It also reduces chronic diseases and conditions including obesity, physical limitations, osteoporosis, NIDDM, hypertension, and coronary heart disease (Gunnarsson and Judge 1997; NCHS 1994c; Simonsick et al. 1993). Exercise improves cardiovascular and respiratory function, and thus reduces the risk of death due to circulatory and respiratory diseases. Our results suggest that the risk of cancer is not substantially reduced through exercise, even though others have found an effect between exercise and cancer (Hakim et al. 1998; Paffenbarger et al. 1986). Perhaps larger sample sizes or a longer follow-up would reveal a greater contribution to exercise in reducing the risk of cancer. Our results also show that fatal accidents are not strongly related to exercise.

The research that revolves around limitations in Activities of Daily Living (ADL) is crucial from policy perspectives, but takes a pessimistic view: that large percentages of individuals are limited in their activities. But most individuals, even at advanced ages, are not functionally limited, and many of those who are can regain their abilities. Individuals who are physically active are more likely to maintain their functional independence (NCHS 1994c). Exercise promotes several beneficial effects, including the reduction of the number and severity of chronic diseases and conditions, of excess weight, and of physical limitations (Simonsick et al. 1993). Thus, we suggest that research focus on increasing people's activities, rather than becoming preoccupied with individual limitations.

Much aging research begins with individuals at older ages, yet many aging problems begin with younger ages. For instance, lack of exercise at young ages can lead to circulatory problems at older ages, which can result in functional limitations. We argue for an optimistic perspective that would encourage individuals of all ages to exercise. Social policies that encourage exercise may have a greater national impact than social policies regarding ADLs. In the long run, exercise policies may be cheaper, affect more people, reduce chronic conditions, further reduce limitations in ADLs, and encourage individuals with limitations to regain and then maintain their abilities. Moreover, the benefits of exercise are touted, even for those who begin exercise programs later in life (Paffenbarger et al. 1993).

This chapter has focused on the benefits of exercise by examining physical activity, type of activity, activity relative to peers, and numbers of different activities. We found strong relations between exercise and mortality. These relations are slightly diminished, but remain with controls for other health behaviors. Indeed, the following chapter, which examines other health behaviors, demonstrates that the effects of exercise on mortality persist, even with controls for demographic factors, economic variables, self-perceived health status, body mass, eating breakfast, eating between meals, efforts to reduce cholesterol, average hours of sleep per night, seat belt use, smoking, and drinking (see chapter 16, Table 16.3).

The five representative sports activities that we selected all significantly relate to mortality. We expect that other activities would exhibit similar relations, and that sex-specific activities should also show clear relations with mortality. For clarity, we examined the actual sports. Future research could, through factor analysis or other similar techniques, examine sets of factors related to mortality. This would be one way to parcel out the effects of social versus physical, aerobic versus anaerobic, or individual versus group forms of exercise. Regardless of the method applied, the results are clear: exercise promotes health, prevents disease, and prolongs life.

16

THE INFLUENCE OF OTHER HEALTH BEHAVIORS ON MORTALITY

Epidemiologic transition theory posits that, over time and in three stages, disease patterns shift so that infections and parasitic diseases are gradually, but not completely, displaced by chronic and degenerative diseases as the leading causes of death in developed countries (Omran 1971, 1983). At the same time, the focus of mortality causation shifts from macro environmental, sanitation, and developmental factors that affect persons of all ages, but particularly infants and children, to more individually based health behaviors, operating in large part among the adult population.

Indeed, a more recent update of epidemiologic transition theory suggests that the United States is now most likely in a fourth stage of epidemiologic transition—the hybristic stage—which focuses on changes in behaviors such as physical activity, dietary practices, sexual behaviors, alcohol use, and cigarette smoking for understanding the current mortality pattern of dominating, but declining, chronic disease mortality (Rogers and Hackenberg 1987; see also Olshansky and Ault 1986).

It is also of note that these health behaviors are seen as critical for nonchronic causes of death as well, such as accidents and homicides (Rogers and Hackenberg 1987). As a consequence, much research in medicine, public health, and demography has focused on health behaviors as precursors of adult mortality in developed nations, and it is widely accepted that such behaviors have important impacts on the length and quality of life for U.S. individuals.

Three of these behaviors—cigarette smoking, alcohol consumption, and exercise—have already been discussed in preceding chapters. We have observed that, to varying degrees, each of these behaviors has a significant relationship to the risks of death. Cigarette smoking is associated with the largest number of deaths in developed countries and is thought to be the single most preventable behavior in the fight against chronic disease (Peto et al. 1995). Our own work shows that mortality variations related to cigarette smoking remain exceptionally wide (Hummer et al. 1998a) and that, if current trends continue, one million excess deaths in the United States could result in each decade between 2020 and 2050 (Nam et al. 1996). Moreover, heavy smoking has profound negative consequences for survival, and light smoking has a deleterious but lesser effect.

Heavy drinking is seen to raise mortality risks, both by endangering the normal function of the liver and other bodily organs and by putting automotive drivers at greater risk of fatal accidents. Light drinking actually produces a positive effect.

Likewise, various forms of exercise have positive effects on health and survival. Several studies have found that physical activity is an important behavioral risk factor for adult mortality (e.g., Blair et al. 1989; Paffenbarger et al. 1986). While the form of activity is less important than the fact a person is active, some forms of exercise appear to exert greater influences than others. For example, compared to those who do not regularly exercise, those who regularly walk are 8% less likely to die, but those who regularly do aerobics are 43% less likely to die over a given time period. These physical behaviors exert associations with mortality net of one another and in multiple forms—such as the number of activities one is involved in or one's self-assessment of activity in comparison to others of the same age.

OTHER HEALTH RISK BEHAVIORS

Heavy cigarette smoking, drinking alcohol excessively, and lack of physical activity are just three of many behavioral risk factors that have been linked to mortality. Widely cited are what is known as the "Alameda 7" behavioral risk factors, which include, in addition to cigarette smoking, alcohol consumption, and lack of physical activity, such factors as obesity, inadequate sleeping habits, not eating breakfast daily, and snacking between meals (Belloc 1973).

Schoenborn (1986), in a 1985 update on these behaviors, reported that, while large numbers of U.S. adults have healthy habits, many do not, and particularly persons in socially and economically disadvantaged groups. Thus, attention should be paid to various kinds of behaviors that can affect health and survival.

In this chapter, we examine the linkages between mortality and several behaviors, some on the Alameda 7 list and others not on this list. Items covered include four measures tied to dietary behavior—body mass index (BMI—the weight divided by the square of height), how regularly breakfast is eaten, how often persons eat between meals, and explicit efforts to reduce cholesterol from the diet—and two other risk behaviors—average amount of sleep at night and use of seat belts.

Several researchers have linked weightedness to mortality risks. Keys (1989) found that body fatness (as indexed by body mass, skinfold thickness, relative girth, and body density) did not discriminate decedents from survivors over a 35-year time span when age, blood pressure, and smoking habits were controlled. However, others have produced different findings. Stevens et al. (1992) discovered that BMI was not associated with mortality of white men but was predictive of all-cause and coronary heart disease mortality for black men.

Waaler (1983) reported a marked U-shaped association between BMI and mortality. He concluded that, if everyone obtained the low mortality at optimum BMI levels, total mortality would be reduced by 15%. Gordon and Doyle (1988) found that cohort mortality over a 27-year period was least at relative weights between 100 and 109% of the desirable weight. Mortality was generally greater at lower and higher weights. In a study of Harvard alumni (Lee et al. 1992), in which there was screening for cardiovascular disease and cancer, both body weight loss and gain were associated with significant increase in mortality from all causes and coronary heart disease but not cancer. In a subsequent analysis of the same population (Lee et al. 1993), with screening for coronary heart disease, stroke, and cancer, and adjusting for age, cigarette habit, and physical activity, the researchers found a J-shaped relationship between BMI and mortality. For current smokers alone, the relationship between BMI and mortality was U-shaped.

Using data from the longitudinal Framingham Heart Study, Garrison and associates (1983) discovered that a higher percentage of smokers were underweight than overweight. Among both smokers and nonsmokers, mortality was lowest for those in the desirable weight group. For cigarette smokers, the highest mortality was among lean men and those most overweight, but even those moderately overweight (about 20% above desirable weight) had appreciably elevated mortality.

In a more recent study (Dorn et al. 1997), the long-term relationship between BMI and mortality from all causes and from specific causes in the population 20–96 years of age in Buffalo, New York, was assessed. The study used a 29-year follow-up of men and women who were originally interviewed in 1960. Data were adjusted for age, education, and cigarette smoking. Investigators found a significant linear association between BMI and all-cause mortality in men less than 65 in 1960, but not in women. In men 65 and older, a quadratic relationship was observed, with lowest risks appearing in the BMI range of 23–27. Moreover, body mass was most strongly related to cardiovascular disease and coronary heart disease mortality in women and younger men, but not in older men. It was not related to an increased risk of death from non-CVD or cancer in either sex.

Sidney et al. (1987) screened white adults for illness at the beginning of a follow-up study and found thinness not related to mortality for never smokers and ex-smokers. Thin men and women who were current smokers did have higher mortality. The U-shaped relationship between BMI and mortality also appeared in data analyzed by Vandenbroucke et al. (1984), but smoking did not explain higher mortality in the lowest BMI category.

Manson et al. (1987) reviewed the literature on the subject and confirmed the inconsistent findings regarding body weight and longevity. Some studies showed a linear, others a J-shaped, and still others a U-shaped relationship. In addition, the inclusion of other variables in the analysis usually altered the relationships observed, and variations were observed by causes of death. Yet, BMI has been established as a risk factor for survival.

Two dietary practices that have been highlighted in attempts to improve people's health conditions are eating regular meals, including breakfast, and not snacking between meals (Berkman et al. 1983). In an early analysis of persons 20 years of age and over in Alameda County in which reports of behaviors of respondents in 1965 were followed up with information on deaths $5\frac{1}{2}$ years later (Belloc 1973; Belloc and Breslow 1972), it was shown that individuals who generally ate breakfast and did not snack between meals reported better health and experienced lower mortality than persons with less regular eating habits. Berkman et al. (1983) repeated the analysis with a 9-year interval for death or survival and found that, for persons 30-69 years old, those who reported eating breakfast almost daily had lower mortality rates than the others who ate breakfast only sometimes, rarely, or never. This finding suggested that it may not be eating breakfast per se that is associated with mortality, but rather the regularity with which one does or does not eat breakfast. Moreover, controlling for level of physical health did not seem to affect the results.

Kaplan et al. (1987) pursued the Alameda County analysis with a focus on persons 60–94 years old in 1965 and a 17-year mortality assessment. The mortality risk of not eating breakfast regularly in this sample was as great as for currently smoking, although there were variations by age.

Berkman et al. (1983) found, however, no consistent relationship between frequency of snacking between meals and mortality. Again, controls for physical health status did not alter that finding. It may be that the nature of the snack is crucial to its health effect. Those who snack on wholesome foods (such as fresh vegetables or low-fat crackers) may have supported their healthfulness, while those who snacked on cakes and sweets may have been affecting their health negatively. Kaplan et al. (1987) also looked at the effects of snacking among those 60–94 years old in Alameda County and found no significant relationship with mortality chances.

In recent years, favorable health practices have included not only regulating one's overall dietary intake, but also being vigilant about the percentage of cholesterol and other fats in the diet. In 1994 the Scandinavian

Simvastatin Survival Study found that lowering cholesterol can prevent heart attacks and reduce death in men and women who already have heart disease and high cholesterol (National Heart, Lung, and Blood Institute 1996). The study found that for those receiving statin (a cholesterol-reducing drug), deaths from heart disease were reduced by 42%, the chance of having a nonfatal heart attack was reduced by 37%, and the need for bypass surgery or angioplasty was reduced by 37%. In the process, deaths from causes other than cardiovascular disease were not increased.

In 1996 the Cholesterol and Recurrent Events Study also showed benefits of cholesterol lowering in coronary heart disease patients. In patients with seemingly normal cholesterol levels, cholesterol lowering with a statin drug lowered the risk of having another heart attack or dying by 24%. Women benefited even more than men, reducing their risk of having another heart attack by 45% (National Heart, Lung and Blood Institute 1996). Because of such research, doctors have advised people with high cholesterol to combine diet and statin drugs to control their cholesterol levels.

Medical specialists frequently caution about the need to get sufficient sleep at night in order to function well during the day. It has not been the case, however, that amount of sleep has been related to mortality prospects. One exception is the Berkman et al. (1983) study, which examined this relationship using the Alameda County study. They discovered that persons who usually slept 7 or 8 hours per night had significantly lower mortality than those reporting 6 or fewer hours of sleep or those with 9 or more hours of sleep. Sleeping 6 or fewer hours was more detrimental than sleeping 9 or more hours. Because amount of sleep could be related to one's physical health status, that variable was controlled in further analysis. The results about amount of sleep and mortality remained relatively unchanged.

In the study by Kaplan et al. (1987) of older persons in Alameda County, the association between amount of sleep and mortality was weak, in contrast to a significant relationship among younger adults. Adjusting for baseline health status did not change the association.

In recent years, high mortality rates due to automobile accidents turned attention to the use of restraining seat belt in cars and their use by passengers. Evans (1987) estimated the effectiveness of three-point lap/shoulder belts in preventing fatalities to drivers and right front passengers in passenger cars of model year 1974 or later. It was reported that, if all presently unbelted drivers and right front passengers were to use the provided lap/shoulder belts, but not otherwise change their behavior, fatalities to this group would decline by an average of 43%. Zador and Ciccone (1993) reported that air bags used in combination with lap/shoulder belts reduced auto fatalities by 44–55%.

Because driver alcohol use and changing automobile safety standards are also involved in car fatality rates, these should be considered in relation to seat belt use when estimating the consequence of using seat belts for auto fatalities. Robertson (1996) conducted such a study for 1961–1990 car models on the road in the period from 1975 through 1991. He found that car occupant deaths had been reduced substantially by improved safety standards and publicized crash tests, but that alcohol use and seat belt use resulted in significant independent effects. The use of seat belts thus remains an important behavior in regard to overall mortality prospects.

DATA AND METHODS

Our study of "other behaviors" and mortality made use of the 1990 Health Promotion and Disease Prevention supplement of the National Health Interview Survey (NHIS-HPDP) (NCHS 1993c) linked to mortality data for these individuals through 1995 (NCHS 1997b). The data included 41,104 individuals aged 18 and over, 2,388 of whom died in the 5-year follow-up period. The HPDP supplement of the NHIS has been identified as the data set with the greatest potential for not only documenting the extent to which people engage in health behaviors, but also for estimating the mortality consequences of such behavior (Schoenborn 1986).

The 1990 HPDP included questions on each of the "Alameda 7" health behaviors as well as other health behaviors. We have selected the variables of body mass, eating breakfast, eating between meals, effort to reduce cholesterol, amount of sleep at night, and use of seat belts to relate to mortality prospects in this chapter. We calculate odds of mortality in the follow-up period, controlling for demographic and social characteristics and baseline health status. In addition to the general analysis, we examine models specific to several cause-of-death categories.

The behavioral variables were constructed as follows:

Body mass index (BMI) was derived in the conventional manner of converting measures of weight and height into metric units and calculating weight/height squared. The distribution of BMIs for the sample were then categorized according to the lowest 10 percent, the 10th to 20th percentiles, the middle 60 percent, the 80th to 90th percentiles, and the highest 10 percent. These categories identify what can be regarded as extreme underweight and overweight, moderately underweight and overweight, and relatively normal weight for height. The "middle 60%" category was regarded as most desirable and used as a reference category in computing the odds ratios of mortality.

Eating breakfast was based on a direct question and categorized into rarely or never, sometimes, and always. The "always" category was regarded as most desirable and used as the reference group in computing the odds ratios of mortality.

Eating between meals (or snacking) was likewise based on a direct question and categorized into rarely or never, sometimes, and always. The "rarely or never" category was regarded as most desirable and used as the reference group in computing the odds ratios of mortality.

Permanently try to reduce cholesterol was based on a direct question that required a yes or no answer. The "yes" category was used as the reference group.

Average sleep per night was obtained in response to a direct question and categorized into 6 or fewer hours, 7 or 8 hours, 9 hours, and 10 or more hours. The "7 or 8 hours" category was used as the reference group.

Use of seat belts in motor vehicles was based on a direct question and categorized into never or almost never, sometimes, and always. The "always" category was used as the reference group.

Demographic, social, health, and basic behavioral (smoking, drinking, and exercise) variables, as well as cause-of-death classifications, were treated as in earlier chapters of this book.

RESULTS

Table 16.1 shows the weighted percentage distributions of several health behaviors, separately for survivors and decedents. By definition, the survivors are divided by body mass into two 10% categories at the highest and lowest BMIs. Those who died in the study interval are slightly more likely to be found at the extremes of the BMI, were more likely to always eat breakfast, were more likely to rarely or never eat between meals, slightly more likely to try to reduce cholesterol in their diet, more likely to sleep longer at night, and slightly more likely to never or almost never use seat belts.

Controlling for age, sex, and race, the odds ratios of mortality for the various health behaviors are shown in Table 16.2, each health behavior examined independent of other behaviors. Persons in the lowest, moderately low, and highest BMI categories have the greatest risk of death, with the most underweight having the highest odds ratio of dying. Those who do not always eat breakfast have a somewhat higher prospect of death than those who always eat breakfast. Persons who always or sometimes eat between meals have a lower mortality risk than those who rarely or never eat between meals. A higher odds ratio of dying is observed for those who do not try to reduce cholesterol. The odds ratio of mortality is highest for those who sleep 9, and especially 10 or more, hours per night. The odds ratio of dying is elevated for individuals who never or almost never use seat belts in vehicles.

Since it is possible that some of these relationships are the consequence of other behaviors, social factors, or health status, the multivariate analysis was repeated taking into account these other variables.

TABLE 16.1   Weighted Percentage Distributions of Various Health
Behaviors Specific to Survival Status, U.S. Adults, 1990–1995

	Survivors	Deaths
Dietary behavior		
Body mass		
Lowest 10%	10.0	12.4
10th to 20th percentile	10.0	9.7
Middle 60%	60.0	56.8
80th to 90th percentile	10.0	9.9
Highest 10%	10.0	11.2
Eat breakfast		
Rarely or never	22.7	12.3
Sometimes	21.3	12.4
Always	56.0	75.3
Eat between meals		
Always	40.7	35.7
Sometimes	34.1	29.0
Rarely or never	25.2	35.3
Try to reduce cholesterol		
No	63.9	61.2
Yes	36.1	38.8
Other behavior		
Average sleep		
6 or fewer hours	24.3	21.8
7–8 hours	66.2	57.3
9 hours	5.6	9.2
10 or more hours	3.9	11.7
Seat belt use		
Never or almost never	16.6	20.4
Sometimes	16.3	16.6
Always	67.1	63.0
Unweighted person-years and deaths	237,929	2,388

Sources: Derived from NCHS 1993c, 1997b.

Model 1 in Table 16.3 presents the results when the other five behaviors
and demographic factors are controlled. The odds ratio for extreme underweight persons is dampened but the general association between BMI and
mortality is unchanged, risks being greatest at the extremes of the BMI.
Further controls for smoking, drinking, and exercise (Model 2) alter the
BMI-mortality relationship very little, but those controls shift the effect for
eating breakfast, reversing the odds ratios from a slightly higher prospect of
dying to a slightly lower one when breakfast is rarely or never eaten. The
controls do not affect the odds ratios for eating between meals, which remain at a more desirable level for those who always or sometimes snack.
Likewise, the controls do not change the slightly more favorable odds for
trying to reduce cholesterol. Sleeping long hours also is associated with

TABLE 16.2   Odds Ratios for Various Health Behaviors and U.S. Adult Mortality, 1990–1995

	Model 1	Model 2	Model 3	Model 4	Model 5	Model 6
Dietary behavior						
Body mass						
Lowest 10%	1.55*					
10th to 20th percentile	1.21*					
Middle 60%	ref					
80th to 90th percentile	1.03					
Highest 10%	1.30*					
Eat breakfast						
Rarely or never		1.18*				
Sometimes		1.17*				
Always		ref				
Eat between meals						
Always			0.91+			
Sometimes			0.89*			
Rarely or never			ref			
Try to reduce cholesterol						
No				1.22*		
Yes				ref		
Other behavior						
Average sleep						
6 or fewer hours					1.07	
7–8 hours					ref	
9 hours					1.23*	
10 or more hours					1.92*	
Seat belt use						
Never or almost never						1.40*
Sometimes						1.17*
Always						ref
Demographic factors						
Age (continuous)	1.08*	1.09*	1.08*	1.08*	1.08*	1.08*
Sex (male)	1.72*	1.73*	1.73*	1.71*	1.69*	1.72*
Race (black)	1.49*	1.48*	1.51*	1.49*	1.43*	1.50*
−2*Log-likelihood	22,086.6	22,280.2	22,268.0	22,013.2	21,939.1	21,920.9

Sources: Derived from NCHS 1993c, 1997b.
$+p \leq .10$; $*p \leq .05$.

higher mortality, even after controls. Persons who never or almost never use seat belts remain at higher odds of dying, after controls, although the effect diminishes when smoking, drinking, and exercise are taken into account.

Introducing education, income, and marital status into the model produces an imperceptible effect on odds ratios of the several health behaviors (Model 3 of Table 16.3). Adding self-reported health (a measure of health selection) into the analysis (Model 4) similarly has a minor effect.

Therefore, beside the deleterious effects on survival of behaviors of smok-

TABLE 16.3   Odds Ratios for the Simultaneous Influence of Various Health Behaviors on U.S. Adult Mortality, 1990–1995

	Model 1	Model 2	Model 3	Model 4
Dietary behavior				
Body mass				
Lowest 10%	1.46*	1.35*	1.32*	1.19*
10th to 20th percentile	1.17*	1.14+	1.14+	1.12
Middle 60%	ref	ref	ref	ref
80th to 90th percentile	0.96	0.97	0.96	0.89
Highest 10%	1.26*	1.29*	1.26*	1.13+
Eat breakfast				
Rarely or never	1.11	0.93	0.93	0.91
Sometimes	1.14+	1.02	1.01	1.00
Always	ref	ref	ref	ref
Eat between meals				
Always	0.91+	0.90*	0.90*	0.88*
Sometimes	0.91+	0.90+	0.90+	0.89*
Rarely or never	ref	ref	ref	ref
Try to reduce cholesterol				
No	1.14*	1.09+	1.06	1.15*
Yes	ref	ref	ref	ref
Other health behavior				
Average sleep				
6 or fewer hours	1.05	1.05	1.04	0.94
7–8 hours	ref	ref	ref	ref
9 hours	1.13	1.10	1.09	1.03
10 or more hours	1.86*	1.80*	1.73*	1.50*
Seat belt use				
Never or almost never	1.32*	1.19*	1.15*	1.11+
Sometimes	1.17*	1.12+	1.09	1.07
Always	ref	ref	ref	ref
Health behavior controls				
Smoking				
Current		2.30*	2.21*	2.03*
Former		1.45*	1.44*	1.38*
Never		ref	ref	ref
Drinking				
Current		0.84*	0.90+	0.95
Former		1.15*	1.15*	1.07
Never		ref	ref	ref
Exercise				
Not regularly		1.41*	1.36*	1.23*
Regularly		ref	ref	ref
Demographic factors				
Age (continuous)	1.08*	1.08*	1.08*	1.08*
Sex (male)	1.64*	1.52*	1.60*	1.62*
Race (black)	1.38*	1.33*	1.23*	1.19*

(*continues*)

TABLE 16.3 (*Continued*)

	Model 1	Model 2	Model 3	Model 4
Social factors				
Education				
Less than 12 years			1.19*	1.04
12 years			1.12+	1.08
13+ years			ref	ref
Income equivalence			0.91*	0.96+
Marital status				
Never married			1.27*	1.36*
Previously married			1.14*	1.17*
Married			ref	ref
Health				
Self-reported health				1.44*
−2*Log-likelihood	21,261.7	20,753.3	20,651.5	20,306.9

Sources: Derived from NCHS 1993c, 1997b.
$+p \leq .10$; $*p \leq .05$.

ing, heavy drinking, and lack of exercise, other behaviors that have a negative effect on survival are being extremely underweight or overweight, sleeping long hours, and not using seat belts. Rarely or never eating breakfast has a negative (but not statistically significant) effect, eating between meals actually is seen to have a positive effect, as does trying to reduce cholesterol.

It is reasonable to expect that some of these measured effects on death or survival of the different behaviors are related to particular types of illness or causes of death. We have, therefore, generated models that incorporate all of the aforementioned controls and relate the six "other behaviors" to the odds ratio of dying for five cause-of-death categories—circulatory diseases (heart or stroke), cancers, respiratory ailments, social pathologies (accidents, suicides, homicides, chronic liver disease, and cirrhosis), and residual causes (Table 16.4).

The effects of body mass vary by cause of death. Extreme underweightedness increases the odds of dying most for respiratory and residual causes, not significantly for circulatory causes or social pathologies. Those with respiratory disease may already have lower BMIs at the time the survey was conducted, due to their poor health. Extreme overweightedness is most strongly related to circulatory and residual causes, not cancers or social pathologies, and seems to provide a significant protective effect for respiratory ailments. Being moderately overweight is also related to a much reduced odds of dying from respiratory diseases.

Rarely or never eating breakfast is associated with significantly lower odds of dying from cancer and much higher odds of dying from respiratory diseases. Eating between meals is also linked to lower odds of dying from cancer and is related to lower odds of dying from social pathologies.

TABLE 16.4 Odds Ratios for the Simultaneous Influence of Various Health Behaviors on Cause-Specific U.S. Adult Mortality, 1990–1995

	Circulatory		Cancer		Respiratory		Social pathologies		Residual causes	
	Model 1	Model 2	Model 3	Model 4	Model 5	Model 6	Model 7	Model 8	Model 9	Model 10
Dietary behavior										
Body mass										
Lowest 10%	1.06	0.95	1.27+	1.20	2.02*	1.69*	1.09	0.97	1.93*	1.56*
10th to 20th percentile	1.01	1.00	1.13	1.14	1.38	1.36	0.82	0.78	1.41+	1.35
Middle 60%	ref	ref	ref	ref	ref	ref	ref	ref	ref	ref
80th to 90th percentile	0.97	0.88	1.10	1.03	0.46*	0.42*	0.79	0.76	1.18	1.08
Highest 10%	1.48*	1.31*	1.14	1.05	0.45*	0.37*	1.13	1.03	1.77*	1.52*
Eat breakfast										
Rarely or never	0.88	0.86	0.77*	0.76*	1.64*	1.48+	1.02	1.02	1.01	1.02
Sometimes	1.04	1.03	1.14	1.14	0.87	0.78	0.90	0.90	0.91	0.88
Always	ref	ref	ref	ref	ref	ref	ref	ref	ref	ref
Eat between meals										
Always	0.92	0.90	0.93	0.91	0.88	0.85	0.61*	0.60*	0.92	0.91
Sometimes	1.07	1.06	0.74*	0.74*	0.82	0.80	0.86	0.85	0.76+	0.76+
Rarely or never	ref	ref	ref	ref	ref	ref	ref	ref	ref	ref
Try to reduce cholesterol										
No	0.98	1.04	1.10	1.19*	1.25	1.30	1.45+	1.43+	1.04	1.10
Yes	ref	ref	ref	ref	ref	ref	ref	ref	ref	ref
Other health behavior										
Average sleep										
6 or fewer hours	0.96	0.86+	1.07	1.01	1.59*	1.32	0.92	0.87	1.10	0.95
7–8 hours	ref	ref	ref	ref	ref	ref	ref	ref	ref	ref
9 hours	1.00	0.93	1.02	0.98	0.90	0.86	2.61*	2.34*	1.06	0.94
10 or more hours	1.72*	1.43*	1.40*	1.26	1.79*	1.46	2.39*	1.85*	2.31*	1.82*
Seat belt use										
Never or almost never	1.09	1.02	1.12	1.11	1.64*	1.58*	1.63*	1.47+	1.12	1.02
Sometimes	1.24*	1.17+	0.94	0.91	1.12	1.08	1.49+	1.39	1.00	0.94
Always	ref	ref	ref	ref	ref	ref	ref	ref	ref	ref

Health behavior controls										
Smoking										
Current	2.40*	2.08*	2.90*	2.66*	4.01*	3.44*	1.22	1.08	1.93*	1.64*
Former	1.34*	1.26*	1.87*	1.78*	3.54*	3.30*	0.46*	0.46*	1.33*	1.29+
Never	ref	ref	ref	ref	ref	ref	ref	ref	ref	ref
Drinking										
Current	0.70*	0.81	1.14	1.18	0.66*	0.75	1.00	1.16	0.87	1.04
Former	1.06	1.00	1.51*	1.43*	1.13	1.02	0.84	0.81	0.98	0.88
Never	ref	ref	ref	ref	ref	ref	ref	ref	ref	ref
Exercise										
Not regularly	1.47*	1.27*	1.26*	1.16	1.74*	1.45+	1.04	0.96	1.74*	1.48*
Regularly	ref	ref	ref	ref	ref	ref	ref	ref	ref	ref
Demographic factors										
Age (continuous)	1.10*	1.10*	1.08*	1.08*	1.11*	1.09*	1.02*	1.02*	1.08*	1.07*
Sex (male)	1.73*	1.84*	1.15	1.13	1.46*	1.66*	3.05*	3.30*	1.35*	1.57*
Race (black)	1.16	1.03	1.31*	1.35*	0.42*	0.39*	1.10	0.90	2.53*	2.03*
Social factors										
Education										
Less than 12 years		1.13		0.93		0.74		1.45		1.01
12 years		1.14		1.12		1.00		0.89		0.99
13+ years		ref		ref		ref		ref		ref
Income equivalence		0.94		1.05		0.93		0.95		0.91
Marital status										
Never married		1.28+		0.74		0.83		1.38		2.43*
Previously married		1.13		0.87		1.35		1.51+		1.62*
Married		ref		ref		ref		ref		ref
Health										
Self-reported health		1.45*		1.35*		1.68*		1.28*		1.59*
−2*Log-likelihood	9,865.6	9,655.9	7,681.6	7,594.4	2,200.4	2,129.0	2,386.8	2,358.5	4,224.7	4,078.1

Sources: Derived from NCHS 1993c, 1997b.

+$p \leq .10$; *$p \leq .05$.

Trying to reduce cholesterol seems to have no effect on the odds of death from circulatory ailments but it is associated with significantly lower odds of dying from cancer or social pathologies.

Sleeping 10 or more hours a night relates to mortality from all causes, while having 6 or fewer hours of sleep nightly is tied to lesser mortality from circulatory diseases and greater mortality from respiratory ailments, after controls for health condition and other behavioral, social, and demographic factors. Having lots of sleep is heavily associated with social pathologies, including suicide, which reflect depression.

The greatest negative effects of not using seat belts are for deaths from respiratory diseases and social pathologies (which include automobile accidents).

CONCLUSION

These findings about the relationship of various health behaviors (other than smoking, drinking, and exercise) to the odds of dying (generally and from specific causes of death) include some expected associations and some unexpected ones. All of the findings must be interpreted in the context of the nature of the variables themselves, the controls that are used, and the possible variables that are not included and may be relevant. We summarize the information produced on each of the behaviors in this way.

Body mass (or relative weight for height) has a definite influence on mortality prospects. When only age, sex, and race are controlled, those who are extremely underweight, moderately underweight, and extremely overweight have the greatest risks of death, with extremely underweight people being most at risk. When smoking, drinking, exercise, and the other behaviors, education, income, and marital status are added to the model, the association of BMI and mortality does not change very much, although the odds of dying are reduced slightly for extremely underweight persons and slightly elevated for extremely overweight persons, the two categories remaining the most risky. When cause of death is taken into account, extreme underweightedness is seen to be linked mainly to deaths from respiratory and residual causes, while overweightedness is related mainly to deaths from circulatory and residual causes. Other causes of death do not seem to be tied to body mass effects.

Although body mass, which is related to both genetic/physiological factors and to dietary practices, has a clear association with odds of dying, the effects on mortality of some eating habits is much less clearcut. We examined both the frequency of eating breakfast and the extent of snacking between meals.

Controlling for age, sex, and race alone, we came up with the expected finding that those who do not always eat breakfast have a higher odds of dying than those who always eat breakfast. However, when smoking, drinking, exercise, other health behaviors, and demographic factors are controlled, the odds ratio of dying shifts for eating breakfast from a slightly higher chance of dying to a slightly lower one when breakfast is rarely or never eaten. When education, income, marital status, and health status are further introduced into the model, a positive effect of not eating breakfast regularly remains, although it is not statistically significant. When causes of death are examined, rarely or never eating breakfast is associated with lower odds of dying from respiratory diseases. These findings are inconsistent with findings on this relationship in other studies, and further study of the topic with additional controls is needed.

Likewise, contrary to expectations, with age, sex, and race controlled, those who eat between meals have a lower expectancy of dying than those who do not. Adding other controls does not change the relationship. Eating between meals is linked to a lower risk of dying from cancer and social pathologies. Thus, our results on snacking and mortality are not consistent with findings from other research.

Trying to reduce cholesterol does result in a lowered chance of mortality, apparently because of successful utilization of the appropriate drugs and diet. Introduction of the various controls used in the analysis does not change this finding. The beneficial effect of trying to reduce cholesterol intake is observed with regard to reductions in deaths from cancers and social pathologies, but not from circulatory diseases. The lack of a linkage between efforts to reduce cholesterol and mortality from circulatory disease is puzzling because other research has shown that high cholesterol is strongly tied to cardiovascular death risks. Perhaps those who are actively trying to reduce their cholesterol are those individuals who have been advised by a doctor that they already have high cholesterol or heart disease, and therefore are attempting to reduce a known elevated risk of death. Thus, the results may assess palliative rather than preventive actions.

Having an optimum amount of sleep is often emphasized as a way of improving one's quality of life as well as a factor in achieving longer life. Our study shows that sleeping long hours is associated with higher mortality, even after the several controls are introduced. Even the inclusion of the health status variable does not alter that finding. Having low amounts of sleep is observed only for deaths due to respiratory ailments. Sleeping excessively (10 or more hours a night) relates to mortality from all causes. Even controls for health status and exercise do not alter these results. It may be that those who are sick sleep more. For example, those who have circulatory diseases, cancer, or respiratory diseases may be physically drained due to the disease and therefore require more rest. Alternatively, excessive sleep may indicate mental problems, like depression, which could also translate into heightened risk of death.

The use of seat belts in motor vehicles does provide a protective effect for survival. Persons who never or almost never use seat belts remain at higher odds of dying, even after controls for other variables are entered into the model. This effect is seen for deaths from social pathologies, which includes motor vehicles accidents, and for mortality from respiratory diseases.

In summary, examination of the effects of other health behaviors on mortality prospects shows some mixed results. BMI, trying to reduce cholesterol, and using seat belts each exhibit associations with the risks of dying that are in line with findings from earlier research. The regularity of eating breakfast or snacking between meals, and the average number of hours of sleep per night are either not related to mortality or are linked in unexpected ways. The three variables with positive effects supplement the smoking, drinking, and exercise variables in demonstrating behavioral ties to mortality risks. Each of those factors shows relationships that remain after controlling for a variety of other variables. The lack of expected associations with regard to the other factors could be due to limitations in how the variables are measured, inadequacies in the inclusion of other variables controlled, or unobserved interactions among variables, which render our study incomplete. Or the lack, in these cases, of consistent findings with other studies may be because our study has a more robust sample that is national in scope and includes more controls than in other research. Further research should examine these possibilities to arrive at a proper judgment.

Our findings support the notion of an hybristic stage to the epidemiologic transition. Earlier chapters showed that smoking, drinking, and exercise were related in significant ways to the risks of death. This chapter reveals a still broader set of behavioral variables—body mass or relative weight for height (resulting in part from dietary habits), amount of sleep at night, use of seat belts in vehicles, and trying to reduce cholesterol—that are added to odds of dying. Thus, one can observe in additional detail the complexity and consequences and connectedness of the factors that produce shorter or longer life.

17

CONCLUSION

Adult mortality levels in the United States have declined rather incredibly over the course of the 20th century, and life expectancy at birth has risen from under 50 years at the turn of the century to nearly 76 years in 1995 (Anderson et al. 1997). Yet, substantial progress can still be achieved, particularly if scientific research can illuminate how the critical demographic, social, behavioral, health, and biological factors are associated with risks of death. Throughout this monograph, we have employed the newest and most innovative national database, moved beyond the descriptive to the multivariate realm, linked findings from other researchers, and included a large set of variables to more fully understand current U.S. adult mortality patterns. We have examined how demographic and sociocultural factors—sex, ethnicity, family composition, religious attendance, and social participation; socioeconomic factors—education, income, employment status, occupational status, and health insurance; health factors—perceived health status, functional limitations, and mental and addictive disorders; and health behaviors—smoking, drinking, exercise, and other behaviors—all relate to the risk of mortality. We have revealed that several factors rarely investigated in related literature—such as religious involvement, functional limitations, and mental and addictive disorders—are strongly related to the risk of overall and cause-specific adult mortality.

Our focus has been on mortality differences across groups, statistically measured in the form of odds ratios using discrete-time hazards modeling, rather than on overall levels of adult mortality. Throughout, we have compared men to women, the uninsured to the insured, the less educated to the more highly educated, smokers to non-smokers, and so on, to best capture the differential risks of mortality suffered by specific subpopulations. While a focus on differential mortality cannot address some important issues in this area—such as those related to the overall mortality prospects and life expectancy for the general population—it allows for the identification of groups that might be targeted for specific programs, policies, and further in-depth research. Moreover, we have broadened our approach from traditional foci on demographic (e.g., Zopf 1992), socioeconomic (e.g., Kitagawa and Hauser 1973), **or** behavioral factors (e.g., Berkman and Breslow 1983) to include simultaneously demographic, social, behavioral, **and** health factors that impact the mortality risks of U.S. individuals.

In the following subsections, we highlight the key findings from each chapter. In so doing, we must remain mindful of the measurement of each variable employed. Some measures are dichotomous and thus represent the presence or absence of a particular characteristic. For example, health insurance is measured in Chapter 9 by whether individuals possess or do not possess health insurance. In reality, health insurance coverage includes a range of categories, including those people who have access to insurance but decline; those who have basic or catastrophic rather than full-coverage health insurance; those who have basic insurance coverage but may not choose to use it because of large deductibles, copayments, and/or exclusions; those who do not have insurance but have access to doctors, clinics, or the health-care system that will care for them in emergencies; those who know of governmental or nongovernmental sources that could help in an emergency; and those who have no insurance, no access to health-care personnel, and no manner to deal with emergency health issues. On the other hand, income is assessed in $10,000 increments. Thus, the comparative strength of these two variables is difficult to directly assess, since they are measured by two separate metrics (e.g., possess/not possess health insurance versus a $10,000 increase in family income equivalence). This and other measurement issues require careful interpretations of the results for each factor and cautiously drawn inferences about the comparative strength of the different variables.

Further, it is extremely important to keep in mind the relative **size** of different population groups when interpreting results. For example, we again highlight the mortality risks of cigarette smoking in Chapter 13. The importance of smoking for adult mortality risk is not only a major public health issue because of the excess risk of death experienced by smokers over the follow-up period in this study, but also because of the large number of people who are smokers or former smokers. Indeed, our data from 1990 (Table 13.1) show that about 29% of the U.S. adult population currently smokes, and another 22% of the population are former smokers. Thus, the excess risk of mortality associated with cigarette smoking, to some degree, affects about one-half of the adult population. In contrast, other covariates of mortality that we investigated are far less prevalent in the population. Thus, the strength of differential mortality risks for each variable must be weighed together with the prevalence of that factor in the population to most fully understand its impact. Note that we have included, in each chapter, the basic distribution of the main variable of interest in the general population.

This book employs an important, new, and innovative data set, but one that is not problem-free. Perhaps most important, the data are not longitudinal and therefore do not allow for time-varying covariates. Second, some variables—for example, detailed information about wealth—are not available. Further, some variables are available, but in less detail than might be preferred. For example, limited data is available on religious involvement, but not religious denomination.

Still, the associations between our central variables and the risk of death individuals experienced over the course of the follow-up period are meaningful and, to a large extent, statistically significant. Changes in effects are often found as we moved from the gross effects of specified variables on mortality, controlling only for demographic factors, to net effects using controls for a host of other pertinent variables. Many factors—such as sex, smoking status, and exercise—display consistently strong associations with mortality on both gross and net bases. The effects of other variables, such as education, show more substantial changes from the gross to the net effect models, indicating that at least part of their influence on mortality operates indirectly through other factors.

DEMOGRAPHIC AND SOCIOCULTURAL CHARACTERISTICS

This book details important relationships between sex, race/ethnicity, nativity, family composition, religious and general social participation, and mortality. Chapter 3 finds that compared to women, men experienced about 1.7 times the odds of mortality over the follow-up period and that this gap persists, even with controls for social and behavioral factors. Nevertheless, we determined that the sex gap in mortality is influenced by male-female differences in social, economic, and behavioral characteristics. Hypothetically, the sex gap in mortality would be larger if females were as likely as males to live in families with high incomes, to obtain high levels of education, and to be employed in the paid labor force. Of course, women have made substantial strides in each of these areas in recent decades, erasing a substantial portion of the gender inequality in socioeconomic status that has characterized U.S. history. Thus, as the wage gap between the sexes closes even further, as women continue to increase their labor force participation rates and gain increased levels of education, female life expectancy should climb even further, and the mortality gap between the sexes, all else being equal, could widen.

However, between 1975 and 1995, the life expectancy at birth sex gap narrowed from a peak of nearly 8 years to 6.4 years, due to rather substantial gains in male life expectancy, coupled with more modest gains in female life expectancy over this time (Anderson et al. 1997). This trend is most likely due to the changing influence of cigarette smoking on sex-specific mortality patterns. While our results suggest that cigarette smoking continues to account for about 25% of the sex mortality gap, young women are now smoking in greater proportions than young men, while older men are quitting in greater proportions (Rogers et al. 1995). A continuation of these smoking trends could further close the sex gap in mortality, as men derive gains in life expectancy by quitting smoking, and women endure somewhat higher mortality due to increased smoking prevalence. But such changes in smoking patterns and the sex gap may be transitory. In time, we are hopeful that the current social and legal action against tobacco use will result in sharp declines in the initiation of smoking for both males and females, along with increases in quit rates for both sexes. To bring about these changes, U.S. social and health policy must continue to be aggressive in fighting the battle against cigarette smoking and other forms of tobacco use, particularly at younger ages, when such behavior is usually learned. Our analysis suggests that lower rates of smoking have the potential to make a strong impact in narrowing the sex mortality differential, particularly for cancers and circulatory and respiratory diseases.

We further revealed that the sex mortality gap varies rather widely across social and economic positions. In particular, men living in high-income families exhibit only moderately higher mortality compared to their high-income female counterparts. Thus, while a male survival disadvantage was evident across all social and economic groups we analyzed, there is evidence that men can achieve a level of mortality much more similar to that of women than currently experienced.

Chapter 4 focuses on race/ethnic adult mortality differences within the context of nativity. While many studies have examined black-white differences, few have examined a broader range of race/ethnic groups and fewer yet have taken into account the nativity of individuals. We found that African Americans exhibited among the highest odds of death among all three broad age groups of adults we specified, with much of the excess mortality attributable to their disadvantaged social and economic characteristics. Puerto Rican mortality, particularly for young and middle-aged adults, was also high, also in large part due to their social and economic circumstances. On the other hand, Asian Americans generally displayed the lowest odds of death of any race/ethnic group, particularly among adults 65 and over. Notably, Mexican Americans and Cubans display odds of mortality similar to Caucasians, a finding that is consistent with the notion of the epidemiologic paradox (Markides and Coreil 1986).

However, race/ethnic differences in mortality are influenced by nativity, because foreign-born persons demonstrated about 20% lower odds of mortality than native-born persons over the follow-up period. Thus, for example, Asian Americans, Mexican Americans, and Other Hispanics enjoy relatively low mortality risks in part because they are disproportionately immigrants. The foreign-born benefit for African Americans, on the other hand, is statistically small, since nearly 95% of the adult African American population is native-born. However, compared to native-born African Americans, their foreign-born counterparts enjoy much lower risks of death (also see Hummer et al. 1999b). Thus, future race/ethnic mortality studies must be cognizant of nativity composition, particularly since immigrants tend to be a select group of hard working, healthy individuals. Further, U.S. policy should consider the beneficial influence of immigrants for the overall health profile of the nation and, particularly, for the Asian and Hispanic subpopulations.

As the National Health Interview Survey (NHIS) collects more information on detailed ethnic groups in the coming years, it will be possible to further disaggregate race/ethnic mortality patterns. Thus, it may be possible to examine the mortality experiences of the diverse Asian and Pacific Islander subpopulations, including Chinese, Filipino, Hawaiian, Korean, Vietnamese, Japanese, Asian Indian, Samoan, and Guamanian Americans. The small number of available deaths and nativity focus of the race/ethnic chapter also precluded the separate examination of Native American mortality, for which there is a need for more in-depth study at the national level (Young 1997). Moreover, future studies may examine other Hispanic subpopulations besides Mexican Americans, Puerto Ricans, and Cubans—including, for example, rather recent entrants from Central American nations and those with ties back to Spain many generations ago. Further, our results suggest the need to investigate the influence of country of origin for immigrant mortality patterns of all race/ethnic groups.

Chapter 5 demonstrates that while individual demographic risk factors are important, so too are those that operate within families. The core NHIS interviews individuals within households, which provides the opportunity to move to another level of analysis. Indeed, we found that family composition is associated with the mortality risks of individuals. For example, individuals who are married and live with two or three children exhibited lower mortality risks over the follow-up period than those who are widowed or divorced, especially if they live with multiple relatives. Thus, family composition can be associated with increased or decreased risks of death for individuals. Similarly, mortality can dramatically change family formation and composition. High mortality can create higher rates of widowhood, single-parent families, and households arranged around extended relations. Thus, future work must consider the complex interplay between family composition, health, and mortality—particularly as the structure of the family in the United States continues to diversify.

Chapter 6 demonstrates that religious attendance, which is rarely examined in studies of adult mortality, exhibits a strong association with mortality similar in magnitude to that of sex and race/ethnicity. For example, our findings indicate that persons who reported never attending religious services exhibited about 1.8 times the odds of mortality in the follow-up period compared to those who reported attending more than once a week (also see Hummer et al. 1999a). Religious involvement is related to health behavior; to emotional, social, instrumental, and financial support; to the reduction of stress; and to improved recovery from illness and surgery (Ellison and Levin 1998). Further, religious involvement takes on added significance when it is demonstrated that it both directly affects mortality prospects, and also indirectly affects mortality through these other mechanisms.

However, religious effects have been viewed with much skepticism in the scientific community, particularly as they relate to health and mortality. The results presented here should work to dispel that notion. Indeed, given our findings and those in recent related work, we recommend that religious items be considered for regular inclusion in health surveys. Such items might not only include formal religious attendance, but also those measuring informal religious involvement, religious denomination, and personal religious beliefs and behavior.

This book does not devote a separate chapter to the influences of age because, while the NHIS-MCD matched data set is superior to its competitors for many purposes, the same is not true when considering the relationship between age and mortality. The relatively small number of deaths at the adult age extremes (e.g., younger than 20 years of age and older than 85 years of age) in these data precludes the in-depth analysis of the black-white mortality crossover, the declining rate of mortality increases among the oldest-old, and mortality among the youngest group of adults—all age-related mortality issues that are of prominence in current literature.

Despite these limitations, our models throughout the book illustrate, as might be expected, that age is strongly and consistently related to the risk of mortality. Generally, each single-year increase in adult age is associated with an increase in the odds of death by 8 to 10%. This relation is only slightly affected by separately examining younger and older adults, by simultaneously examining all adults, or by introducing other covariates. We measure age by single-years in this book, but have also examined the association between 5-year age groups and mortality (results not shown). Five-year age groups generally display the same effects as those from cumulating 5 single years; in other words, each 5-year increase in age increases the odds of death by between 40 and 50%. In short, the effect of age on overall mortality is unyielding through most of the life course, although we do note that important recent work suggests a decreasing influence of age on the mortality of the oldest-old (e.g., Carey 1997; Olshansky and Carnes 1997). Age effects are, however, stronger for certain causes of death. The effects of age on mortality are greater for degenerative diseases—circulatory and respiratory diseases and cancer, and weaker for social pathologies—suicides, homicides, and accidents. That is, the odds of dying due to social pathologies are only weakly associated with increasing age.

SOCIOECONOMIC FACTORS

Chapters 7 through 9 examine socioeconomic status, a multidimensional construct that includes education, income, employment status, occupation, and health insurance (see also Pappas et al. 1993; Preston and Elo 1995; Sorlie et al. 1995; Williams and Collins 1995). The analysis of basic socioeconomic effects in Chapter 7 shows that education, income, and employment status influence mortality in interrelated ways; that is, controlling for any two measures dampens the effect of the other measure on the risk of dying. In fact, controlling for income and employment status eradicates a separate effect of education on mortality. This suggests that education operates through employment and income to influence mortality. But income and employment status retain separate independent effects on mortality, even with a variety of controls. Indeed, those not in the labor force suffer especially high mortality, suggesting that such individuals may not have a choice in working: they may be forced out of the labor force due to poor physical health, disabling chronic conditions, or mental or addictive disorders.

Chapter 8 demonstrates that mortality is related to occupational status as well as to overall employment status. Indeed, there is a larger gap between the high-status occupations and those who have never worked or who quit working than there is between high- and low-status occupations. This occupational effect remains significant even when education, income, and employment status are introduced into the analysis. These results also confirm the healthy worker effect: those who work, even in low-status jobs, are generally healthier than those not in the labor force.

The low mortality risks witnessed by those who enjoy high levels of education and income and among those who are employed are due in part to the indirect benefits bestowed on high socioeconomic status. That is, such individuals may have more knowledge, skills, training, and ability; are more likely to possess wealth and assets; and are more likely to qualify for and to purchase private health insurance (Chapter 9). Education reduces the risk of death by providing the knowledge necessary to secure employment with benefits; to find insurance coverage, either private or governmental; to know what is covered and what insurance gaps exist; and to engage in health promoting activities. There is concern about the relatively high mortality among the uninsured, who may number 40 million individuals in the United States (Franks et al. 1993). Uninsured individuals have limited access to preventive and curative health care, may delay seeking medical care for current health conditions, are more likely to receive improper diagnosis and treatment, are more likely to sustain injury through substandard medical care, and may forego treatment, all of which cumulates into increased chances that their health conditions will persist, worsen, and possibly become fatal (see also Burstin et al. 1992).

Thus, the cluster of socioeconomic factors—income, education, employment status, occupational status, and health insurance—are interrelated and interact to influence mortality. Kitagawa and Hauser's (1973) classic differential mortality study provided some needed documentation of national patterns of socioeconomic differentials. By linking death records to prior census reports for the decedents, the authors were able to describe mortality variations by education and income. Yet, their study did not use a multivariate approach, is now over 25 years old, and was not able to examine the interrelationships of several socioeconomic indicators in their effects on mortality. More recent studies have made advances with regard to analytical methods and theoretical orientations (see Pappas et al. 1993), but our analysis goes beyond these studies by introducing the effects of other demographic, sociocultural, behavioral, and health variables. Income and occupational influences signify the economic underpinnings of opportunities for obtaining health insurance, working in healthful environments, and experiencing desirable living conditions. Education is a critical variable in the chain of influences, but it seems to operate indirectly through other socioeconomic factors to affect survival prospects.

HEALTH FACTORS

Health status is a crucial connector in relating various demographic, socioeconomic, and behavioral factors to mortality. Our interest in health status is twofold—as an indicator of the bodily risks that individuals experience throughout their lifetimes that capture their relative illness or wellness, and as a selective force that indicates which persons enter certain categories of other variables of interest (such as favorable education or occupation statuses or particular marital statuses). In many of the chapters of this book, the second interest is satisfied by including a health status measure as a control in studying the effects of other variables on mortality. In Chapter 10, we focus on the first interest by examining health status in relation to mortality, controlling for other factors.

While recognizing that health status incorporates several dimensions of physical well-being and can be determined by medical as well as lay evaluators of health, we adopted a single health status measure that is based on a judgment of a person's overall health as it is perceived by the respondent (or a family member of the respondent) in the NHIS. A recent review of a range of studies using such a variable (Idler and Benyamini 1997) validates the use of this measure as a strong predictor of mortality in follow-up studies. The measure indicates whether one's health is perceived as poor, fair, good, very good, or excellent.

Our analysis supports the notion that self-reported health status is strongly related to the risk of mortality. Moreover, the relationship persists despite the inclusion of demographic, socioeconomic, and behavioral variables in the analysis. The linkage between health status and mortality is observed for all cause-of-death categories and for younger and older adults, but was not statistically significant for deaths due to social pathologies.

Functional limitations are important to understand because they indicate the ability of individuals to remain independent, to live in their residences, and to interact in the community (see Chapter 11). Individuals who are functionally limited may become institutionalized and thereby lose contact with their neighborhood friends, local businesses, social service agencies, and the church. Activities of Daily Living (ADLs) and Instrumental Activities of Daily Living (IADLs) are crucial indicators of peoples' functional independence. These measures assess the ability to perform uncomplicated motions with low physical demands that are required to maintain a household on a daily basis. Our results suggest that, although younger adults possess fewer limitations than older adults, the limitations of young adults are associated with comparatively higher odds of death. These findings warrant further investigation into the severity and mortality implications of functional limitations for young adults. Indeed, much of the literature in this area has examined only the elderly.

Our results also contribute to the literature by examining single and joint contributions of functional limitations. We found a functional health gradient such that individuals with more limitations experience a greater risk of death than those with fewer limitations. For example, compared to young adults with no limitations in IADLs, comparable individuals with one limitation experienced about 60% higher odds of death in the follow-up period, those with three limitations exhibited 85% higher odds of death, and those with five or six limitations displayed almost 300% higher odds of death. Thus, it is important to include both the type and number of functional limitations in mortality analyses.

Mental and addictive disorders can prevent people from working full time, working at optimum capacity, maintaining clear judgement, forming and retaining strong social ties, remaining healthy and independent, and ultimately from living a long life (Chapter 12). Individuals who reported a mental or addictive disorder exhibited twice the risk of death in the follow-up period compared to those who reported that they are free of such disorders, even controlling for demographic, familial, and socioeconomic factors. Compared to those free of a disorder, those who have cognitive disorders, affective disorders, alcohol abuse, or drug abuse each exhibited higher odds of death than those free from disorders. Fortunately, many mental and addictive disorders have declined in prevalence over time, in part because of improved treatments with drug and psychosocial therapies. Furthermore, exercise and other interventions can help reduce the effects of mental disorders, including depression.

Mental and addictive disorders can increase the risk of death through multiple avenues. Compared to individuals without disorders, those with disorders often have more difficulty maintaining functional independence—managing money, performing household chores, shopping, and getting around outside their home. They also have more difficulty in social relations, such as in forming and keeping friendships. Further, their concentration and ability to cope with stress may exacerbate their risk of death. Individuals with mental and addictive disorders may also place others at greater risk of death. For example, alcoholics and persons addicted to drugs may place others at risk for homicides, accidents, and AIDS. Thus, mental disorders, while not receiving the attention in the literature that they might deserve, are a major contributing factor to an increased risk of death for those affected.

HEALTH-RELATED BEHAVIORS

Health-related behaviors are often studied from public health and medical perspectives, but rarely from a demographic perspective. Indeed, it is surprising that relatively little national-level research has investigated the relationships between health behavior and the risk of adult mortality. Chapter 13 shows that cigarette smoking still dominates the behavioral factors known to affect adult mortality, even controlling for other important variables. Heavy smokers especially, but also those who were heavy smokers before quitting, are at significantly higher risk of premature death than those who never smoked, quit early, or smoked few cigarettes. We found that, compared to never smokers, smokers are more likely to die during the follow-up period from a range of diseases, including not only cancer, but heart, respiratory, and other diseases, in addition to social pathologies. For instance, compared to never smokers, current pack-a-day or heavier smokers are 3.6 times more likely to die from cancer in the follow-up period, but also twice as likely to die from circulatory diseases, the major causes of death in the United States, 3.7 times more likely to die from respiratory diseases, and 1.6 times more likely to die from social pathologies. Moreover, as we have previously shown, smokers are more likely to die from multiple causes of death, an indication that smokers may suffer from more complex and functionally limiting illnesses than nonsmokers (Rogers et al. 1994).

Future research could extend our analyses by examining additional details about smoking, including the age at smoking initiation, age at time of quitting, types of cigarette smoked, amount of tar and nicotine, and the extent of inhaling. Moreover, smoking research is complicated by the fact that smokers can quit and resume smoking multiple times. Thus, an interesting extension of our research would be the examination of smoking and mortality from a multistate perspective, taking into account transitions between smoking statuses. Additionally, new research could delve into the use of other tobacco products—cigars, pipes, snuff, chewing tobacco, or smokeless tobacco—to determine the interactive and individual contributions of tobacco use and mortality. For example, the prevalence of cigar smoking has recently increased, due in part to individuals switching from cigarettes to cigars. Generally, cigar smokers do not inhale the smoke, but cigarette smokers and former cigarette smokers who switch to cigar smoking are more apt to inhale. Thus, mortality may be highest for current cigarette smokers, next highest for cigarette smokers who switched to cigar smoking, and lower for individuals who only smoke cigars (see Wald and Watt 1997).

The relationship between alcohol use and mortality risk is affected by the amount of consumption, past problems with drinking, and the presence of other health conditions and health behaviors (see Chapter 14). Our results demonstrate that heavy drinking increases the risk of death for cancers and social pathologies. For instance, compared to abstainers and infrequent drinkers, those who drink more than three drinks a day are about 50% more likely to die from cancer and about 90% more likely to die from social pathologies in the follow-up period. Other studies have substantiated these findings by showing that heavy drinking can increase the risk of death due to cirrhosis of the liver, alcoholism, some cancers, and home, automobile, industrial, and recreational accidents. On the other hand, our results also showed that light to moderate drinking is associated with a reduced risk of death, most likely through its association with improved food digestion and increase in cholesterol-reducing lipids (DeLabry et al. 1992; Thun et al. 1997).

Exercise is an important factor in improving health and reducing the risk of death (Chapter 15). Exercise benefits individuals of all ages, even people who begin exercise programs late in life. There are social, physiological, and psychological advantages to exercise: it increases physical functioning, mental health, lung functioning, muscle strength, and flexibility. Generally, the type of activity is less important than the fact that a person is active. Because exercise encapsulates so many benefits, including the prolongation of healthy lives, we highlight the importance of exercise in increasing health and length of life.

Being extremely under- or over-weight, sleeping long hours, and not using seat belts are each associated with an increase in the risk of death over the follow-up period (Chapter 16). As expected, some health behaviors directly translate into heightened risk of death from specific causes: obesity increases the risk of circulatory diseases; seat belt use protects against the risk of social pathologies, especially automobile accidents; and cigarette smoking increases the risk of death due to circulatory diseases, cancer, and respiratory diseases. Some health behaviors may also protect against mortality in indirect ways, but especially through their emphasis on health promotion. Thus, one health behavior may spill into other health behaviors. For example, our results show that seat belt use is associated with lower respiratory disease mortality; most likely, those individuals who wear seat belts also engage in other health practices to prevent respiratory illness.

What is sometimes overlooked in the mortality literature is the magnitude of mortality effects. For instance, compared to individuals who are average weight-for-height and adjusting for other health factors, obese individuals are 12% more likely to die in the follow-up period; compared to those who always wear their seat belts, those who never wear their them are 11% more likely to die during follow-up; but compared to those who never smoke those who currently smoke are twice as likely to die over the follow-up period. Thus, compared to other behaviors, cigarette smoking is the most life-threatening behavior that we examined. In addition, about 29% of the U.S. adult population were current smokers in 1990. Thus, this risk factor is not only strongly associated with mortality, but also numerically widespread.

FACTORS RELATED TO ADULT MORTALITY

In Chapter 1, we identified important demographic, sociocultural, socioeconomic, behavioral, and health variables that were thought to be related to mortality in meaningful ways. Of necessity, we limited the topics included to those for which we had strong reason to expect important relations and had adequate data from the matched data set. Clearly, there are other variables for which we do not have adequate data that would enhance our analysis. Nevertheless, we have been able to amass a large and diverse set of covariates to more fully understand current adult mortality differentials.

Based on the research done in this book, we can say that most all of the variables studied are important ones and work to inform mortality patterns. Moreover, the simultaneous examination of the variables included herein underscores the fact that, while some of the variables have greater explanatory power than others, most factors contribute in some way to the overall chances of death among U.S. adults. Indeed, the picture that emerges is one of adult mortality prospects being influenced by a host of factors, each of which adds incrementally to the explanation of overall mortality. No analysis of mortality that focuses on one or a few of these variables as determinants of the chances of dying captures sufficiently the sense of the broad range of factors that affect survival chances.

Conceptual frameworks are intended to be outlines of the variables and their interrelationships that portray a particular explanatory pattern. Our interest in understanding the forces that influence adult mortality outcomes led us to devise the framework that was used for this study. Clearly, however, the search for greater insights into explanations of phenomena require us to continually revise and expand conceptual frameworks. It was our intent to focus our analysis on demographic, sociocultural, socioeconomic, health, and behavioral factors. While we do cover a range of variables under those rubrics, we recognize that there are others that come under those headings that we have not included, and that some we do include could be measured differently. Also, some may argue that our focus creates the impression that a set of variables not included in our analysis is not relevant or important. In particular, there is a host of factors that can be labeled "biological" whose inclusion in the framework would elaborate the kinds of understandings we can achieve about mortality risks. We expect that broader and more informative conceptual frameworks will emerge as researchers carry on this line of inquiry, and that appropriate data sets will enable analysis that simultaneously examines the more elaborate span of variables in their multivariate effect on adult mortality.

DIRECTIONS FOR FUTURE DATA COLLECTION AND RESEARCH

This book has demonstrated the power and flexibility of the NHIS-MCD for research on U.S. adult mortality. Important strengths of the data set include its recent release, large size, the breadth of available factors, the relatively small amount of missing data, and the high quality of matches between the NHIS and MCD files. Moreover, the use of a single source for numerator (death) and denominator (survival) information eliminates the inconsistency that plagues mortality analyses which use two different sources of data. Thus, we are confident that our results are as methodologically sound as most, if not all, other large-scale mortality studies of the U.S. population to date. Further research could incorporate additional factors contained in various years of the Current Health Topic Questionnaires of the NHIS, including supplements focusing on cancer and diabetes. There are also additional available data on parents' longevity, on women's health, and on AIDS-related knowledge and attitudes. Thus, while we have examined in detail many demographic, social, behavioral, and health factors that affect mortality, this rich data source provides additional opportunities for new and innovative analyses.

We uncovered some variables that are important factors to consider in mortality analyses, but are not regularly included in the NHIS. For example, religious attendance was asked only in the Cancer Risk Factor Supplement in 1987. Nevertheless, we found a strong association between religious attendance and mortality risk during follow-up. Clearly, these results call for additional information to more fully understand the mechanisms by which religious involvement affects mortality. A series of items related to stress and the ability to cope with stress is just one example. Additional sets of questions could also be posed related to religious denominations; strength of religious beliefs; frequency of prayer or meditation; reasons for attending church or synagogue; and resources, support, and services that are provided by the person's church, temple, or synagogue. We also recommend increased inclusion of important, but infrequently used variables, including more supplements and questions on mental health. In addition to questions on specific disorders, the NHIS could pose questions on broader mental and emotional concerns, including confusion, distress, daily hassles, and alienation (see Mirowsky and Ross 1989a).

It is of paramount importance that the NHIS continue to be matched with new deaths from the National Death Index (NDI). The NHIS-MCD data set, based on matches between the NHIS and NDI, is of recent origin and will gain power with additional death matches. With additional years of mortality data, it will be possible to provide more detailed analyses of social, economic, cultural, and behavioral factors that are associated with the risk of mortality. For example, we showed that the Asian and Pacific Islander group had the lowest odds of mortality of any race/ethnic group over the follow-up period. However, this umbrella group actually is composed of a diverse set of ethnic groups, including some with seemingly very high mortality (e.g., Hawaiians and Samoans) and others with seemingly very low mortality (e.g., Chinese and Japanese Americans) (Hoyert and Kung 1997). The NHIS only began collecting information on specific Asian and Pacific Islander group membership in 1992, and it will take several years of matches to the NDI before the detailed analysis of Asian and Pacific Islander subgroup mortality can be accomplished. Thus, it is with much enthusiasm that we recommend the ongoing match of the NHIS with the NDI.

Further, future research with the NHIS-MCD data set might explore how individual-level characteristics—such as education, employment, and health behaviors—impinge on the risk of death for other individuals in the household. With such household-level information, it would be possible to examine, say, the effects of problem drinking or drug abuse on other family members, or to parse the effects of direct and passive smoking. More detailed measures of passive smoking could be obtained by linking the smoking status of an individual in the household to other household members. Unfortunately, many of the health behaviors are ascertained in NHIS supplements that are based on sample persons rather than on household sets. In these supplements, one person was selected from each sampled household, and NCHS ascertains information from that single person. We recommend that, similar to the core NHIS, some subsequent NHIS detailed supplements include the same rich detailed covariates for all adults in the household, rather than only for single sample persons. This could be accomplished with the entire sample, or with samples of households (i.e., where households instead of individuals were sampled).

Although we have focused mainly on individual-level associations with adult mortality, future research could expand the existing literature by including variables from the contextual level, including those of the local neighborhood and larger community (see LeClere et al. 1997, 1998). Individuals are not socially isolated but are surrounded and influenced by others. Contextual factors include the social, political, health service, cultural, and physical environments that individuals experience in their daily lives. These forces exert some influence on health and survival conditions beyond those impinging on the individual by operating in neighborhoods, communities, and other geographic units. However, most demographic and public health mortality research has been grounded in an individualistic paradigm (Hummer et al. 1998b; Kunitz 1987). Moreover, few health and mortality data sources contain information on both individuals and the larger settings in which they live (Moss and Krieger 1995). However, individuals are affected not only by their action and the actions of their family and friends, but also by actions of others in the community and the structure of the community itself. Neighborhoods characterized by high poverty, high unemployment, family disruption, and high rates of crime can place people at a heightened risk of death apart from the individual characteristics of those people. For example, recent analyses describe the extreme mortality consequences for individuals who live in areas of highly concentrated poverty (Geronimus et al. 1996; McCord and Freeman 1990). NCHS could move toward allowing more contextual links with the NHIS-MCD data; the current use of contextual data is severely limited because of confidentiality concerns.

The confidentiality concerns could be addressed in a number of ways. First, geocoded information could be released to researchers who could protect the data. It is now possible to include sensitive information on a single workstation that would not be networked or accessible to other users or stations. Second, NCHS could link contextual information to the data set and release broad rather than detailed values of variables. Last, NCHS could experiment with including neighborhood information that is not provided by the interviewers, but is produced by qualitative or quantitative researchers. Such researchers could collect information that is normally collected by the Census, but could also glean information that the Census does not collect, for example, the level of social organization, community integration, and family solidarity. This neighborhood information could be provided as a separate data file and would be like another NHIS supplement, but might be cheaper to produce because the level of analysis would be the neighborhood instead of the individual.

The NHIS was originally established as a national survey of the U.S.

population's health, not mortality risks. Full exploitation of the data for mortality analyses would require some changes in the structure of data collection. For example, the NHIS currently oversamples the elderly to ensure robust estimates of health status. But the elderly experience higher risks of death than do adults at other ages. Thus, a focus on mortality suggests that the NHIS should oversample younger ages, especially ages 18 to 44.

Despite the tremendous benefits of this new and exciting data set, our analysis is influenced by data limitations. The data were collected for particular years and so are bound by period effects; include only individuals aged 18 and over; provide detailed single years of age only to 98, with ages aggregated at 99 and above—which limits the analysis of centenarians; initially includes only noninstitutionalized individuals, but then includes those individuals who may become institutionalized over the course of the mortality follow-up; do not oversample high risk individuals (e.g., alcoholics, drug addicts, or the homeless), which creates problems in investigating rare and life-threatening statuses (e.g., mental and addictive disorders); and are not longitudinal and therefore do not include time-varying covariates (e.g., changes in income, marital status, or smoking status). We offer these caveats because the data and methods are far from perfect, but we maintain that our findings, despite these shortcomings, remain robust, critical, and informative.

UNDERLYING AND MULTIPLE-CAUSE MORTALITY

We have presented an integrated approach to mortality research, with a focus on overall and underlying cause-specific mortality. Future research can also elaborate and extend our findings through different analytic techniques involving the outcome variables. One such way could be through the analysis of different underlying cause of death schemes. Our focus here has been on a rather broad underlying cause of death classification because we wished to paint a general picture of U.S. mortality differentials. Certainly, however, the analysis of more specific, detailed causes is also warranted. Two such foci include HIV/AIDS and Alzheimer's Disease. Each of these causes has made its way to the top 15 of all U.S. causes of death in recent years; indeed, the underlying cause death rate for Alzheimer's Disease has increased substantially since it was first given a separate title in the International Classification of Diseases in 1979 and is now the eighth leading cause of death among adults 65 and over (Hoyert and Rosenberg 1997). However, relatively little work has examined the detailed differentials in mortality associated with these causes, particularly since the reporting of these causes has only recently improved.

Another important aim will be to employ multiple-cause mortality specifications, which refers to deaths in terms of all identifiable medical conditions entered on the death certificate (Nam 1990). Combinations of conditions can be more lethal than single conditions, can affect the timing of death, and can influence the mortality differentials between subpopulations (Wrigley and Nam 1987). Again, Alzheimer's Disease may be an important example of why multiple cause specifications are desired. U.S. Vital Statistics data from 1995 demonstrate that the total number of death certificates on which Alzheimer's Disease was either listed as the underlying cause of death or mentioned as a contributing cause was twice the number for which it was recorded only as the underlying cause (Hoyert and Rosenberg 1997: 112). Thus, an underlying cause analysis of Alzheimer's Disease mortality might seriously underestimate the extent to which this disease affects the U.S. population. Indeed, similar arguments might be made regarding other causes, such as respiratory diseases, which are most often listed as a contributing rather than an underlying cause on death certificates (Israel et al. 1986; Manton and Stallard 1984).

POLICY AND APPLICATION

Our findings with regard to forces affecting adult mortality in the United States are useful not only for explaining the social context of differential mortality and in the development of theory concerning mortality levels and changes, but also contain policy implications. What we have found has consequences for social and health policies, as well as for more practical applications in government and business.

Our chapter summaries identify critical findings that suggest public and private actions, some amenable to policy initiatives and others not, that would help improve survival prospects for the U.S. adult population. The pervasive effect of some socioeconomic factors (especially occupation and income) argues for strengthening economic policies to provide an adequate level of living for everyone to permit better health standards and more widespread access to health care. People seem to be at greater risk of dying when they are not part of an intact family and when social support systems do not sustain them. Policies facilitating health-related assistance to single, divorced, and separated parents and those living alone would go a long way toward insuring longer life. Programs providing for social networks (religious or otherwise) to which people can get attached may help achieve needs not met when people are not so connected. The survival advantages that are experienced by foreign-born groups in the United States suggest that attention should be given to the health aspects of immigration policy. Is there an element of health selection with regard to who immigrates, or are immigrants to the United States subjected to harsher patterns of life only after they have lived in the country for awhile? More focused research can inform future immigration policy in this respect.

That those with functional limitations or mental and addictive disorders exhibited higher risks of mortality in our follow-up period is not surprising. Yet, even persons with those handicaps can live longer and more satisfying lives if programs to improve their conditions are expanded. Recent emphasis on genetic and medical research to identify and correct negative health conditions bodes well for easing the problem, and policies and programs to further pursue these initiatives can be helpful. Above all, our study shows that individual behaviors can be negative or positive in their mortality consequences, apart from demographic and socioeconomic statuses. There is no doubt that heavy smoking is a major deterrent to longer life, as are heavy drinking, lack of adequate exercise, obesity, and failure to secure one's safety (as in the case of using seat belts when in motor vehicles). We already have public and private programs that advise people about some of the attendant health and survival risks, but often these do not flow from specific governmental policies and do not have the force that such policies would engender. Moreover, the public is sometimes uninformed about the nature of risks involved. For instance, while great emphasis is placed on smokers being subject to higher risks of cancer, much less emphasis is placed on the cardiovascular, stroke, and respiratory consequences of smoking. Similarly, while exercise is put forth as a virtue for a healthy life, broad policies and programs are lacking that would not only encourage but facilitate exercise in the community as well as at home.

While a considerable dialogue concerning health policy has been carried out in the United States, often the debate gets mired in issues of program types and costs and who exerts control over the programs. Less consideration is given to the set of factors that are the principal contributors to poorer health and mortal risks and how to integrate this knowledge within a general health policy. Our study, along with others, can provide empirical results for assessing the important factors and stipulating ways in which actions with regard to those factors should be integrated into the policy for particular target groups who are most at risk.

In addition to policy consequences, there are implications of our analysis for practical applications undertaken by federal, state, and local governments, as well as by private agencies. A few examples will suffice as illustrations. Because mortality is one of the principal components of population change, a better understanding of what contributes to changing mortality levels can introduce more refined assumptions about that component in making population estimates and projections used by public and private agencies. To cite another example, those who calculate insurance risks generally base their rates on observed mortality conditions for specific groups. The inclusion in our analysis of such factors as family composition and work statuses can enable actuaries to introduce added elements of precision to those calculations. Finally, the medical profession is attentive to research findings of this type for developing recommendations to patients. Our study sharpens the profiles of persons who are at high risk of premature death, and can assist doctors in giving sounder advice to those for whom they are providing preventive or curative care.

FUTURE OUTLOOK

Until the late 20th century, demographic and social research on mortality was confined to descriptions of existing conditions and measurement of the extent of differences among population categories in death rates and, sometimes, life expectancies. Advances in data collection arising from the expansion of large-scale surveys and improvements in analytical techniques and the use of large-scale computers permitted more refined study of factors affecting mortality. It then became possible to develop more complex conceptual frameworks and apply them to newer data, some involving record linkages, to arrive at explanations of mortality patterns and changes.

The movement from description to explanation in mortality research has gained momentum as we approach the 21st century. For a while, the emphasis was on explaining infant mortality patterns (Mosley and Chen 1984; Eberstein et al. 1990). More recently, population aging has encouraged studies in many parts of the world to be oriented toward understanding adult mortality and, even more specifically, to focusing on explaining differentials in adult mortality (Lopez et al. 1995). Because the vast majority of deaths in developed countries are at adult ages, we would expect the volume and quality of relevant research on adult mortality to continue to be increased.

As we enter a new century, it is natural to take stock of where we have been, where we are, and where we would like to go. An examination of the mortality patterns of the population is one such area where this is possible in an in-depth manner. Although the United States has no clear social policy regarding demographic events, the U.S. Government in 1990 specified National Objectives for Health Promotion and Disease Prevention, with targets for certain health goals for the year 2000 (Stoto 1995). These served as monitoring devices for noting changes in health and mortality, but they have not led to more-clearly formulated policies. Individuals generally agree that the nation should progress toward increasing life expectancy while improving health and the quality of life. And this seems to be the path on which we are heading; indeed, the United States is now experiencing the lowest overall mortality and highest ever life expectancy in our history. This is good news. Moreover, the oldest-old segment of the U.S. population probably experiences the lowest death rate worldwide (Manton and Vaupel 1995).

However, the news is not all positive. Although this book elevates mortality to a central variable, our results carry a larger role. In a more general sense, we are concerned with social inequality. And death is one of the most basic and central indicators of social inequality. Moreover, our book has pointed to different arenas wherein social inequality has not only a central role, but also an immense effect. We have identified inequalities in socioeconomic conditions, family arrangements, health behaviors, and health conditions that can lead to vastly different chances of life or death. Thus, understanding, documenting, and explaining social inequality permeates much of our research and resides at the heart of many of our analyses. Moreover, if U.S. social inequality widens over time (see Massey 1996), the gap in mortality for many social and economic characteristics—race, income, employment status, and occupational status—may also widen. Thus, increasing inequality has the potential to hinder future improvements in mortality.

We have specified factors that lead to short abbreviated lives, and the alternate paths to longer, extended lives. Some of these paths simply require individual choice; individuals can chose to live healthy, active lives, or lives filled with inactivity and risky health behaviors. But some of these paths are laden with structural obstacles. Because of the social structure, some individuals are not completely free to make their own choices. Some individuals, through peer pressure, influences from family members, advertising, or environmental stresses may resort to excessive drinking, smoking, inactivity, and poor diets. Choices are filtered through structural lenses. Not everyone has the opportunity to make unfettered choices. But individuals can make more informed choices based on our identification of areas that lead to long lives, and by balancing the magnitudes that contribute to the risk of death. In short, this book has revealed the broad range of forces that impinge on living and dying in the USA.

Epilogue

Our results counter the central notion presented in "The Triumph of Death," depicted on the book's frontispiece. The force of death is not the same for everyone. Instead, the force of death in the contemporary United States is stronger for the poor, the less educated, the unemployed, and the uninsured rather than for the rich, the highly educated, and the insured; for males rather than for females; for those who rarely attend religious services rather than for those who frequently attend; for those with mental and functional disorders and limitations rather than for those who are disorder- and limitation-free; and for those who smoke, drink heavily, and are inactive rather than for those who have never smoked, who drink moderately, and exercise regularly. Thus, our results carve an updated version of the fifteenth century metal-cut: still trapped beneath the wheels of death are the socially disadvantaged, the sick, and those who engage in destructive health behaviors. But becoming more and more removed from the all-encompassing threat of the wheels, sometimes by great distances, are those with life-promoting behavioral, health, and social characteristics.

REFERENCES

Adams, Patricia F., and Veronica Benson. 1990. "Current Estimates from the National Health Interview Survey, 1989." Vital and Health Statistics. 10(176): National Center for Health Statistics.

Adams, Patricia F., and M. A. Marano. 1995. "Current Estimates from the National Health Interview Survey, 1994." Vital and Health Statistics. 10(193): National Center for Health Statistics.

Adler, Nancy, Thomas Boyce, Margaret Chesney, Sheldon Cohen, Susan Folman, Robert Kahn, and Leonard Syme. 1994. "Socioeconomic Status and Health: The Challenge of the Gradient." American Psychologist. 49(1):15–24.

Aldrich, John H., and Forrest D. Nelson. 1984. Linear Probability, Logit, and Probit Models. Beverly Hills: Sage.

Allison, Paul D. 1984. Event History Analysis: Regression for Longitudinal Event Data. Beverly Hills, CA: Sage Publications.

Alreck, Pamela L., and Robert B. Settle. 1985. The Survey Research Handbook. Homewood, IL: Irwin.

American Psychiatric Association. 1994. Diagnostic and Statistical Manual of Mental Disorders. Fourth edition. Washington, DC: American Psychiatric Association.

Anderson, Robert N., Kenneth D. Kochanek, and Sherry L. Murphy. 1997. "Report of Final Mortality Statistics, 1995." Monthly Vital Statistics Report. 45(11), supplement 2. Hyattsville, MD: National Center for Health Statistics.

Angel, Jacqueline L., Ronald J. Angel, and Kristin J. Henderson. 1997. "Contextualizing Social Support and Health in Old Age: Reconsidering Culture and Gender." International Journal of Sociology and Social Policy. 17(9–10):83–116.

Antonucci, Toni C. 1990. "Social Supports and Social Relationships." Pp. 205–216 in Handbook of Aging and the Social Sciences, Third Edition, edited by Robert H. Binstock and Linda K. George. NY: Academic Press.

Atchley, Robert C. 1991. Social Forces and Aging: An Introduction to Social Gerontology. Belmont, CA: Wadsworth Publishing Company.

Barringer, Herbert R., Robert W. Gardner, and Michael J. Levin. 1993. Asians and Pacific Islanders in the United States. NY: Russell Sage.

Bean, Frank D., and Marta Tienda. 1987. The Hispanic Population of the United States. NY: Russell Sage Foundation.

Belloc, N. B. 1973. "Relationship of Health Practices and Mortality." Preventive Medicine. 2(1):67–81.

Belloc, N. B., and L. Breslow. 1972. "Relationship of Physical Health Status and Health Practices." Preventive Medicine. 1(3):409–421.

Berkman, Lisa F., and Lester Breslow. 1983. Health and Ways of Living. NY: Oxford University Press.

Berkman, Lisa F., Lester Breslow, and Deborah Wingard. 1983. "Health Practices and Mortality Risk." Pp. 61–112 in Berkman, Lisa F. and Lester Breslow, eds. 1983. Health and Ways of Living. New York: Oxford University Press.

Berkman, Lisa F., and S. Leonard Syme. 1979. "Social Networks, Host Resistance, and Mortality: A Nine-Year Follow-up Study of Alameda County Residents." American Journal of Epidemiology. 109:186–204.

Biraben, J. N. 1982. "Morbidity and the Major Processes Culminating in Death." In Samuel Preston, ed., Biological and Social Aspects of Mortality and the Length of Life, pp. 385–392. Liege: Ordina Editions.

Blackwelder,William C., K. Yano, C. G. Rhodes, A. Kagan, T. Gordon. 1980. "Alcohol and Mortality: The Honolulu Heart Study." American Journal of Medicine 68(2):164–169.

Blair, Steven N., Harold W. Kohl, Ralph S. Paffenbarger, Debra G. Clark, Kenneth H. Cooper, and Larry W. Gibbons. 1989. "Physical Fitness and All-Cause Mortality: A Prospective Study of Health Men and Women." Journal of the American Medical Association. 262(17):2395–2401.

Blane, David, George Davey Smith, and Mel Bartley. 1993. "Social Selection: What Does It Contribute to Social Class Differences in Health?" Sociology of Health and Illness. 15(1):1–15.

Blau, Peter M., and Otis Dudley Duncan. 1967. The American Occupational Structure. NY: John Wiley and Sons.

Bradley, Don E. 1995. "Religious Involvement and Social Resources:Evidence from the Dataset American Changing Lives." Journal for the Scientific Study of Religion. 34(2):259–267.

Bradshaw, Benjamin S., and Karen A. Liese. 1991. "Mortality of Mexican-Origin Persons in the Southwestern United States." Pp. 81–94 in Mortality of Hispanic Populations, edited by I. Rosenwaike. New York: Greenwood Press.

Brown, A. S., and J. Birthwhistle. 1996. "Excess Mortality of Mental Illness." British Journal of Psychiatry. 169(3):361–368.

Bruce, Martha Livingston, and Philip J. Leaf. 1989. "Psychiatric Disorders and 15-Month Mortality in a Community Sample of Older Adults." American Journal of Public Health. 79(6):727–730.

Bryant, Sharon, and William Rakowski. 1992. "Predictors of Mortality among Elderly African Americans." Research on Aging. 14(1):50–67.

Buhmann, Brigitte, Lee Rainwater, Guenther Schmans, and Timothy M. Smeeding. 1988. "Equivalence Scales, Well-being, Inequality, and Poverty: Sensitivity Estimates Across Ten Countries Using the Luxembourg Income Study (LIS) Database." Review of Income and Wealth. 34(2):115–142.

Bumpass, Larry L., James A. Sweet, and Andrew J. Cherlin 1991. "The Role of Cohabitation in Declining Rates of Marriage." Journal of Marriage and the Family. 53:913–927.

Burstin, Helen R., Stuart R. Lipsitz, Troyen A. Brennan. 1992. "Socioeconomic Status and Risk for Substandard Medical Care." Journal of the American Medical Association. 268(17):2383–2387.

Butz, Roger H., and W. John Elder. 1996. "Drug Abuse, Alcohol, and Tobacco." Chapter 30 in Medical Selection of Life Risks. Third edition. Edited by R. D. C. Brackenridge and W. John Elder. NY: Stockton Press. Pp. 895–906.

Cabral, Howard, Lise E. Fried, Suzette Levenson, Hortensia Amaro, and Barry Zuckerman. 1990. "Foreign-Born and U.S.-Born Black Women: Differences in Health Behaviors and Birth Outcomes." American Journal of Public Health. 80(1):70–72.

Caetano, Raul. 1991. "Findings from the 1984 National Survey of Alcohol Use Among US Hispanics," pp. 293–307 in Walter B. Clark and Michael E. Hilton, eds., Alcohol in America: Drinking Practices and Problems. Albany: State University of New York Press.

Calnan, Michael. 1987. Health and Illness: the Lay Perspective. London: Tavistock.

Camacho, Terry C., George A. Kaplan, and Richard D. Cohen. 1987. "Alcohol Consumption and Mortality in Alameda County." Journal of Chronic Disease. 40:229–236.

Campbell, Robert J. 1981. Psychiatric Dictionary. Fifth edition. NY: Oxford University Press.

Carey, James R. 1997. "What Demographers Can Learn from Fruit Fly Actuarial Models and Biology." Demography. 34: 17–30.

Carter, Lawrence R., and Ronald D. Lee. 1992. "Modeling and Forecasting U.S. Sex Differentials in Mortality." International Journal of Forecasting. 8: 393–411.

Casselli, Graziella, and Alan D. Lopez. 1996. Health and Mortality Among Elderly Populations. Oxford: Clarendon Press.

Castro, Felipe G., Lourdes Baezconde-Garbanati, and Hector Beltran. 1985. "Risk Factors for Coronary Heart Disease in Hispanic Populations: A Review." Hispanic Journal of Behavioral Sciences. 7(2):153–175.

Centers for Disease Control. 1993. "Cigarette Smoking Attributable Mortality and Years of Potential Life Lost—U.S., 1980." Morbidity and Mortality Weekly Report 42:645–649.

Christenson, Bruce A., and Nan E. Johnson. 1995. "Educational Inequality in Adult Mortality: An Assessment with Death Certificate Data from Michigan." Demography. 32(May): 215–230.

Chyba, Michele M., and Linda R. Washington. 1993. "Questionnaires from the National Health Interview Survey, 1985–89." Vital and Health Statistics. 1(31):1–412.

Coale, Ansley J. 1996. "Age Patterns and Time Sequence of Mortality in National Populations with the Highest Expectation of Life at Birth." Population and Development Review. 22(1): 127–135.

Cobas, Jose A., Hector Balcazar, Mary B. Benin, Verna M. Keith, and Yinong Chong. 1996. "Acculturation and Low Birthweight Infants among Latino Women: A Reanalysis of HHANES Data with Structural Equation Models." American Journal of Public Health. 86(3):394–96.

Cobb, Sidney. 1976. "Social Support as a Moderator of Life Stress." Psychosomatic Medicine. 38(5):300–14.

Cockerham, William C. 1988. "Medical Sociology." In Handbook of Sociology, edited by Neil J. Smelser. Beverly Hills, CA: Sage.

Comstock, George W., and Kay B. Partridge. 1972. "Church Attendance and Health." Journal of Chronic Diseases. 25: 665–672.

Comstock, George W., and James A. Tonascia. 1977. "Education and Mortality in Washington County, Maryland." Journal of Health and Social Behavior. 18(1):54–61.

Crimmins, Eileen M. 1997. "Trends in Mortality, Morbidity, and Disability: What Should We Expect for the Future of Our Ageing Population?" pp. 317–325 in International Population Conference: Beijing 1997. Vol. 1. Liege: International Union for the Scientific Study of Population.

Day, J. C. 1993. Population Projections of the United States, by Age, Sex, Race, and Hispanic Origin: 1993 to 2050. Current Population Reports, P25–1104.

DeLabry, Lorraine O., et al. 1992. "Alcohol Consumption and Mortality Among Men Enrolled in an American Cancer Society Prospective Study." Epidemiology. 53:25–32.

Demers, Raymond Y., C. William Michaels, Robert Frank, Kathy Fagan, Melissa McDiarmid, and Theresa Rohr. 1990. "Termination of Health Benefits for Pittston Mine Workers: Impact on the Health and Security of Miners and Their Families." Journal of Public Health Policy. 11(4):474–480.

DeVita, Carol J. 1996. "The United States at Mid-Decade." Population Bulletin. 50(4). Washington, D.C.: Population Reference Bureau.

Dey, Achintya N. 1997. "Characteristics of Elderly Nursing Home Residents: Data from the 1995 National Nursing Home Survey." Advance Data from Vital and Health Statistics. 289. Hyattsville, MD: NCHS.

Donahue, Ricard P., Robert D Abbot, Dwayne M. Reed, and Katsuhiko Yano. 1988. "Physical Activity and Coronary Heart Disease in Middle-Aged and Elderly Men: The Honolulu Heart Program." American Journal of Public Health. 78(6):683–685.

Dorn, Joan M., Enrique F. Schisterman, Warren Winklestein, Jr., and Maurizio Trevisan. 1997. "Body Mass Index and Mortality in a General Population Sample of Men and Women: The Buffalo Study." American Journal of Epidemiology. 148(11): 919–931.

Duncan, Otis Dudley. 1961. "A Socioeconomic Index for All Occupations." In A. J. Reiss, Jr., ed., Occupations and Social Status. NY: The Free Press of Glencoe.

Durkheim, Emile. 1951. Suicide: A Study in Sociology. New York: Free Press. (Original work published 1897.)

Dwyer, Jeffrey W., Leslie L. Clarke, and Michael K. Miller. 1990. "The Effect of Religious Concentration and Affiliation on County Cancer Mortality Rates." Journal of Health and Social Behavior 31(2):185–202.

Eastwood, M. Robin, Susan Stiasny, H.M. Rosemary Meier, and Caroline M. Woogh. 1982. "Mental Illness and Mortality." Comprehensive Psychiatry. 23(4):377–385.

Eberstein, Isaac W., Charles B. Nam, and Robert A. Hummer. 1990. "Infant Mortality by Cause of Death: Main and Interactive Effects." Demography. 27(Aug):413–30.

Ellison, Christopher G. 1991. "Religious Involvement and Subjective Well-Being." Journal of Health and Social Behavior. 32: 80–99.

———. 1994. "Religion, the Life Stress Paradigm, and the Study of Depression." Pp. 78–124 in Religion in Aging and Health: Theoretical Foundations and Methodological Frontiers, edited by J. Levin. Thousand Oaks, CA: Sage Productions.

Ellison, Christopher G., and Linda K. George. 1994. "Religious Involvement, Social Ties, and Social Support in a Southeastern Community." Journal for the Scientific Study of Religion. 33(Mar): 46–61.

Ellison, Christopher G., and Jeffrey S. Levin. 1998. "The Religion-Health Connection: Evidence, Theory, and Future Directions." Health Education and Behavior. 25:700–720.

Elo, Irma T., and Samuel H. Preston. 1992. "Effects of Early-Life Conditions on Adult Mortality: A Review." Population Index. 58(2):186–212.

———. 1996. "Educational Differentials in Mortality: United States, 1979–85." Social Science and Medicine. 42(1):47–57.

———. 1997. "Racial and Ethnic Differences in Mortality at Older Ages." Pp. 10–42 in Racial and Ethnic Differences in the Health of Older Americans, edited by L. Martin and B. Soldo. Washington, D.C.: National Academy Press.

Engels, Friedrich. [1845] 1958. The Condition of the Working Class in England. Translated by W.O. Henderson and W.H. Chaloner. Stanford, CA: Stanford University Press.

Evans, Leonard. 1987. "Fatality Risk Reduction from Safety Belt Use." The Journal of Trauma. 27(7): 746–749.

Fang, Jing, Shantha Madhavan, and Michael H. Alderman. 1997. "The Influence of Birthplace on Mortality among Hispanic Residents of New York City." Ethnicity and Disease. 7: 55–64.

Feldman, J., D. Makuc, J. Kleinman, and J. Cornoni-Huntley. 1989. "National Trends in Educational Differences in Mortality." American Journal of Epidemiology. 129(5): 919–933.

Felker, Bradford, J. Joe Yazel, and Delmar Short. 1996. "Mortality and Medical Comorbidity among Psychiatric Patients: A Review." Psychiatric Services. 47(12):1356–1363.

Fernandez, Nelson A. 1975. "Nutrition in Puerto Rico." Cancer Research. 35(11):3272–3291.

Fingerhut, Lois A., Cheryl Jones, and Diane M. Makuc. 1994. "Firearm and Motor Vehicle Injury Mortality—Variations by State, Race, and Ethnicity: United States, 1990–91." Advance Data from Vital and Health Statistics. 242:112.

Forthofer, R. 1992. "Complex Surveys and Their Analysis." Prepared for the National Institute of Dental Research.

Fox, J. 1984. Linear Statistical Models and Related Methods. NY: Wiley.

Franks, Peter, Carolyn M. Clancy, and Marthe R. Gold. 1993. "Health Insurance and Mortality." JAMA. 270(6):737–741.

Fraser, G. E. 1988. "Determinants of Ischemic Heart Disease in Seventh-day Adventists: A Review." American Journal of Clinical Nutrition. 48: 833–836.

Friend, K., A. Belanger, R. D'Agostino, and W. Kannel. 1993. "The Health Risks of Smoking: The Framingham Study: 34 Years of Follow-Up." Annual Epidemiology. 3:417–424.

Friedman, Howard S. (editor). 1998. Encyclopedia of Mental Health. NY: Academic Press.

Gage, Timothy B. 1994. "Population Variation in Cause of Death: Level, Gender, and Period Effects." Demography. 31(May): 271–296.

Gardner, John W., and Joseph L. Lyon. 1982a. "Cancer in Utah Mormon Women by Church Activity Level." American Journal of Epidemiology. 116(2): 258–265.

———. 1982b. "Cancer in Utah Mormon Men by Lay Priesthood Level." American Journal of Epidemiology. 116(2): 243–257.

Garrison, Robert J., et al. 1983. "Cigarette Smoking as a Confounder of the Relationship Between Relative Weight and Longterm Mortality: the Framingham Heart Study." Journal of the American Medical Association. 249(16):2199–2203.

Geronimus, Arline T., John Bound, Timothy A. Waidmann, Marianne M. Hillemeier, and Patricia B. Burns. 1996. "Excess Mortality among Blacks and Whites in the United States." New England Journal of Medicine. 335:1552–1558.

Goldstein, Sidney. 1996. "Changes in Jewish Mortality and Survival, 1963–1987." Social Biology. 43(1–2):72–97.

Gordon, Tara and Joseph T. Doyle. 1988. "Weight and Mortality in Men: The Albany Study." International Journal of Epidemiology. 17(1):77–81.

Gottlieb, Nell H., and Lawrence W. Green. 1984. "Life Events, Social Network, Life-Style, and Health: An Analysis of the 1979 National Survey of Personal Health Practices and Consequences." Health Education Quarterly. 11: 91–105.

Gove, Walter R. 1973. "Sex, Marital Status, and Mortality." American Journal of Sociology. 79: 45–66.

Grodstein, Francine, Meir J. Stampfer, Graham A. Colditz, Walter C. Willett, JoAnn E. Manson, Marshall Joffe, Bernard Rosner, Charles Fuchs, Susan E. Hankinson, David J. Hunter, Charles H. Hennekens, and Frank E. Speizer. 1997. "Postmenopausal Hormone Therapy and Mortality." New England Journal of Medicine. 336: 1769–1775.

Groenbaek, Morten, A. Dies, T.I.A. Sorenson, U. Becker. 1994. "Influence of Sex, Age, Body Mass Index, and Smoking on Alcohol Intake and Mortality." British Medical Journal. 308(6924):302–306.

Guendelman, Sylvia, and Paul B. English. 1995. "Effect of United States Residence on Birth Outcomes among Mexican Immigrants: An Exploratory Study." American Journal of Epidemiology. 142: S30–S38.

Gunnarsson, Olafur T., and James O. Judge. 1997. "Exercise at Midlife: How and Why to Prescribe it for Sedentary Patients." Geriatrics. 52(5):71–80.

Hahn, Robert A., and Donna F. Stroup. 1994. "Race and Ethnicity in Public Health Surveillance: Criteria for the Scientific Use of Social Categories." Public Health Reports. 109(1):715.

Hahn, Robert A. 1995. Life Expectancy in Four U.S. Racial/Ethnic Populations: 1990. Epidemiology. 6:350–355.

Hakim, Amy A., Helen Petrovitch, Cecil M. Burchfiel, G. Webster Ross, Beatriz L. Rodriguez, Lon R. White, Katsuhiko Yano, J. David Curb, and Robert D. Abbott. 1998. "Effects of Walking on Mortality Among Nonsmoking Retired Men." The New England Journal of Medicine. 338(2):94–99.

Hansen, Kristin A., and Carol S. Faber. 1997. "The Foreign-Born Population of the United States: 1996." Current Population Reports: Population Characteristics, P20–494.

Hanushek, E., and J. Jackson. 1977. Statistical Methods for Social Scientists. Orlando, FL: Academic Press.

Haug, Marie R. 1977. "Measurement in Social Stratification." Annual Review of Sociology. 3:51–77.

Hauser, Robert M. 1994. "Measuring Poverty and Socioeconomic Status in Studies of Health and Well-Being." Paper prepared for the NICHD Conference, "Measuring Social Inequalities in Health," Annapolis, Maryland.

Hayward, Mark D., Melissa A Hardy, and William R. Grady. 1989. "Labor Force Withdrawal Patterns among Older Men in the United States." Social Science Quarterly. 70(2):425–448.

Heligman, Larry, and J. H. Pollard. 1980. "The Age Pattern of Mortality." Journal of the Institute of Actuaries 10: 49–75.

Helmrich, Susan P., David R. Ragland, Rita W. Leung, and Ralph S. Paffenbarger, Jr. 1991. "Physical Activity and Reduced Occurrence of Non-Insulin-Dependent Diabetes Mellitus." The New England Journal of Medicine. 325(3):147–152.

Hilton, Michael E. 1991a. "The Demographic Distribution of Drinking Patterns in 1984," pp. 73–86 in Walter B. Clark and Michael E. Hilton, eds., Alcohol in America. Albany: State University of New York Press.

———. 1991b. "Trends in U.S. Drinking Patterns: Further Evidence from the Past Twenty Years," pp. 121–138 in Walter B. Clark and Michael E. Hilton, eds., Alcohol in America. Albany: State University of New York Press.

Hilton, Michael E., and Walter B. Clark. 1991. "Changes in American Drinking Patterns and Problems, 1967–1984," pp. 105–120 in Walter B. Clark and Michael E. Hilton, eds., Alcohol in America. Albany: State University of New York Press.

Himes, Christine L. 1994. "Age Patterns of Mortality and Cause of Death Structures in Sweden, Japan, and the United States." Demography. 31(Nov): 633–650.

Horiuchi, Shiro. 1997. "Postmenopausal Acceleration of Age-Related Mortality Increase." Journal of Gerontology: Biological Sciences. 52A(1):B78–B92.

Horiuchi, Shiro, and John R. Wilmoth. 1997. "Age Patterns of the Life Table Aging Rate for Major Causes of Death in Japan, 1951–1990." Journal of Gerontology: Biological Sciences. 52A(1):B67–B77.

———. 1998. "Deceleration in the Age Pattern of Mortality at Older Ages." Demography. 35(4):391–412.

Horm, John. 1993. "The National Health Interview Survey and the National Death Index." Presentation to the National Center for Health Statistics. May 19. Hyattsville, MD.

———. 1996. "Linkage of the National Health Interview Survey with the National Death Index: Methodologic and Analytic Issues." Paper presented at the annual meeting of the Population Association of America, New Orleans.

Hosmer, David W. and Stanley Lemeshow. 1989. Applied Logistic Regression. NY: John Wiley and Sons.

House, James S. 1987. "Social Support and Social Structure." Sociological Forum. 2(1):135–146.

House, James S., Karl R. Landis, and Debra Umberson. 1988. "Social Relationships and Health." Science. 241(4865): 540–545.

House, James S., Cynthia Robbins, and Helen L. Metzner. 1982. "The Association of Social Relationships and Activities with Mortality: Prospective Evidence from the Tecumseh Community Health Study." American Journal of Epidemiology. 116(1): 123–140.

House, James S., Victor Strecher, Helen L. Metzner, and Cynthia Robbins. 1986. "Occupational Stress and Health among Men and Women in the Tecumseh Community Health Study." Journal of Health and Social Behavior. 27(1):62–77.

Hoyert, Donna L., and Hsiang-Ching Kung. 1997. "Asian or Pacific Islander Mortality, Selected States, 1992." Monthly Vital Statistics Report. 46(1): Supplement.

Hoyert, Donna L., and Harry M. Rosenberg. 1997. "Alzheimer's Disease as a Cause of Death in the United States." Public Health Reports. 112: 497–505.

Hummer, Robert A. 1996. "Black-White Differences in Health and Mortality: A Review and Conceptual Model." The Sociological Quarterly. 37(1):105–125.

Hummer, Robert A., Charles B. Nam, and Richard G. Rogers. 1998a. "Adult Mortality Differentials Associated with Cigarette Smoking in the United States." Population Research and Policy Review. 17:284–304.

Hummer, Robert A., Richard G. Rogers, and Isaac W. Eberstein. 1998b. "Sociodemographic Differentials in Adult Mortality: Review of Analytic Approaches." Population and Development Review. 24(3):553–578.

Hummer, Robert A., Richard G. Rogers, and Charles B. Nam. 1995. "Smoking and Premature Adult Mortality: Combined Effects of Drinking, Weight Status, and Sociodemographic Background." Paper presented at the Population Association of America.

Hummer, Robert A., Richard G. Rogers, Charles B. Nam, and Christopher G. Ellison. 1999a. "Religious Involvement and U.S. Adult Mortality." Demography. 36(2):273–285.

Hummer, Robert A., Richard G. Rogers, Charles B. Nam, and Felicia B. LeClere. 1999b. "Race/Ethnicity, Nativity, and U.S. Adult Mortality." Social Science Quarterly. 80(1):136–153.

Idler, Ellen. 1987. "Religious Involvement and the Health of the Elderly: Some Hypotheses and an Initial Test." Social Forces. 66(Sept): 226–238.

———. 1995. "Religion, Health, and Nonphysical Senses of Self." Social Forces. 74(Dec):683–704.

Idler, Ellen, and Yael Benyamini. 1997. "Self-Rated Health and Mortality: A Review of Twenty-Seven Community Studies." Journal of Health and Social Behavior. 39 (Mar):21–37.

Idler, Ellen L., and Stanislav V. Kasl. 1991. "Health Perceptions and Survival: Do Global Evaluations of Health Status Really Predict Mortality?" Journal of Gerontology: Social Sciences. 46(Mar):S55–S65.

———. 1992. "Religion, Disability, Depression, and the Timing of Death." American Journal of Sociology. 97(Jan):1052–1079.

Illsley, Raymond. 1980. Professional or Public Health? Sociology in Health and Medicine. London: Nuffield Provincial Hospitals Trust.

———. 1986. "Occupational Class, Selection, and the Production of Inequalities." Quarterly Journal of Social Affairs. 2(2):151–161.

Ingram, Rick E., and Christin Scher. 1998. "Depression." Pp. 723–732 in Encyclopedia of Mental Health. Edited by Howard S. Friedman. Volume 1. NY: Academic Press.

Institute of Medicine. 1985. "Research on Mental Illness and Addictive Disorders: Progress and Prospects. A Report of the Board on Mental Health and Behavioral Medicine." American Journal of Psychiatry. 142(7 Suppl):1–41.

Israel, Robert A., Harry M. Rosenberg, and Lester R. Curtin. 1986. "Analytical Potential for Multiple Cause-of-Death Data." American Journal of Epidemiology. 124: 161–179.

Jarvis, George K., and Herbert C. Northcott. 1987. "Religion and Differences in Morbidity and Mortality." Social Science and Medicine. 25(7): 813–824.

Jasso, Guillermina, and Mark Rosenzweig. 1990. The New Chosen People: Immigrants in the United States. NY: Russell Sage.

Jones, Camara Phyllis, Thomas A. LaVeist, and Marsha Lillie-Blanton. 1991. "Race in the Epidemiologic Literature: An Examination of the 'American Journal of Epidemiology', 1921–1990." American Journal of Epidemiology. 134: 1079–1084.

Kahn, Ada P., and Jan Fawcett. 1993. The Encyclopedia of Mental Health. NY: Facts on File.

Kaplan, George A., and Terry Camacho. 1983. "Perceived Health and Mortality: A Nine Year

Follow-up of the Human Population Laboratory Cohort." American Journal of Epidemiology. 117(3):292–304.

Kaplan, George A., Teresea E. Seeman, Richard D. Cohen, Lisa P. Knudsen, and Jack Guralnick. 1987. "Mortality among the Elderly in the Alameda County Study: Behavioral and Demographic Risk Factors." American Journal of Public Health. 77(3):307–312.

Kaplan, George A., and Julian E. Keil. 1993. "Socioeconomic Factors and Cardiovascular Disease: A Review of the Literature." Circulation. 88(4):1973–1998.

Kark, Jeremy D., Galia Shemi, Yechiel Friedlander, Oz Martin, Orly Manor, and S. H. Blondheim. 1996. "Does Religious Observance Promote Health? Mortality in Secular vs Religious Kibbutzim in Israel." American Journal of Public Health. 86(3): 341–346.

Katz, Sidney, Laurence G. Branch, Michael H. Branson, Joseph A. Papsidero, John C. Beck, and David S. Greer. 1983. "Active Life Expectancy." The New England Journal of Medicine. 309(20):1218–224.

Katz, Sidney, et al. 1963. "Studies of Illness in the Aged. The Index of ADL: A Standardized Measure of Biological and Psychosocial Function." Journal of the American Medical Association. 185:94–101.

Kaufman, Jay S., and Richard S. Cooper. 1995. "In Search of the Hypothesis." Public Health Reports. 110: 662–666.

Kestenbaum, Bert. 1986. "Mortality by Nativity." Demography. 23: 87–90.

———. 1997. "Recent Mortality of the Oldest Old, from Medicare Data." Paper presented at the annual meeting of the Population Association of America, Washington, DC.

Keys, Ancel. 1989. "Longevity of Men: Relative Weight and Fatness in Middle Age." Annals of Medicine. 21(3): 163–168.

Kisker, Ellen E., and Noreen J. Goldman. 1987. "Perils of Single Life and Benefits of Marriage." Social Biology. 34:135–152

Kitagawa, Evelyn M., and Phillip M. Hauser. 1973. Differential Mortality in the United States: A Study in Socioeconomic Epidemiology. Cambridge, MA: Harvard University Press.

Kitano, H., and R. Daniels. 1995. Asian Americans: Emerging Minorities. NY: Prentice-Hall.

Klatsky, Arthur L., Mary Anne Armstrong, and Gary D. Friedman. 1992. "Alcohol and Mortality." Annals of Internal Medicine. 117(8):646–654.

Klatsky, Arthur, and Gary Friedman. 1995. "Annotation: Alcohol and Longevity." American Journal of Public Health. 85(1): 16–18.

Kleinman, Joel C., Lois A. Fingerhut, and Kate Prager. 1991. "Differences in Infant Mortality by Race, Nativity Status, and Other Maternal Characteristics." American Journal of Diseases of Children. 145(2):194–99.

Knudsen, Christin, and Robert McNown. 1993. "Changing Causes of Death and the Sex Differential in the USA: Recent Trends and Projections." Population Research and Policy Review. 12: 27–42.

Krieger, N., D. Rowley, A. Herman, B. Avery, and M. Phillips. 1993. "Racism, Sexism, and Social Class: Implications for Studies of Health, Disease, and Well-Being." American Journal of Preventive Medicine. 9 (6 supplement): 82–122.

Kunitz, Stephen J. 1987. "Explanations and Ideologies of Mortality Patterns." Population and Development Review. 13:379–408.

Lawson, James J., and Deborah Black. 1993. "Socioeconomic Status: The Prime Indicator of Premature Death in Australia." Journal of Biosocial Science. 25(4):539–552.

Leavitt, Judith Walzer, and Ronald L. Numbers. 1997. Sickness and Health in America. Madison, WI: University of Wisconsin Press.

LeClere, Felicia, Richard G. Rogers, and Kimberley Peters. 1998. "Neighborhood Social Context and Racial Differences in Women's Heart Disease Mortality." Journal of Health and Social Behavior. 39(2):91–107.

———. 1997. "Ethnicity and Mortality in the United States: Individual and Community Correlates." Social Forces. 76:169–198.

Lee, I-Min, J. E. Manson, C. H. Hennekens, R. S. Jr. Paffenbarger 1993. "Body Weight and

Mortality: a 27-Year Follow-up of Middle-aged Men." Journal of the American Medical Association. 270(23):2823–2828.

Lee, I-Min, and R. S. Paffenberger, Jr. 1992. "Change in Body Weight and Longevity." Journal of the American Medical Association. 268(15) : 2045–2828.

Lee, P. 1995. "Measuring Social Inequalities in Health: Introduction." Public Health Reports. 110: 302–305.

Levin, Jeffrey S. 1994a. "Introduction: Religion in Aging and Health." Pp. xv–xxiv in Religion in Aging and Health: Theoretical Foundations and Methodological Frontiers, edited by J. S. Levin. Thousand Oaks, CA: Sage Publications.

———. 1994b. "Investigating the Epidemiologic Effects of Religious Experience: Findings, Explanations, and Barriers." Pp. 3–17 in Religion in Aging and Health: Theoretical Foundations and Methodological Frontiers, edited by Jeffrey S. Levin. Thousand Oaks, CA: Sage Publications.

———. 1994c. "Religion and Health: Is There an Association, Is it Valid, and Is it Causal?" Social Science and Medicine. 38(11):1475–1482.

Levin, Jeffrey S., and Kyriakos S. Markides. 1986. "Religious Attendance and Subjective Health." Journal for the Scientific Study of Religion. 25: 31–39.

Levin, Jeffrey S., and Preston L. Schiller. 1987. "Is There a Religious Factor in Health?" Journal of Religion and Health. 26: 9–36.

Levin, Jeffrey S., and H.Y. Vanderpool. 1987. "Is Frequent Religious Attendance Really Conducive to Better Health?: Toward an Epidemiology of Religion." Social Science and Medicine. 24(7): 589–600.

Lewis, M. A., B. Leake, M. Leal-Sotelo, and V. Clark. 1990. "First Nursing Home Admissions: Time Spent at Home and in Institutions after Discharge." American Journal of Public Health. 80(1):22–24.

Liao, Youlian, Richard S. Cooper, Guichan Cao, Ramon Durazo-Arvizu, Jay S. Kaufman, Andrew E. Long, and Daniel L. McGee. 1997. "Mortality from Coronary Heart Disease among Adult U.S. Hispanics: Findings from the National Health Interview Survey (1986 to 1994)." Journal of the American College of Cardiology. 30: 1200–1205.

Liao, Youlian, Richard S. Cooper, Guichan Cao, Ramon Durazo-Arvizu, Jay S. Kaufman, Amy Luke, and Daniel L. McGee. 1998. "Mortality Patterns among Adult Hispanics: Findings from NHIS, 1986–1990." American Journal of Public Health. 88(2):227–232.

Liberatos, Penny, Bruce G. Link, and Jennifer L. Kelsey. 1988. "The Measurement of Social Class in Epidemiology." Epidemiologic Reviews. 10:87–121.

Lillard, Lee A., and Constantijn W. Panis. 1996. "Marital Status and Mortality: The Role of Health." Demography. 33(3):313–327.

Lillard, Lee A., and Linda Waite. 1995. "Til Death Do Us Part: Marital Disruption and Mortality." American Journal of Sociology. 100(Mar):1131–1156.

Link, Bruce G., and Jo C. Phelan. 1995. "Social Conditions as Fundamental Causes of Disease." Journal of Health and Social Behavior. Extra Issue. Pp. 80–94.

———. 1996. "Editorial: Understanding Sociodemographic Differences in Health—The Role of Fundamental Social Causes." American Journal of Public Health. 86(4):471–473.

Lipsedge, Maurice. 1996. "Psychiatric Disorders." Pp. 782–804 in Medical Selection of Life Risks. Chapter 24. Third edition. Edited by R. D. C. Brackenridge and W. John Elder. NY: Stockton Press.

Longino, C. F., Jr., G. J. Warheit, and J. A. Green. 1989. "Class, Aging, and Health." In K. S. Markides (Ed.), Aging and Health: Perspectives on Gender, Race, Ethnicity, and Class. Pp. 70–109). Newbury Park, CA: Sage.

Lopez, Alan D. 1983. "The Sex Mortality Differential in Developed Countries." In Sex Differentials in Mortality. Edited by A. D. Lopez and L. T. Ruzicka. Pp. 53–120. Australian National University, Canberra.

Lopez, Alan D., Graziella Caselli, and Tapani Valkonen. 1995. Adult Mortality in Developed Countries: From Description to Explanation. Oxford: Clarendon Press.

Loscocco, Karyn A., and Glenna Spitz. 1990. "Working Conditions, Social Support, and the Well-Being of Female and Male Factory Workers." Journal of Health and Social Behavior. 31(Dec):313–327.

Lyon, Joseph L., John W. Gardner, Melville R. Klauber, and Charles R. Smart. 1977. "Low Cancer Incidence and Mortality in Utah." Cancer. 39(6): 2608–2618.

Lyon, Joseph L., Melville R. Klauber, John W. Gardner, and Charles R. Smart. 1976. "Cancer Incidence in Mormons and non-Mormons in Utah, 1966–1970." New England Journal of Medicine. 294(3):129–133.

Maddala, G. 1983. Limited-Dependent and Qualitative Variables in Econometrics. NY: Cambridge University Press.

Madigan, Francis C. 1957. "Are Sex Mortality Differentials Biologically Caused?" Milbank Memorial Fund Quarterly. 35: 202–223.

Manson, JoAnn E., M. J. Stampfer, C. H. Hennekens, W. C. Willett. 1987. "Body Weight and Longevity: A Reassessment." Journal of the American Medical Association. 257: 353–358.

Manton, Kenneth G. 1988. "A Longitudinal Study of Functional Change and Mortality in the United States." Journal of Gerontology. 43(5):S153–S161.

Manton, Kenneth G., and E. Stallard. 1984. Recent Trends in Mortality Analysis. Orlando: Academic Press.

Manton, Kenneth G., and James W. Vaupel. 1995. "Survival After the Age of 80 in the United States, Sweden, France, England, and Japan." New England Journal of Medicine. 333: 1232–1235.

Mare, Robert D. 1990. "Socio-economic Careers and Differential Mortality among Older Men in the United States." In Measurement and Analysis of Mortality—New Approaches, ed. J. Vallin, S. D'Souza, and A. Palloni. Pp. 362–87. Oxford: Clarendon.

Markides, Kyriakos S., and Jeanine Coreil. 1986. "The Health of Hispanics in the Southwestern United States: An Epidemiological Paradox." Public Health Reports. 101(3): 253–265.

Markush, Robert E, John J. Schwab. Patricia Farris, Paula A. Present, and Charles E. Holzer. 1977. "Mortality and Community Mental Health." Archives of General Psychiatry. 34(12):1393–1401.

Marmot, Michael G., and Eric Brunner. 1991. "Alcohol and Cardiovascular Disease: The Status of the U-Shaped Curve." British Medical Journal. 303:565–568.

Marmot, Michael G., M. Kogevinas, and M. A. Elston. 1987. "Social/Economic Status and Disease." Annual Review of Public Health. 8:111–135.

Marmot, Michael G., G. Rose, M. J. Shipley, B. J. Thomas. 1981. "Alcohol and Mortality: A U-Shaped Curve." Lancet. 1(8220):580–583.

Marmot, Michael G., M. J. Shipley, and G. Rose. 1984. "Inequalities in Death—Specific Explanations of a General Pattern." Lancet. 1:1003–1006.

Marmot, Michael G., and Tores Theorell. 1988. "Social Class and Cardiovascular Disease: The Contribution of Work." International Journal of Health Services. 18(4):659–674.

Massey, Douglas. 1996. "The Age of Extremes: Concentrated Affluence and Poverty in the Twenty-First Century." Demography. 33: 395–412.

Massey, James T., Thomas F. Moore, Van L. Parsons, and William Tadros. 1989. "Design and Estimation for the National Health Interview Survey, 1985–94." Vital and Health Statistics. 29(110):1–33.

McDonough, Peggy, Greg Duncan, Donald Williams. 1994. "Income Dynamics and Adult Mortality in the U.S., 1972–1989." American Journal of Public Health. 87(Sept):1476–1483.

McGee, Daniel L., Youlian Liao, Guichan Cao, and Richard S. Cooper. 1999. "Self-reported Health Status and Mortality in a Multiethnic U.S. Cohort." American Journal of Epidemiology. 149:41–46.

McKeown, Thomas. 1976a. The Modern Rise of Population. London:Edward Arnold.

———. 1976b. The Role of Medicine: Dream, Mirage, or Nemesis. London: Nuffields Provincial Hospitals Trust.

Menchik, P. 1993. "Economic Status as a Determinant of Mortality among Black and White Older Men: Does Poverty Kill?" Population Studies. 47(3): 427–436.

Metropolitan Life Insurance Company. 1990. "Deaths from Chronic Obstructive Pulmonary Disease in the United States, 1987." Statistical Bulletin. 71(3): 20–26.

Midanik, Lorraine T., and Walter B. Clark. 1994. "The Demographic Distribution of US Drinking Patterns in 1990: Description and Trends from 1984." American Journal of Public Health. 84(8):1218–1222.

Mirowsky, John, and Catherine E. Ross. 1989a. "Psychiatric Diagnosis as Reified Measurement." Journal of Health and Social Behavior. 39(1):11–25.

———. 1989b. Social Causes of Psychological Distress. NY: Aldine De Gruyter.

———. 1992. "Age and Depression." Journal of Health and Social Behavior. 33(3):187–205.

Moen, Phyllis, Donna Dempster-McClain, and Robin Williams. 1992. "Successful Aging: A Life Course Perspective on Women's Multiple Roles and Health." American Journal of Sociology. 97(6):1612–1638.

Monson, Richard R. 1986. "Observations on the Healthy Worker Effect." Journal of Occupational Medicine. 28(6):425–433.

Montgomery, L., J. Kiely, and G. Pappas. 1996. "The Effects of Poverty, Race, and Family Structure on U.S. Children's Health: Data From the NHIS, 1978 through 1980 and 1989 through 1991." American Journal of Public Health. 86(10):1401–1405.

Moore, David E., and Mark D. Hayward. 1990. "Occupational Careers and Mortality of Elderly Men." Demography. 27(1):31–53.

Morris, N. M. 1996. "The Influence of Socioeconomic Position on Health—and Vice Versa." American Journal of Public Health. 86(11): 1649–50.

Moser, K. A., P. O. Goldblatt, A. J. Fox, and D. R. Jones. 1987. "Unemployment and Mortality: Comparison of the 1971 and 1981 Longitudinal Study Census Samples." British Medical Journal. 294:86–90.

Mosley, W. H., and L. C. Chen (eds.). 1984. "Child Survival: Strategies for Research." Population and Development Review. 10 (Supplement).

Moss, N., and N. Krieger. 1995. "Measuring Social Inequalities in Health: Report on the Conference of the National Institutes of Health." Public Health Reports. 110(3): 302–305.

Mossey, Jana M., and Evelyn Shapiro. 1982. "Self-Rated Health: A Predictor of Mortality among the Elderly." American Journal of Public Health. 72(8):800–808.

Musick, Marc A. 1996. "Religion and Subjective Health among Black and White Elders." Journal of Health and Social Behavior. 37(3): 221–237.

Mutchler, Jan E., and Dudley L. Poston, Jr. 1983. "Do Females Necessarily Have the Same Occupational Status Scores as Males? A Conceptual and Empirical Examination of the Duncan Socioeconomic Status Index and Nam-Powers Occupational Status Scores." Social Science Research. 12(4):353–362.

Nam, Charles B. 1990. "Mortality Differentials from a Multiple Cause-of-Death Perspective." Pp. 328–342 in Stan D'Souza, Alberto Palloni, and Jacques Vallin, eds. Measurement and Analysis of Mortality. London: Oxford Press.

———. 1995. "Another Look at Mortality Crossovers." Social Biology. 42(1–2): 133–142.

———. 1996. "Comparison of Three Occupational Scales." Unpublished paper.

Nam, Charles B., and Thomas M. Harrington. 1986. "Factors Shaping the Morbidity-Mortality Expectations of Youth: A Socialization Model." Pp. 302–313 in Fertility and Mortality: Theory, Methodology, and Empirical Issues, edited by K. Mahadevan. New Delhi: Sage.

Nam, Charles B., Robert A. Hummer, and Richard G. Rogers. 1994. "Underlying and Multiple Causes of Death Related to Smoking." Population Research and Policy Review. 13: 305–325.

———. 1995a. "Underlying and Multiple Causes of Death Related to Smoking." Population Research and Policy Review. 13:305–25.

Nam, Charles B., and Mary G. Powers. 1983. The Socioeconomic Approach to Status Measurement. Houston: Cap and Gown Press.

Nam, Charles B., Richard G. Rogers, and Robert A. Hummer. 1995b. "The Impact of Smoking Trends on Future Life Expectancy and Population Age Structure in the U.S." Paper presented at the REVES (Network on Health Expectancy) Meetings, Chicago.

———. 1996. "Impact of Future Cigarette Smoking Scenarios on Mortality of the Adult Population in the U.S.: 2000–2050." Social Biology. 43(3–4): 155–168.

Nam, Charles B., and Chingfa Wu. 1994. "Occupational Socioeconomic Status and Premature Adult Mortality: United States, Early 1980's." Paper presented to the Southern Demographic Association, October 20–22, Atlanta, GA.

Nathanson, Constance A. 1984. "Sex Differences in Mortality." Annual Review of Sociology. 10: 191–213.

———. 1995. "Mortality and the Position of Women in Developed Countries." Pp. 135–157 in Adult Mortality in Developed Nations, edited by A. Lopez, G. Caselli, and T. Valkonen. Oxford: Clarendon Press.

Nathanson, Constance A., and Alan D. Lopez. 1987. "The Future of Sex Mortality Differentials in Industrialized Societies: A Structural Hypothesis." Population Research and Policy Review. 6(1) :123–136.

National Center for Health Statistics. 1980. DHEW Publication No (PHS) 80–1247. Hyattsville: NCHS.

———. 1988. National Health Interview Survey, 1987. Computer file and documentation. Hyattsville, MD: Public Health Service.

———. 1989a. National Health Interview Survey, 1986: Functional Limitations Supplement. Computer file and documentation. Hyattsville, MD: Public Health Service.

———. 1989b. National Health Interview Survey, 1986: Health Insurance Supplement. Computer file and documentation. Hyattsville, MD: Public Health Service.

———. 1989c. National Health Interview Survey, 1987: Cancer Risk Factor Supplement, Epidemiology Study. Computer file and documentation. Hyattsville, MD: Public Health Service.

———. 1991a. Monthly Vital Statistics Report. 39(13). Hyattsville: NCHS.

———. 1991b. National Health Interview Survey, 1989. Computer file and documentation. Hyattsville, MD: Public Health Service.

———. 1991c. National Health Interview Survey, 1990, Field Representative's Manual. Hyattsville, MD: Public Health Service.

———. 1991d. Vital Statistics of the United States, 1988: Life Tables. Vol. II, Sec. 6. Washington: USGPO.

———. 1992a. National Health Interview Survey, 1989: Mental Health Supplement. Computer file and documentation. Hyattsville, MD: Public Health Service.

———. 1992b. National Health Interview Survey, 1990. Computer file and documentation. Hyattsville, MD: Public Health Service.

———. 1992c. National Health Interview Survey, 1991: Field Representative's Manual. Hyattsville, MD: NCHS.

———. 1993a. "Advance Report of Final Mortality Statistics, 1990." Monthly Vital Statistics Report. 41(7):1–52.

———. 1993b. National Health Interview Survey, 1988: Occupational Health Supplement. Computer file and documentation. Hyattsville, MD: Public Health Service.

———. 1993c. National Health Interview Survey, 1990: Health Promotion and Disease Prevention Sample Person Supplement. Computer file and documentation. Hyattsville, MD: Public Health Service.

———. 1993d. National Health Interview Survey, 1991. Computer file and documentation. (Distributed by ICPSR).

———. 1993e. National Health Interview Survey, 1991: Health Promotion and Disease Prevention Supplement. Computer file and documentation. (Distributed by ICPSR).

———. 1994a. Current Estimates from the National Health Interview Survey, 1992. Vital and Health Statistics. Hyattsville, MD: PHS.

———. 1994b. Health, United States, 1993. Hyattsville, MD: USGPO.

———. 1994c. Healthy People 2000 Review, 1993. Hyattsville, MD: PHS.

———. 1994d. National Health Interview Survey, 1992. Computer file and documentation. Hyattsville, MD: Public Health Service.

———. 1995a. "Advance Report of Final Mortality Statistics, 1992." Monthly Vital Statistics Report 43:176.

———. 1995b. Health, United States, 1994. Hyattsville, MD: Public Health Service.

———. 1995c. Healthy People 2000 Review, 1994. Hyattsville, MD: Public Health Service.

———. 1995d. National Health Interview Survey, 1990: Family Resources Supplement. Computer file and documentation. Hyattsville, MD: Public Health Service.

———. 1995e. National Health Interview Survey, 1993. Computer file and documentation. Hyattsville, MD: Public Health Service.

———. 1996a. "Advance Report of Final Mortality Statistics, 1994." Monthly Vital Statistics Report. 44(3):Supplement.

———. 1996b. Health, United States, 1995. Hyattsville, MD: Public Health Service.

———. 1996c. National Health Interview Survey, 1994. Computer file and documentation. Hyattsville, MD: Public Health Service.

———. 1996d. Vital Statistics of the United States, 1992. Hyattsville, MD: NCHS.

———. 1997a. Health, United States, 1996–97 and Injury Chartbook. Hyattsville, MD.

———. 1997b. National Health Interview Survey: Multiple Cause of Death Public Use Data File, 1986–1994 Survey Years. Computer file and documentation. Hyattsville, MD: Public Health Service.

———. 1998. Vital Statistics of the United States, 1994 Preprint of Vol II, Mortality, Part A, Section 6, Life Tables. Hyattsville, MD.

National Heart, Lung, and Blood Institute. 1996. Live Healthier, Live Longer: Lowering Cholesterol for the Person with Heart Disease. Document H34, No. 5. Washington: U.S. Government Printing Office.

National Research Council. 1989. A Common Destiny: Blacks and American Society, edited by G. Jaynes and R. Williams. Washington, DC: National Academy Press.

Olds, Clifton C., and Ralf G. Williams. 1976. Images of Love and Death in Medieval and Renaissance Art. Catalogue by William R. Levin. Ann Arbor: University of Michigan.

Olshansky, S. Jay, and Brian Ault. 1986. "The Fourth Stage of the Epidemiologic Transition: The Age of Delayed Degenerative Diseases." The Milbank Quarterly. 64(3): 355–391.

Olshansky, S. Jay, and Bruce A. Carnes. 1997. "Ever Since Gompertz." Demography. 34(Feb): 115.

Omran, Abdel R. 1971. "The Epidemiologic Transition: A Theory of the Epidemiology of Population Change." Milbank Memorial Fund Quarterly. 49(4): 509–538.

———. 1983. "The Epidemiologic Transition Theory: A Preliminary Update." Journal of Tropical Pediatrics. 29: 305–316.

Orshansky, M. 1963. "Children of the Poor." Social Security Bulletin. 26:3–13.

Otten, Mac W. Jr., Steven M. Teutsch, David F. Williamson, and James S. Marks. 1990. "The Effect of Known Risk Factors on the Excess Mortality of Black Adults in the United States." JAMA. 263: 845–850.

Paffenbarger, Ralph S., Robert T. Hyde, Alvin L. Wing, and Chung-Cheng Hsieh. 1986. "Physical Activity, All-Cause Mortality, and Longevity of College Alumni." The New England Journal of Medicine. 314(10):605–613.

Paffenbarger, Ralph S., Robert T. Hyde, Alvin L. Wing, Dexter Jung, and James K. Kampert. 1993. "The Association of Changes in Physical Activity Level and Other Lifestyle Characteristics with Mortality among Men." The New England Journal of Medicine. 328(8):538–545.

Pappas, Gregory, Susan Queen, Wilber Hadden, and Gail Fisher. 1993. "The Increasing Disparity in Mortality Between Socioeconomic Groups in the United States, 1960 and 1986." New England Journal of Medicine. 329(2): 103–109.

Patterson, Blossom H., and Robert Bilgrad. 1986. "Use of the National Death Index in Cancer Studies." Journal of the National Cancer Institute. 77(4):877–881.

Pavalko, Eliza K., Glen H. Elder, Jr., and Elizabeth C. Clipp. 1993. "Worklives and Longevity: Insights from a Life Course Perspective." Journal of Health and Social Behavior. 34(4):363–380.

Pearce, Neil. 1996. "Traditional Epidemiology, Modern Epidemiology, and Public Health." American Journal of Public Health. 86(5):678–683.

Pearl, Raymond. 1938. "Tobacco Smoking and Longevity." Science. 87:216–217.

Peters, Kimberley, Kenneth D. Kochanek, and Sherry L. Murphy. 1998. "Deaths: Final Data for 1996." National Vital Statistics Reports. 47(9):1–100.

Peters, Kimberley, and Richard G. Rogers. 1997. "The Effects of Perceived Health Status and Age on Elder's Longevity." International Journal of Sociology and Social Policy. 17(9/10):117–141.

Peto, R., A. Lopez, J. Boreham, M. Thun, and C. Heath. 1995. Mortality from Smoking in Developed Countries, 1950–2000: Indirect Estimates from National Statistics. Oxford: Oxford Press.

Phillips, David, and Daniel Smith. 1990. "Postponement of Death until Symbolically Meaningful Occasions." Journal of the American Medical Association. 263(14): 1947–1951.

Phillips, Roland L., J.W. Kuzma, W.L. Benson, and T. Lotz. 1980. "Influence of Selection Versus Lifestyle on Risk of Fatal Cancer and Cardiovascular Disease among Seventh-Day Adventist Men." American Journal of Epidemiology. 112(2): 296–314.

Population Reference Bureau. 1998. World Population Data Sheet. Washington, DC: Population Reference Bureau.

Potter, Lloyd B. 1991. "Socioeconomic Determinants of White-Black Male Life Expectancy." Demography. 28(2):303–321.

Preston, Samuel H. 1970. Older Male Mortality and Cigarette Smoking: A Demographic Analysis. Berkeley: Institute of International Studies, University of California.

Preston, Samuel, and Irma Elo. 1995. "Are Educational Differentials in Adult Mortality Increasing in the United States?" Journal of Aging and Health. 7: 476–496.

Preston, Samuel, and Paul Taubman. 1994. "Socioeconomic Differences in Adult Mortality and Health Status." Pp. 279–318 in Demography of Aging, edited by Linda Martin and Samuel Preston. Washington, D.C.: National Academy Press.

Rakowski, William, Vincent Mor, and Jeffrey Hiris. 1991. "The Association of Self-Rated Health with Two-Year Mortality in a Sample of Well Elderly." Journal of Aging and Health. 3:527–545.

Ravenholt, R. T. 1984. "Addiction Mortality in the U.S., 1980: Tobacco, Alcohol, and Other Substances." Population and Development Review. 10(4):697–724.

Retherford, R. D. 1975. The Changing Sex Differential in Mortality. Westford: Greenwood Press.

Rice, D. P., and J. J. Feldman. 1983. "Living Longer in the United States: Demographic Changes and Health Needs of the Elderly." Milbank Memorial Fund Quarterly/Health and Society. 61(3):362–96.

Riley, James C., and George Alter. 1989. "The Epidemiologic Transition and Morbidity." Annales de Demographie Historique, 199–213.

Roberts, Robert E., George A. Kaplan, and Terry C. Camacho. 1990. "Psychological Distress and Mortality: Evidence from the Alameda County Study." Social Science and Medicine. 31(5):527–536.

Robertson, Leon S. 1996. "Reducing Death on the Road: The Effects of Minimum Safety Standards, Publicized Crash Tests, Seat Belts, and Alcohol." American Journal of Public Health. 86(1):31–34.

Robine, J. M., and J. P. Michel. 1992. "Toward International Harmonization of Health Expectancy Indices." Paper presented to the 6th International REVES Workshop. October, Montpellier, France.

Rogers, Richard G. 1991a. "Demographic Characteristics of Cigarette Smokers in the United States." Social Biology. 38(1–2):1–12.

———. 1991b. "Health-Related Lifestyles among Mexican-Americans, Puerto Ricans, and Cubans in the United States." Chapter 9 in Ira Rosenwaike, ed. Mortality of Hispanic Populations: Mexicans, Puerto Ricans, and Cubans in the United States and in the Home Countries. NY: Greenwood Press.

———. 1992. "Living and Dying in the USA: Sociodemographic Determinants of Death among Blacks and Whites." Demography. 29(2):287–303.

———. 1995a. "Marriage, Sex, and Mortality." Journal of Marriage and the Family. 57:515–526.

———. 1995b. "Sociodemographic Characteristics of Long-Lived and Healthy Individuals." Population and Development Review. 21(1):33–58.

———. 1996. "The Effects of Family Composition, Health, and Social Support Linkages on Mortality." Journal of Health and Social Behavior. 37(4):326–338.

Rogers, Richard G., Jacqueline A. Carrigan, and Mary Grace Kovar. 1996a. "Income, Education, and Mortality." Unpublished paper.

Rogers, Richard G., Jacqueline A. Carrigan, and Mary Grace Kovar. 1997. "Comparing Mortality Estimates Based on Different Administrative Records." Population Research and Policy Review. 16:213–224.

Rogers, Richard G., and Robert Hackenberg. 1987. "Extending Epidemiologic Transition Theory: A New Stage." Social Biology. 34(3–4): 234–243.

Rogers, Richard G., Robert A Hummer, Charles B. Nam, and Kimberley Peters. 1996b. "Demographic, Socioeconomic, and Behavioral Factors Affecting Ethnic Mortality by Cause." Social Forces. 74(June):1419–1438.

Rogers, Richard G., Charles B. Nam, and Robert A. Hummer. 1994. "Activity Limitation and Cigarette Smoking in the United States: Implications for Health Expectancies." In Advances in Health Expectancies. Edited by C. D. Mathers, J. McCallum, and J. M. Robine. Canberra, ACT: Australian Institute of Health and Welfare. Pp. 337–344.

———. 1995. "Demographic and Socioeconomic Links to Cigarette Smoking." Social Biology. 42:12.

Rogers, Richard G., and Eve Powell-Griner. 1991. "Life Expectancies of Cigarette Smokers in the United States." Social Science and Medicine. 32(10):1151–1159.

Rogers, Richard G., Andrei Rogers, and Alain Belanger. 1989. "Active Life among the Elderly in the United States: Multistate Life-table Estimates and Population Projections." The Milbank Quarterly. 67(3–4):370–411.

Rogot, Eugene, Paul D. Sorlie, and Norman J. Johnson. 1986. "Probabilistic Methods in matching Census Samples to the National Death Index. Journal of Chronic Diseases. 39:719–734.

———. 1992. "Life Expectancy by Employment Status, Income, and Education in the National Longitudinal Mortality Study." Public Health Reports. 107(4):457–461.

Rogot, Eugene, Paul D. Sorlie, Norman J. Johnson, and Claudia. Schmitt. 1992. A Mortality Study of 1.3 Million Persons by Demographic, Social, and Economic Factors: 1979–1985 Followup. Washington, DC: USGPO.

Rosenberg, Harry M., Carol Burnett, Jeff Maurer, and Robert Spirtas. 1993. "Mortality by Occupation, Industry, and Cause of Death: 12 Reporting States, 1984." Monthly Vital Statistics Report. 42(4):1–64.

Rosenberg, Harry M., and Eve Powell-Griner. 1991. "New Data on Socioeconomic Differential Mortality in the United States." Proceedings of the Social Statistics Section. American Statistical Association.

Rosenwaike, Ira. 1987. "Mortality Differentials among Persons Born in Cuba, Mexico, and Puerto Rico Residing in the United States, 1979–81." American Journal of Public Health. 77(5):603–606.

———. 1991. Mortality of Hispanic Populations. Westport, CN: Greenwood Press.

Ross, Catherine E. 1995. "Reconceptualizing Marital Status as a Continuum of Social Attachment." Journal of Marriage and the Family. 57(February)129–140.

Ross, Catherine E., and John Mirowsky. 1989. "Explaining the Social Patterns of Depression: Control and Problem Solving or Support and Talking?" Journal of Health and Social Behavior. 30(June):206–219.

———. 1995. "Does Employment Affect Health?" Journal of Health and Social Behavior. 36(Sept):230–243.

Rowe, John W., and Robert L. Kahn. 1987. "Human Aging: Usual and Successful." Science. 237(4811):143–149.

Ruggles P. 1990. Drawing the Line: Alternative Poverty Measures and Their Implications for Public Policy. Washington, DC: Urban Institute Press.

Rumbaut, Ruben G., and John R. Weeks. 1989. "Infant Health among Indochinese Refugees: Patterns of Infant Mortality, Birthweight, and Prenatal Care in Comparative Perspective." Research in the Sociology of Health Care. 8:137–196.

Rumbaut, Ruben G., and John R. Weeks. 1996. "Unraveling a Public Health Enigma: Why do Immigrants Experience Superior Perinatal Health Outcomes?" Research in the Sociology of Health Care. 13B: 337–391.

Schoenborn, Charlotte A. 1986. "Health Habits of U.S. Adults, 1985: The 'Alameda 7' Revisited." Public Health Reports. 101(6):571–580.

Schoenfeld, David E., Lynda C. Malmrose, Dan G. Blazzer, Deborah T. Gold, and Teresa E. Seeman. 1994. "Self-Rated Health and Mortality in the High-Functioning Elderly—A Closer Look at Health Individuals: MacArthur Field Study of Successful Aging." Journal of Gerontology. 49(3):M109–M115.

Scribner, Richard S. 1996. "Paradox as Paradigm: The Health Outcomes of Mexican Americans." American Journal of Public Health. 86(3):303–304.

Scribner, Richard S., and James H. Dwyer. 1989. "Acculturation and Low Birthweight among Latinos in the Hispanic HANES." American Journal of Public Health. 79(9): 1263–1267.

Seeman, Teresa E., George A. Kaplan, Lisa Knudsen, Richard Cohen, and Jack Guralnik. 1987. "Social Network Ties and Mortality among the Elderly in the Alameda County Study." American Journal of Epidemiology. 126(4): 714–723.

Sells, C. Wayne, and Robert W. Blum. 1996. "Morbidity and Mortality among U.S. Adolescents: An Overview of Data and Trends." American Journal of Public Health. 86(4): 513–519.

Seltzer, Carl C., and Seymour Jablon. 1977. "Army Rank and Subsequent Mortality by Cause: 23-Year Follow-up." American Journal of Epidemiology. 105(6):559–566.

Shah, Babubhai V., Beth G. Barnwell, and Gayle S. Bieler. 1996. SUDAAN User's Manual, Release 7.0. Research Triangle Park, NC: Research Triangle Institute.

Shaper, A. G. 1990. "Alcohol and Mortality: A Review of Prospective Studies." British Journal of Addiction. 85(7):837–847.

Shaper, A. G., Goya Wannamethee, and Mary Walker. 1988. "Alcohol and Mortality in British Men: Explaining the U-shaped Curve." Lancet. 2(8623):1267–1273.

Sidney, Stephen, Gary D. Friedman, and Abraham B. Siegelaub. 1987. "Thinness and Mortality." American Journal of Public Health. 77(3):317–322.

Simonsick, Eleanor M., Marry E. Lafferty, Caroline L. Phillips, Carlos F. Mendes de Leon, Stanislav V. Kasl, Teresa E. Seeman, Gerda Fillenbaum, Patricia Hebert, and Jon H. Lemke. 1993. "Risk Due to Inactivity in Physically Capable Older Adults." American Journal of Public Health. 83(1):1443–1450.

Singer, Eleanor, Robin Garfinkel, Steven M. Cohen, and Leo Srole. 1976. "Mortality and Mental Health: Evidence from the Midtown Manhattan Restudy." Social Science and Medicine. 10(11–12):517–525.

Singh, Gopal K., and Stella M. Yu. 1996a. "Adverse Pregnancy Outcomes: Differences Between U.S. and Foreign-Born Women in Major U.S. Racial and Ethnic Groups." American Journal of Public Health. 86(6): 837–843.

———. 1996b. "Trends and Differentials in Adolescent and Young Adult Mortality in the United States, 1950–1993." American Journal of Public Health. 86(4):560–564.

Smith, Adam. 1937. The Wealth of Nations. NY: Modern Library. (Original work published in 1776.)

Smith, D. G., J. Neaton, D. Wentworth, R. Stamler, and J. Stamler. 1996. "Socioeconomic Differentials in Mortality Risk among Men Screened for the Multiple Risk Factor Intervention Trial: 1. White Men." American Journal of Public Health. 86(4):486–96.

Smith, Kenneth R. 1996. "All-Cause and Cause-Specific Mortality and Marital Status: Findings from the NHIS-NDI Merged File, 1986–1991." Paper presented at the annual meeting of the Population Association of America, New Orleans, LA.

Smith, Kenneth R. and Norman J. Waitzman. 1994. "Double Jeopardy: Interaction Effects of Marital and Poverty Status on the Risk of Mortality." Demography. 31(3):487–507.

Smith, Kenneth R., and Cathleen D. Zick. 1994. "Linked Lives, Dependent Demise? Survival Analysis of Husbands and Wives." Demography. 31(Feb):81–93.

Sorlie, Paul D., Eric Backlund, Norman J. Johnson, and Eugene Rogot. 1993. "Mortality by Hispanic Status in the United States." The Journal of the American Medical Association. 270(2):2464–2468.

Sorlie, Paul, Eric Backlund, and J. Keller. 1995. "U.S. Mortality by Economic, Demographic, and Social Characteristics: The National Longitudinal Mortality Study." American Journal of Public Health. 85(7): 949–956.

Sorlie, Paul D., and Eugene Rogot. 1990. "Mortality by Employment Status in the National Longitudinal Mortality Study." American Journal of Epidemiology. 132(4):983–992.

Sorlie, Paul D., Eugene Rogot, Roger Anderson, Norman J. Johnson, and Eric Backlund. 1992a. "Black-White Mortality Differences by Family Income." Lancet. 340(8815): 346–350.

Sorlie, Paul D., Eugene Rogot, and Norman J. Johnson. 1992b. "Validity of Demographic Characteristics on the Death Certificate." Epidemiology. 3(2):181–184.

Sournia, Jean-Charles. 1990. A History of Alcoholism. Oxford: Basil Blackwell.

Speare, Alden Jr., and Roger Avery. 1993. "Who Helps Whom in Older Parent-Child Families." Journals of Gerontology. 48:S64–73.

Stafford, M. Therese, and Mark A. Fossett. 1991. "Measuring Occupational Sex Inequality Over Time Using Nam-Powers SES Scores." Texas Population Research Center Papers, Number 12.01.

Stevens, J., J. E. Keil, P. F. Rust, R. R. Verdugo, C. E. Davis, H. A. Tyroler, P. L. Guzes. 1992. "Body Mass Index and Body Girths as Predictors of Mortality in Black and White Men." American Journal of Epidemiology. 135(10): 1137–1146.

Stoto, Michael A. 1995. "Setting Objectives for Preventable Mortality and Promoting Healthful Behaviors: Experiences from the United States." In Lopez, Alan D., Graziella Caselli, and Tapani Valkonen. Adult Mortality in Developed Countries: From Description to Explanation. Oxford: Clarendon Press.

Strawbridge, W. J., R. D. Cohen, S. J. Shema, and G. J. Kaplan. 1997. "Frequent Attendance at Religious Services and Mortality over 28 Years." American Journal of Public Health. 87(6):957–961.

Susser, Mervyn, and Ezra Susser. 1996. "Choosing a Future for Epidemiology: I. Eras and Paradigms." American Journal of Public Health. 86(5):668–673.

Susser, Mervyn, William Watson, and Kim Hopper. 1985. Sociology in Medicine. New York: Oxford University Press.

Taylor, Robert J., and Linda M. Chatters. 1986. "Church Based Informal Support Among Elderly Blacks." The Gerontologist. 26:637–642.

Teachman, Jay D., Lucky Tedro, and Daniel Hill. 1994. "A Note on Discrete Time Hazard Rate Models: Estimated parameters and Standard Errors." Unpublished manuscript.

Terrie, E. Walter, and Charles B. Nam. 1994. "1990 and 1980 Nam-Powers-Terrie Occupational Status Scores." Working Paper Series 94–118. Center for the Study of Population. Tallahassee: Florida State University.

Thun, Michael J., Richard Peto, Alan D. Lopez, Jane H. Monaco, S. Jane Henley, Clark W. Heath Jr., and Richard Doll. 1997. "Alcohol Consumption and Mortality among Middle-Aged and Elderly U.S. Adults." The New England Journal of Medicine. 337(24): 1705–1714.

Torres-Gil, Fernando M. 1992. The New Aging: Politics and Change in America. Westport, CT: Auburn House.

Trovato, Frank. 1985. "Mortality Differences Among Canada's Indigenous and Foreign-Born Populations, 1951–1971." Canadian Studies in Population. 12:49–80.

Trovato, Frank, and G. Lauris. 1989. "Marital Status and Mortality in Cananda:1951–1981." Journal of Marriage and the Family. 51:907–922.

Trovato, Frank, and N.M. Lalu. 1998. "Contribution of Cause-Specific Mortality to Changing Sex Differences in Life Expectancy: Seven Nations Case Study." Social Biology 45: 1–20.

United Nations. 1991. "Social Statistics and Indicators." The World's Women, 1970–1990: Trends and Statistics, Series K, No. 8. New York: United Nations.

U.S. Bureau of the Census. 1987. Statistical Abstract of the United States: 1988 (108th edition.) Washington, DC: USGPO.

———. 1991. Poverty in the United States: 1990. Current Population Reports, Series P–60, No. 175. Washington, D.C.: U.S. Government Printing Office.

———. 1992. Population Trends in the 1980's. Series P–23, No.175. Washington, DC: Government Printing Office.

———. 1993. Statistical Abstract of the United States: 1993. Washington, DC: Government Printing Office.

———. 1994. Statistical Abstract of the United States: 1994 (114th edition). Washington, DC: USGPO.

———. 1996. Statistical Abstract of the United States, 1996, 116th Edition. Washington, D.C.: Government Printing Office.

U.S. Bureau of Labor Statistics. 1995. Employment and Earnings. 42(1). Washington, DC: USGPO.

U.S. Department of Health, Education, and Welfare. 1979. Healthy People: The Surgeon General's Report on Health Promotion and Disease Prevention. Washington, DC: USGPO.

U.S. Department of Health and Human Services. 1990. International Classification of Diseases. Vol. 1, 9th Revision, 3rd Edition. DHHS Publication (PHS) 891–260. Washington, DC: USGPO.

U.S. Surgeon General's Advisory Committee on Smoking and Health. 1964. Smoking and Health: Report of the Advisory Committee to the Surgeon General of the Public Health Service. Washington, DC: USGPO.

Vallin, Jacques. 1995. "Can Sex Differentials in Mortality be Explained by Socioeconomic Mortality Differentials?" Pp. 179–200 in Adult Mortality in Developed Nations, edited by A. Lopez, G. Caselli, and T. Valkonen. Oxford: Clarendon Press.

Vandenbroucke, Jan P., Bernard J. Mauritz, and Agnes de Bruin. 1984. "Weight, Smoking, and Mortality." Journal of the American Medical Association. 252(Nov 23/30):2859–2860.

Van der Gaag, Jacques, and Eugene Smolensky. 1982. "True Household Equivalence Scales and Characteristics of the Poor in the United States." Review of Income and Wealth. 28(1):17–28.

Vaupel, James W. 1998. "Summary Comments on the German-American Academic Council Summer Institute on the Biological and Social Determinants of Longevity," August 3–13. Max Planck Institute: Rostock, Germany.

Vega, William A., and Hortensia Amaro. 1994. Latino Outlook: Good Health, Uncertain Prognosis. Annual Review of Public Health. 15: 39–68.

Ventura, Stephanie J., Robert N. Anderson, Joyce A. Martin, and Betty L. Smith. 1998. "Births and Deaths: Preliminary Data for 1997." National Vital Statistics Reports. 47(4). Hyattsville, MD: National Center for Health Statistics.

Verbrugge, Lois M. 1989. "The Twain Meet: Empirical Explanations of Sex Differences in Health and Mortality." Journal of Health and Social Behavior. 30(3): 282–304.

———. 1990. "The Iceberg of Disability." In The Legacy of Longevity, Health and Health Care in Later Life. Edited by Sidney M. Stahl. Newbury Park: Sage Publications. Pp. 55–75.

Vogt, Thomas, Clyde Pope, John Mullooly, and Jack Hollis. 1994. "Mental Health Status as a Predictor of Morbidity and Mortality: A 15-Year Follow-Up of Members of a Health Maintenance Organization." American Journal of Public Health. 84(2):227–231.

Waaler, H. 1983. "Height, Weight and Mortality: The Norweigan Experience." Acta Medica Scandinavica Supplementum 679.

Wald, N. J., and H. C. Watt. 1997. "Prospective Study of Effect of Switching from Cigarettes to Pipes or Cigars on Mortality from Three Smoking Related Diseases." British Medical Journal. 314:1860–1863.

Waldron, Ingrid. 1983. "Sex Differences in Human Mortality: The Role of Genetic Factors." Social Science and Medicine. 17(6): 321–333.

———. 1986. "The Contribution of Smoking to Sex Differences in Mortality." Public Health Reports. 101(2):163–173.

———. 1995. "Contributions of Biological and Behavioural Factors to Changing Sex Differences in Ischaemic Heart Disease Mortality." Pp. 161–178 in Adult Mortality in Developed Nations, edited by A. Lopez, G. Caselli, and T. Valkonen. Oxford: Clarendon Press.

Wei, Ming, Rodolfo A. Valdez, Braxton D. Mitchell, Steven M. Haffner, Michael P. Stern, and Helen P. Hazuda. 1996. "Migration Status, Socioeconomic Status, and Mortality Rates in Mexican Americans and non-Hispanic Whites: The San Antonio Heart Study." Annals of Epidemiology. 6:307–313.

Wilkinson, Richard G. 1986. "Socio-economic Differences in Mortality: Interpreting the Data on Their Size and Trends." In Class and Health, edited by Richard G. Wilkinson. NY: Tavistock Publications.

Williams, David R. 1990. "Socioeconomic Differentials in Health: A Review and Redirection." Social Psychology Quarterly. 53(2):81–99.

———. 1994. "The Measurement of Religion in Epidemiologic Studies: Problems and Prospects." Pp. 125–148 in Religion in Aging and Health: Theoretical Foundations and Methodological Frontiers, edited by J. S. Levin. Thousand Oaks, CA: Sage Publications.

Williams, David R., and Chiquita Collins. 1995. "U.S. Socioeconomic and Racial Differences in Health: Patterns and Explanations." Annual Review of Sociology. 21:349–386.

Williams, David, Risa Lavizzo-Mourey, and Rueben C. Warren. 1994. "The Concept of Race and Health Status in America." Public Health Reports. 109(1):26–41.

Wingard, Deborah L. 1982. "The Sex Differential in Mortality Rates: Demographic and Behavioral Factors." American Journal of Epidemiology. 115(2): 205–216.

Wingard, Deborah. L., L. Suarez, and E. Barrett-Connor. 1983. "The Sex Differential in Mortality From all Causes and Ischemic Heart Disease." American Journal of Epidemiology. 117(2):165–172.

Wolinsky, Fredric D., and Robert J. Johnson. 1991. "The Use of Health Services by Older Adults." Journals of Gerontology: Social Sciences. 46(6):S345–S357.

The 1998 World Book Multimedia Encyclopedia. 1998. San Diego, CA.

World Health Organization. 1980. International Classification of Impairments, Disabilities, and Handicaps. Geneva: World Health Organization.

Wrigley, J. Michael, and Charles B. Nam. 1987. "Underlying vs. Multiple Causes of Death: Effects on Interpreting Cancer Mortality Differentials by Age, Sex, and Race." Population Research and Policy Review. 6:149–160.

Young, T. Kue. 1997. "Recent Health Trends in the Native American Population." Population Research and Policy Review. 16: 147–167.

Yu, E., C. F. Chang, W. Liu, and S. Kan. 1985. Asian-White Mortality Differences: Are There

Excess Deaths? Pp. 209–251 in Report of the Secretary's Task Force on Black and Minority Health, Volume II. Washington.

Zador, Paul L., and Michael A. Ciccone. 1993. Automobile Driver Fatalities in Frontal Impacts: Air Bags Compared with Manual Belts. American Journal of Public Health. 83(5): 661–666.

Zane, Nolan, and Jeannie Huh Kim. 1994. "Substance Use and Abuse." In Nolan Zane, David Takeuchi, and Kathleen Young, eds. Confronting Critical Health Issues of Asian and Pacific Islander Americans. Thousand Oaks, CA: Sage Publications.

Zheng, Deyi, Caroline A. Macera, Janet B. Croft, Wayne H. Giles, Dorothy Davis, and William K. Scott. 1997. "Major Depression and All-Cause Mortality Among White Adults in the United States." Annals of Epidemiology. 7(3):213–218.

Zopf, Paul. 1992. Mortality Patterns and Trends in the U.S. Westport, CN: Greenwood Press.

Zuckerman, Diana M., Stanislav V. Kasl, and Adrian M. Ostfeld. 1984. "Psychosocial Predictors of Mortality among the Elderly Poor: The Role of Religion, Well-Being, and Social Contacts." American Journal of Epidemiology. 119(3): 410–423.

AUTHOR INDEX

SUBJECT INDEX